PHYSICAL THERAPY
of the
FOOT and ANKLE

CLINICS IN PHYSICAL THERAPY
VOLUME 15

PHYSICAL THERAPY
of the
FOOT and ANKLE

Edited by
Gary C. Hunt, M.A., P.T.

Deputy Chief
Physical Therapy Department
Medical Center for Federal Prisoners
Springfield, Missouri
Formerly, Rehabilitation Department
Physical Therapy Service
National Institutes of Health
Bethesda, Maryland

CHURCHILL LIVINGSTONE

NEW YORK, EDINBURGH, LONDON, MELBOURNE

1988

Library of Congress Cataloging-in-Publication Data

Physical therapy of the foot and ankle.

  (Clinics in physical therapy; v. 15)
  Includes bibliographies and index.
    1. Foot—Diseases—Treatment. 2. Ankle—Diseases—
Treatment. 3. Physical therapy. I. Hunt, Gary C.
II. Series. [DNLM: 1. Ankle Joint—injuries.
2. Foot Diseases—therapy. 3. Physical Therapy.
W1 CL831CN v.15 / WE 800 P578]
RC951.P39 1988   617′.585062   87-24235
ISBN 0-443-08467-X

© **Churchill Livingstone Inc. 1988**

Distributed in the United Kingdom by Churchill Livingstone,
Robert Stevenson House, 1-3 Baxter's Place, Leith Walk,
Edinburgh EH1 3AF, and by associated companies,
branches, and representatives throughout the world.

Accurate indications, adverse reactions, and dosage
schedules for drugs are provided in this book, but it is
possible that they may change. The reader is urged to review
the package information data of the manufacturers of the
medications mentioned.

Acquisitions Editor: *Kim Loretucci*
Copy Editor: *Ozzievelt Owens*
Production Designer: *Gloria Brown*
Production Supervisor: *Jocelyn Eckstein*

Printed in the United States of America

First published in 1988

Contributors

James A. Birke, M.S., P.T.
Chief, Physical Therapy Department, Gillis W. Long Hansen's Disease Center, Carville, Louisiana

Ronald S. Brocato, P.T.
Director, Southside Rehabilitation Inc., Farmville, Virginia

William A. Fromherz, P.T., M.S.
Chief Professional and Placement Officer, Therapist Category, Division of Commissioned Personnel, Office of the Surgeon General, United States Public Health Service, Rockville, Maryland

Lynn H. Gerber, M.D.
Chief, Rehabilitation Department, Physical Therapy Service, National Institutes of Health, Bethesda, Maryland

Damien W. Howell, M.S., P.T.
President, Damien Howell Physical Therapy, Richmond, Virginia

Gary C. Hunt, M.A., P.T.
Deputy Chief, Physical Therapy Department, Medical Center for Federal Prisoners, Springfield, Missouri; Formerly, Rehabilitation Department, Physical Therapy Service, National Institutes of Health, Bethesda, Maryland

Shepard Hurwitz, M.D.
Assistant Professor, Department of Orthopedic Surgery, George Washington University School of Medicine and Health Sciences, Washington, D.C.

Charles L. McGarvey III, M.S., P.T.
Rehabilitation Department, Physical Therapy Service, National Institutes of Health, Bethesda, Maryland

Trudy Culotta McGarvey, M.S., P.T., A.T.C.
Staff Therapist, Josephs, Phillips, and Green P.A., Fort Washington, Maryland

Thomas G. McPoil, Ph.D., P.T., A.T.C.
Teaching Associate, Department of Physical Therapy, University of Illinois; Clinical Instructor, Department of Dermatology, University of Illinois Abraham Lincoln School of Medicine, Chicago, Illinois

Andrew Novick, P.T.
Rehabilitation Medicine Department, Physical Therapy Service, National Institutes of Health, Bethesda, Maryland

Joseph K. Reed, Ed.M., P.T.
Clinical Consultant, Pensacola, Florida

Susan D. Ryerson, M.A., P.T.
Clinical Consultant and Lecturer, Washington, D.C.

Marie A. Schroeder, M.S., P.T.
Center for Devices and Radiological Health, Office of Device Evaluation, Division of Surgical and Rehabilitation Devices, Food and Drug Administration, Silver Spring, Maryland

David S. Sims, M.S., P.T.
Biomechanics, Pennsylvania State University, University Park, Pennsylvania; Formerly, Deputy Chief, Physical Therapy Department, Gillis W. Long Hansen's Disease Center, Carville, Louisiana

Stacy Theriot, P.T.
Physical Therapy Department, Gillis W. Long Hansen's Disease Center, Carville, Louisiana

Preface

Problems of the lower extremity, particularly of the foot and ankle, have become the subject of renewed interest. One needs only to look at the variety of symposia addressing topics related to the foot to appreciate this observation. In spite of the foot's recognized effect on lower extremity function, little has been written in the clinical literature about this important anatomical structure. I hope this volume will increase that body of knowledge.

Physical therapy has had a significant impact on the care of foot related problems. One physical therapist who has stood out as a model by striving for clinical excellence through innovative evaluation and management is Joseph K. Reed. He has directly or indirectly influenced each contributor in this volume. Without Joe's dedication to his profession and his interest in sharing his knowledge, the role of physical therapy in foot care would not be what it is today. Anyone associated with physical therapy and foot care owes Joe Reed a huge debt of gratitude.

This text addresses three main areas: (1) basic foot science and examination, (2) pathologic categories, and (3) management tools and approaches.

Chapter 1 covers normal anatomic and biomechanical issues, which are important in order to establish a frame of reference. Chapter 2 presents the commonly recognized deviations from the norm and how they affect gait. Chapter 3 outlines an examination schema that is based on observed gait deviations and anatomically relevant relationships.

Chapters 4 through 8 cover specific pathologic categories, skin and toenail problems, and concerns of the athlete. These chapters address a variety of commonly faced problems ranging from the painful arthritic foot to the injury-prone insensitive foot. Particular problems observed in the adult with hemiplegia and in the athlete are discussed.

Chapters 9 through 12 cover management considerations and approaches. Physical agents, therapeutic exercise, orthotic management principles, and surgical intervention are presented to stimulate thought and suggest possible treatment options.

We, the contributors, hope that we have provided the clinician with a reference that will facilitate the decision-making process for foot-related problems.

I would like to thank Kim Loretucci and the staff of Churchill Livingstone for their help in making this volume possible.

Gary C. Hunt, M.A., P.T.

Contents

1 | Anatomy and Biomechanics

Andrew Novick

An appreciation for disorders that affect the foot requires an understanding of normal foot structure and resultant biomechanical interrelationships. The introductory section of this chapter examines the articulations, axes of motion, type and amount of motion available, and requirements for proper function within the four major joint complexes of the foot. Associated soft tissue structures are likewise discussed, specifically regarding how they influence motion at each joint. Lastly, specific aspects relating the dynamic function of the foot as a whole to those biomechanical principles discussed earlier are presented as a precursor for the following chapter on gait analysis.

BIOMECHANICS

A discussion concerning movement about any joint should not begin until the reference system in which this motion occurs has been defined. Regardless of the body's position in three-dimensional space, motion is defined in relation to prescribed body planes. These are the three cardinal planes, each perpendicular to the other two and each dividing the body into halves.[1,2] The frontal plane is a flat, vertical plane that divides the body into an anterior and posterior half[2] (Fig. 1-1). The sagittal plane is also a flat, vertical plane but divides the body into a right and left half. The transverse plane is a flat horizontal plane that divides the body into an upper and lower half. All three planes pass through the body's center of mass, but only the sagittal plane creates symmetrical halves.[2]

Motion of a rigid body within the defined reference system may be of two types. The first is termed translation and occurs when all particles contained

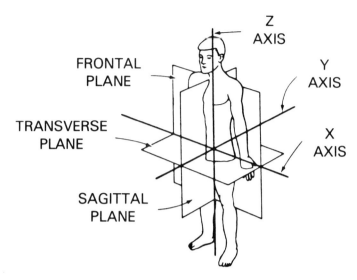

Fig. 1-1.   Frontal, sagittal and transverse planes. Intersection of these planes define the X, Y, and Z coordinate axes of the body's reference system. (Adapted from Kelley DL: Kinesiology: Fundamentals of Motion Description. Prentice-Hall, Englewood Cliffs, NJ, 1971.)

within that body undergo an equal linear displacement during a specified time interval.[3] The second, rotation, describes angular motion and occurs when all particles contained within that body move in a circular path around the same center, termed the axis of rotation.[3] During a specified time, each particle will rotate an equal number of degrees. These two motions may also occur simultaneously. As is discussed in the following section, motions of the foot are primarily those of rotation around a specific joint axis.

The motions of translation and rotation may each occur in all three planes. The coordinate axes, the X, Y, and Z axes which identify the coordinates of all points contained within the reference system, are formed by the intersection of the cardinal planes (Fig. 1-1). It is around these coordinate axes that the rotational motion of a rigid body in each plane is defined. Rotation in the frontal plane around the *Y* axis (the intersection of the sagittal and transverse planes) includes inversion and eversion. Inversion of the foot occurs around an axis parallel to the Y axis and requires that the plantar aspect of the foot turn inward toward the midline of the body, whereas it moves away from the midline during eversion. Rotation in the sagittal plane around the X axis (the intersection of the frontal and transverse planes) includes plantarflexion and dorsiflexion. Plantarflexion of the foot occurs around an axis parallel to the X axis such that the forefoot moves inferiorly and correspondingly moves superiorly during dorsiflexion. Transverse plane rotation around the Z axis (the intersection of the frontal and sagittal planes) includes adduction and abduction. Adduction of the foot occurs around an axis parallel to the Z axis such that the forefoot moves inward toward the midline, with abduction resulting in an outward motion of the forefoot away from the midline. This nomenclature differs from that of the hip, where rotation around the Z axis is termed internal and external rotation.

The preceding description of how a rigid body moves within the reference system is called kinematics. The study of those corresponding forces that act on a rigid body and result in translational or rotational motion is termed kinetics. As is discussed later in the chapter, numerous forces are exerted on the foot. A brief definition of force and the resultant motion produced will be presented.

A force, F, can be described as the influence of the environment acting on a rigid body, with a mass, M, that produces a linear change in velocity, termed acceleration, a.[3] Derived from Newton's Second Law of Motion, this relationship is as follows:

$$F(\text{Newtons}) = M(\text{kg}) \; a(m/s^2).$$

Forces are vector quantities having both magnitude and direction. Common examples of forces acting on the human body include gravity, the upward force of the ground (ground reaction force), and contraction of muscles. Forces can be applied to a rigid body to produce either translation, rotation, or a combination of both. When a force creates rotation of a body around an axis, the result is a torque, T. As with the linear force, torque is a vector quantity and is defined as follows:

$$T = Fd,$$

where F is the force exerted on the body and d is the perpendicular distance between the applied force and the axis of rotation (also termed the lever arm or moment arm.)[3]

When a muscle contracts, a linear tensile force is generated, which then acts on the osseous components of the joint, resulting in the appropriate rotatory movement. The muscle has therefore generated a moment, or torque, around the respective joint axis. The magnitude of the force generated by a muscle is proportional to the cross-sectional area of its fibers.[4] Recalling that torque (T) is the product of the force (F) multiplied by the perpendicular distance (d) between the joint axis and the applied force, termed the lever arm, it is apparent that position of the muscle forms an important relationship. The proximity of each muscle tendon to the joint axis determines the length of the lever arm through which the muscle force can act. Those muscles having a greater distance to the axis will consequently have a larger lever arm. This allows a muscle with a smaller cross-sectional area to produce equivalent or greater amounts of torque than those of larger size through the application of a larger, more efficient, mechanical lever. Perry[5] illustrates the interaction of force and lever arm in the production of torque. The anterior tibialis, for example, generates slightly less force than does the flexor hallucis longus, but is able to produce greater torque due to the more efficient lever.

Major Joint Complexes

The foot will be considered as a structure containing four major joint complexes. They are, from proximal to distal, the (1) ankle joint, (2) subtalar joint, (3) midtarsal joint, and (4) metatarsophalangeal (MTP) joints. Included within the discussion of each joint will be relevant articular anatomy, orientation of the resultant axes of motion, definition of the motion available in relation to the reference system, and supplementary information to describe the biomechanical functioning of the foot.

Ankle Joint

The ankle joint consists of the articulations between the distal tibia, trochlea of the talus, and distal fibula, forming the corresponding tibiotalar, fibulotalar, and distal tibiofibular joints. The tibiotalar joint contains both the articulation between the large, convex surface of the trochlea with the concave, distal tibia, and the proximal facet on the medial surface of the body of the talus with the inner aspect of the medial malleolus.[6] A superior view of the talus shows the wedge-shaped configuration of the talus, such that the articulating surface is usually wider anteriorly than posteriorly by 2.4 mm on the average.[7] Inman[8] examined the tali of 100 cadavers and concurs that most tali have a wedge-shaped trochlea, although the difference between the anterior and posterior widths ranges from 0 to 6 mm. This suggests that some tali are not wedge-shaped. Barnett and Napier[9] however, explain that the small facet at the posteromedial aspect of the trochlear surface that articulates with the inferior transverse ligament can be misleading when the actual functional reduction in width is considered. This wedge shape will be shown later to influence both stability and orientation of the ankle joint axis during dorsiflexion and plantarflexion. The fibulotalar joint consists of the articulation between the large facet on the lateral surface of the talus with the inner aspect of the lateral malleolus. The distal, or inferior, tibiofibular joint, is composed of the convex articulating surface of the inner aspect of the distal fibula with the corresponding concave surface along the inner aspect of the distal tibia.[6]

Alignment of the articular surfaces at the ankle joint, as with all joints, defines the orientation of the resultant axis of motion. From a functional viewpoint, the ankle joint can be considered a hinge or ginglymus, joint, allowing motion in one plane about a single, stationary axis.[6,10] The defined rotational motion is that of dorsiflexion/plantarflexion occurring in the sagittal plane around an axis similar in orientation to the previously defined X axis of the reference system. The exact location, however, is defined by the articulations between the talus and the inner aspects of the malleoli. Malleolar alignment in the transverse plane shows a more anterior placement of the medial than the lateral, and a more caudal position of the lateral malleolus than the medial in the frontal plane. The actual axis originates just distal to the tip of the medial malleolus, passes distally and posteriorly through the body of the talus, and exits at a point just distal and anterior to the tip 'of the lateral malleolus.[11] Quantitatively the ankle joint axis measures 80° on the average from a vertical reference and 84° from a longitudinal axis of the foot (Fig 1-2A and B). Because this axis deviates from a true frontal plane orientation of the foot by 6° and from a true transverse plane orientation by 10°, motion around the ankle joint cannot be uniplanar, but is triplanar. These are the motions of pronation and supination, such that pronation includes dorsiflexion of the foot in the sagittal plane, eversion in the frontal plane, and abduction in the transverse plane. Supination, conversely, consists of plantarflexion, inversion, and adduction. Dorsiflexion and plantarflexion are the principle components of these triplanar movements and subsequently account for most of the motion occurring at the ankle joint.

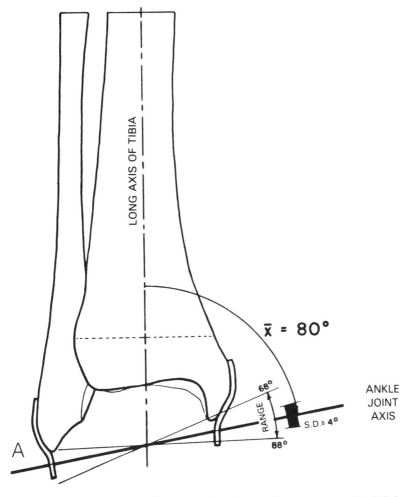

Fig. 1-2. Orientation of the ankle joint axis. Mean values measure (**A**) 80° from a vertical reference. (*Figure continues.*)

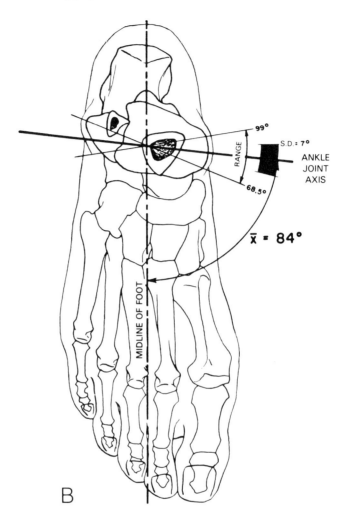

Fig. 1-2 (*Continued*). (**B**) 84° from the longitudinal reference of the foot. (Adapted from Isman RE, Inman VT: Anthropometric Studies of the Human Foot and Ankle: Technical Report No. 58, University of California, San Francisco, 1968.)

Closer examination of the ankle joint axis reveals that it is not stationary during dorsiflexion and plantarflexion. Sammarco et al[12] constructed instant centers of rotation from consecutive x-ray views of normal male subjects for movement of the tibia over the fixed talus from a position of extreme plantarflexion to maximal dorsiflexion. They found that the location of the instant centers for each of the five time intervals selected was quite variable. Parlasca et al[13] state that 96% of the instant centers fell within a circle with a radius of 1.2 cm, with the center located in the distal aspect of the talus (Fig. 1-3). This is in contrast to the instant center locations for a painful ankle secondary to rheumatoid arthritis, showing a much greater variability and a larger number of posi-

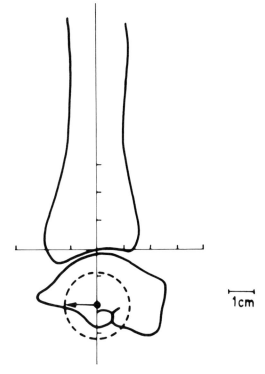

Fig. 1-3. Location of instant centers for normal male ankle joint movement from maximal plantarflexion to full dorsiflexion. (Parlasca R, Shoji H, D'Ambrosia RD: Effects of ligamentous injury on ankle and subtalar joints: a kinematic study. Clin Orthop Rel Res 140: 266, 1979.)

1cm

tions outside the talar body (Fig. 1-4). Barnett and Napier[9] identified two distinct axes, one each for dorsiflexion and plantarflexion, owing to the curvature of the articulating trochlear surface. A side view of the talus shows the convex, lateral joint surface to be an arc of one continuous circle. The medial profile, however, can be described by arcs of two separate circles of differing radii. The anterior one-third of the medial joint surface has a radius less than the corresponding anterior lateral aspect, whereas the radius for the posterior two-thirds of the medial surface is larger than the lateral profile. Therefore, since the anterior one-third of the trochlear surface makes contact with the distal tibia during dorsiflexion, the dorsiflexion axis can be defined as passing through the centers of the large lateral and small medial circles. Correspondingly, the posterior two-thirds makes contact during plantarflexion, allowing the plantarflexion axis to be defined by the centers of the large lateral and larger medial circles. The result is two axes with inclination in opposite directions. Barnett and Napier[9] further state that the shift from one axis to the other occurs within a few degrees of neutral.

Reports of maximal ankle joint range of motion (ROM) vary. Morris[7] states that "normal" ROM is 70°, consisting of 20° dorsiflexion and 50° plantarflexion. Sammarco et al[12] however, using x-ray studies and examining only tibiotalar motion, report a much smaller value. The mean total range for the weight-bearing foot was 40°, including 21° dorsiflexion and 23° plantarflexion.

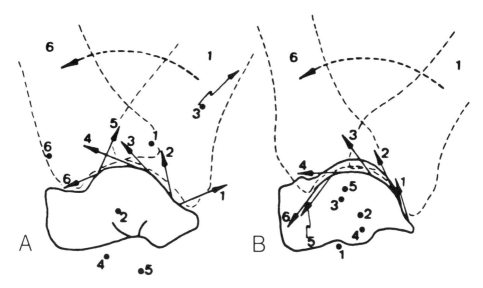

Fig. 1-4.   Instant centers and surface velocities of a (**A**) right and (**B**) left weightbearing ankle in a subject with painful rheumatoid arthritis. Both show deviations in the location of the instant centers and direction of surface velocities from normal, with the more painful right ankle showing the greatest variability. (Sammarco GJ, Burnstein AH, Frankel VH: Biomechanics of the ankle: a kinematic study. Orthop Clin North Am 4(1): 75, 1973. Reprinted with permission from WB Saunders Co.)

Nonweightbearing values were similar, measuring 42°, 23°, and 23°, respectively. They explain this discrepancy in reported ranges by noting that external measurements may include error created by movement of the tarsal bones, evident on cineroentgenography, during dorsiflexion and plantarflexion.

Reports citing required ankle ROM to allow proper foot function during the stance phase of gait are variable. Thirty degrees of total motion is generally accepted as necessary, including 8 to 10° of dorsiflexion and 20° plantarflexion.[14] Stauffer et al[15] report a mean total range value of 24.4° for five normal male subjects wearing regular street shoes consisting of 10.2° dorsiflexion and only 14.2° plantarflexion. Jordan et al[16] examined 50 normal male subjects walking barefoot and concluded that a mean value of only 4° dorsiflexion was required for normal gait. Clearly, the amount of functional ankle motion is variable and dependent on the conditions of gait.

A closer examination of ankle motion at the joint surfaces during stance from heel-strike to heel-off reveals two distinct patterns. During the interval from heel-strike to foot-flat, the first 15 percent of the gait cycle, the motion is essentially that of the talus plantarflexing under a relatively stable tibia. This talar motion allows the foot to become flat on the floor and is the necessary motion required for pronation of the foot. The arthrokinematics, which describes motion occurring at the joint surface, is similar to any convex or concave joint arrangement, such that the convex trochlear joint surface of the talus moves anteriorly in the concave tibial articulation. This is opposite in direction

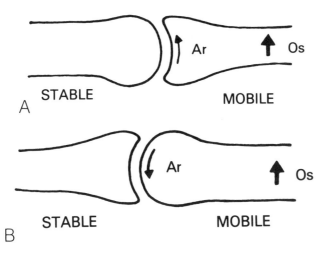

Fig. 1-5. Arthrokinematics (Ar) and osteokinematics (Os) of articulating surfaces. (**A**) A mobile concave joint surface moving over a stable convex surface results in movement at the joint surface (Ar) to be in the same direction as that of the corresponding bone (Os). (**B**) This relationship is reversed when the convex joint surface becomes the mobile segment.

to the osteokinematic movement of the talus itself, which describes movement of the bone (Fig. 1-5). Following foot-flat, the situation reverses, so that the tibia is advancing over the relatively fixed talus. The arthrokinematic motion also changes, so that the direction of motion of the concave tibial joint surface is now in the same direction as the osteokinematic motion of the tibia. Examination of the velocity vectors within the ankle joint during this period of stance indicates sliding between the joint surfaces, as shown by the tangential orientation of the vectors at the joint surface.[12] Observation of the velocity vectors from maximal plantarflexion to maximal dorsiflexion, however, shows that at the beginning of motion, there is a slight distraction of the joint. Sliding then continues until the limits of dorsiflexion, when compression, or jamming of the joint surfaces exist.[12] In support of this compression theory, Sammarco et al[12] state that osteophyte formation can be found along the anterior aspect of the talar articulation in baseball catchers who are subjected to prolonged, forced dorsiflexion, and reports describing skeletons of human races who frequently squat showed that articular facets had actually formed in the anterior aspect of the distal tibia and the corresponding location on the talar neck. As previously stated, the dorsiflexion axis is described by two circles with unequal radii, the largest being lateral; thus, the configuration is essentially that of a cone. This is confirmed by Morris[7] (Fig. 1-6) who adds that as the lower leg is advancing over the convex trochlea, the larger lateral radius (lesser curvature) results in a greater anteroposterior displacement of the lateral malleolus than of the medial malleolus. This results in an internal rotation movement imparted from the leg to the talus and ultimately into the foot. This internal rotation of the talus is possible due to the wedge-shape configuration of the superior surface of talus

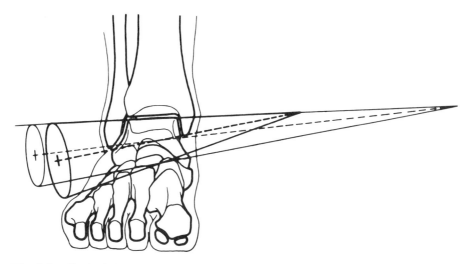

Fig. 1-6. Conical shape of the trochlear surface of the talus. The base of the cone, the segment having the largest radius, is positioned laterally. The perpendicular within the cone represents the ankle joint axis. (Morris JM: Biomechanics of the foot and ankle. Clin Orthop Rel Res 122: 10, 1977.)

and resultant freedom from blockage by the inner aspect of the lateral malleolus.[9]

Actual joint contact between the trochlear surface and distal tibia predominantly occurs laterally on the talus.[17] Across this contact area, each ankle supports approximately one-half of the body weight during static standing.[10] This weightbearing function increases to five times body weight later in stance phase due to contraction of the gastrocnemius and soleus as the large plantarflexion moment is produced for push-off.[10,15] This would oppose the equal and opposite dorsiflexion moment produced from ground reaction force. Ramsey and Hamilton[17] calculate the mean contact area to be 4.4 cm when the talus is in proper alignment. Trauma, however, such as fractures or ligamentous injuries, can result in displacement of the talus within the joint. Ramsey and Hamilton[17] demonstrate that a lateral displacement of only 1 mm can result in a 42 percent reduction in surface contact area, from 4.4 to 2.5 cm^2. This will greatly increase the pressure across those areas still making contact, since the force (body weight) remains constant but the surface area decreases by almost one-half.

Intraarticular joint pressure within the ankle joint is dependent on position of the joint. Eyring and Murray[18] maintained the subtalar joint in neutral position and found joint pressure to be least when the ankle was in 15° plantarflexion and maximal at the limits of plantarflexion. They also examined the effects of subtalar pronation and supination to the ankle joint. While maintaining the ankle in 15° plantarflexion, ankle joint intraarticular pressure was least in subtalar neutral and maximal at the limits of calcaneal inversion (supination).

The fibula plays both a kinetic and kinematic role in ankle joint function.

Weightbearing responsibilities of the fibula include the transmission of one-sixth of the weightbearing force in each leg to the ankle joint, beginning at the proximal tibiofibular joint and ending distally at its point of application on the lateral articulating surface of the talus.[10] Accessory motion of the fibula is demonstrated during dorsiflexion and plantarflexion. Although no studies describing accessory fibular motion were found, Kapandji[19] states that during dorsiflexion the fibula moves superiorly, the lateral malleolus moves outward away from the medial malleolus, and the fibula rotates internally. The motions are reversed for plantarflexion. The outward movement of the malleolus during dorsiflexion is necessary to accommodate the larger width of the anterior aspect of the wedge-shaped talus, which makes contact with the distal tibia during dorsiflexion. This greater surface contact ensures greatest ankle joint stability in the mortise while in the dorsiflexed position. Inman[8] concedes that although this outward malleolar motion does occur, the magnitude is very small, showing a range of only 0.13–1.8 mm. Barnett and Napier[9] agree that the fibula rotates during dorsiflexion, but state that it rotates externally. They maintain that this outward rotation is necessary for the articular surface of the fibula to maintain proper alignment with the lateral side of the talus. Clearly, the exact nature of the rotational accessory motion is questionable.

Subtalar Joint

The subtalar joint includes the distal talar articulations between the inferior talus and superior aspect of the calcaneus. The superior calcaneal surface generally has three articular facets: anterior, middle, and posterior. Bunning and Barnett[20] have shown, however, that three distinct facet arrangements are possible, classified into type A with three facets as previously described, type B in which the anterior and middle facets become one larger facet but the posterior remains separate, and type C in which all three facets are contiguous, such that the superior calcaneal surface presents with only one large articulation. Bunning and Barnett[20] described the differences as genetic, with no significant correlations between facet type and either foot features or amount of subtalar joint motion. The posterior calcaneal facet is the largest of the three and has a varying joint contour. It is typically convex in an upward direction, facing slightly anteriorly.[6,21] The anterior and middle facets, on the other hand, both have a concave joint surface, but their orientation is similar to that of the posterior facet.[21] The middle facet is most medial, located on the superior aspect of the sustentaculum tali. Situated between the middle and posterior facets is the sulcus calcanei, which together with the corresponding sulcus tali of the talus forms the sinus tarsi. The corresponding joint surfaces of the talus that articulate with the calcaneus are located on the inferior surface of the talar body. As with the calcaneus, the posterior talar facet is largest, but here has a concave surface contour.

Subtalar joint function is generally believed to be a rotational motion around a single axis functioning as an oblique hinge.[22–24] There is disagreement, however, concerning the existence of an anterior/posterior translation of the talus accompanying the rotational subtalar motion. This is discussed later in the chapter. Orientation of the subtalar joint axis, as defined by Isman and Inman,[11] shows a mean, medial deviation of 23° from the longitudinal reference of the foot when viewed superiorly (Fig. 1-7A). This reference passes from the center of the calcaneus to a point between the second and third metatarsal heads (MTHs). The range varies between 4 and 47°. A lateral view shows a mean deviation upward from the transverse plane of 41° having a range between 20.5 and 68.5° (Fig. 1-7B). It passes through the talus and enters the calcaneus just anterior to the posterior calcaneal facet, which is responsible for most of the subtalar jotion.[25] Manter[26] reports mean values of 16° from the longitudinal foot reference and 42° from the transverse plane. The discrepancy between the reported means of 23° and 16° can be explained by differing longitudinal reference lines, the initial passing between the second and third toes and the latter falling between the first and second. The wide ranges reported illustrate the individual variations in subtalar axis orientation. These differing profiles of the foot result in different subtalar joint function, both in terms of the actual motion produced and in the ability of the subtalar joint to transmit transverse plane rotation of the lower limb into the foot. This is discussed later.

Motion around the subtalar joint axis consists of the triplanar motions of

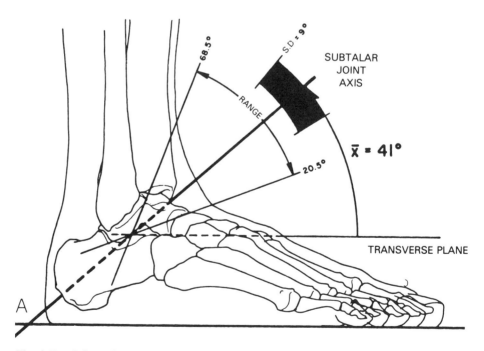

Fig. 1-7. Orientation of the subtalar joint axis. Mean values measure (**A**) 41° from the transverse plane and (**B**) 23° medially from the longitudinal reference of the foot. (Adapted from Isman RE, Inman VT: Anthropometric Studies of the Human Foot and Ankle: Technical Report No. 58. University of California, San Francisco, 1968.)

pronation and supination. Many different combinations of talar and calcaneal motion, however, can result in these identical movements. For example, in the nonweightbearing position, pronation is defined as dorsiflexion, abduction, and eversion of the calcaneus and foot under the fixed talus and lower limb, with supination including the trio of motions in the opposite directions. The mechanics change with weightbearing, in which either the calcaneus, talus, or both can become the moving segment. Green et al[27] illustrate that in the weightbearing condition, pronation can accurately be described as plantarflexion, adduction, and inversion of the talus over the fixed calcaneus. The resultant alignment of the calcaneus and foot in relation to the talus and lower leg is identical for both the weightbearing and nonweightbearing conditions. These two examples illus-

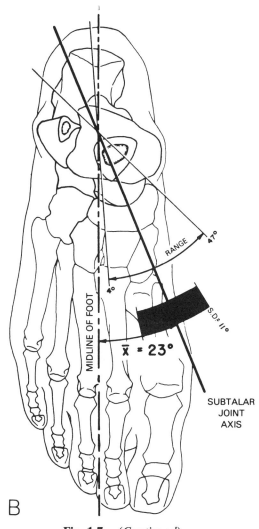

Fig. 1-7.   (*Continued*).

trate either calcaneal or talar movement exclusive of the other. Weightbearing function actually incorporates motion of both segments, such that the principle movements of pronation are plantarflexion and adduction of the talus combined with frontal plane eversion of the calcaneus (Fig. 1-8).[27] These movements combine to produce the required motion in three planes. Normal weightbearing supination incorporates the opposite motions of talar dorsiflexion and abduction with calcaneal inversion.

Angular ROM of the subtalar joint was measured by Inman et al[24] with a spherical goniometer, who reported an average total range of 40° in living subjects, with a range between 20 and 65°. Noting that subtalar joint function includes motion of the calcaneus in the frontal plane, mobility of this joint can be assessed by the degree of calcaneal inversion and eversion. Normal ROM values for calcaneal motion are 20° of inversion during supination and 10° of eversion with pronation, establishing a 2:1 ratio. Movement of the calcaneus is not purely in the frontal plane. This could only occur if the subtalar joint axis were perpendicular to the frontal plane (parallel to the Y axis from the earlier section). The actual motion is rotation of the calcaneus around the subtalar axis, which deviates from this perpendicular axis by 41°. The observed frontal plane excursion does, however, functionally reflect subtalar joint motion.

Reports of required subtalar joint ROM for normal function during gait

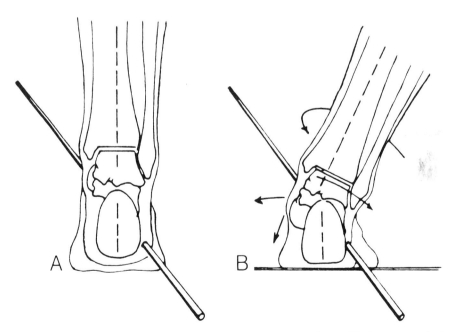

Fig. 1-8. (**A** and **B**) Normal subtalar joint pronation while weightbearing includes plantarflexion and adduction of the talus coupled with eversion of the calcaneus. (Green DR, Whitney AK, Walters P: Subtalar joint motion. J Am Podiatry Assoc 69(1): 83, 1979.)

vary. Wright et al[28] placed a potentiometer over the dorsum of the foot and aligned the device so that it rotated about the theoretical subtalar axis. They then recorded 8 to 10° of total pronation/supination ROM. Mann[22] reports a total range of 8° for calcaneal inversion and eversion during the stance phase of gait. Subotnick[29] also examined excursion of the calcaneus and states that 18° of total motion is required for proper subtalar function of the 2:1 ratio of inversion to eversion is to be maintained.

As mentioned previously, there is disagreement regarding actual function of the subtalar joint. It is generally believed that subtalar function is similar to that of an oblique, mitered hinge joint, whereby the only motion occurring is rotation around the joint axis (Fig. 1-9). Proponents of this hypothesis state that the axis of motion is basically perpendicular to the plane of motion and that no other motion of the mobile talus over the relatively fixed calcaneus occurs.[22,23] The resultant paired motions are simply internal rotation of the lower leg/talus segment creating the rotational motion of pronation of the calcaneus/foot segment. External rotation imparts a supinatory rotation on the calcaneus/foot segment.

Others describe subtalar joint function as "screw-like" in nature, such that

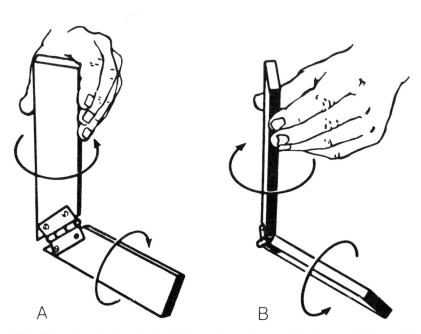

A   B

Fig. 1-9. Function of the subtalar joint axis can be described as an oblique mitered hinge. (**A**) External rotation of the upper segment, analogous to the shank, results in an outward rotation of the lower segment, analogous to supination of the foot. (**B**) Similarly, internal rotation of the upper segment produces inward rotation of the lower segment, or pronation of the foot. (Reproduced with permission from Mann RA: Biomechanics of the foot. p. 257. In American Academy of Orthopedic Surgeons' Atlas of Orthotics: Biomechanical Principles and Application. CV Mosby, St. Louis, 1975.)

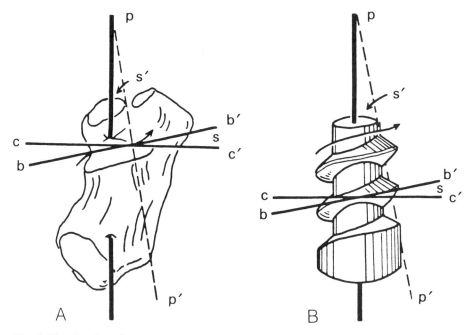

Fig. 1-10. Analogy between (**A**) right-handed subtalar joint function and (**B**) a right-handed screw. The helix of the screw, s, is equal to the angle between the plane of the posterior calcaneal facet, bb′, and the perpendicular to the subtalar joint axis, cc′. The helix angle, s, equals angle s′, which is derived by dropping a perpendicular from the subtalar joint axis to the plane bb′. (Adapted from Sammarco GJ: Biomechanics of the foot. p. 193. In Frankel VH, Nordin M (eds): Basic Biomechanics of the Skeletal System. Lea & Febiger, Philadelphia, 1980.)

translation of the talus accompanies the previously described rotational motion. Manter[26] reported an anterior talar migration of 1.5 mm/10° of rotation. This type of motion was confirmed in observation of cadavers by Close et al,[30] and Imhauser[31] reports a translatory shift of more than 5 mm between the articulating surfaces of the talus and calcaneus during the rotation. The basis for the screw-like function is the spiral orientation, or helix, formed between the plane of motion at the joint surface with the plane perpendicular to subtalar joint axis.[26] In Figure 1-10A, line bb′ represents the plane of motion at this articulation, which is essentially parallel to the joint surface. Line cc′ corresponds to the plane perpendicular to the subtalar joint axis. The helix is calculated as the angle between these two planes. Inman[24] reports a mean angle of 25 ± 6°, with a range of 0 to 40°, whereas Manter[26] reported a value half as large, measuring an average of 12°. This illustrates the wide variability in alignment of the hindfoot. Figure 1-10B shows how this helix forms the "screw-like" mechanism, which is a right-handed screw in the right foot and a left-handed screw in the left foot.[32]

Studies by Inman et al,[24] however, indicate that subtalar joint function can be either "hinge-like" or "screw-like" in nature. He reports that 58 percent of 102 specimens examined showed an anterior translation of the talus when the subtalar joint was moved from full supination to full pronation. The remaining specimens exhibited either no translation, a posterior translation along the subtalar joint axis, or translations that oscillated between anterior and posterior directions. The latter represents an additional classification of joint behavior, termed "unscrew-like." It is reasonable to conclude, then, that subtalar function is quite variable and dependent on such varying factors as helix angle and contour of the posterior articulating surfaces, and intrinsic forces such as ligamentous and capsular structures.[24]

The subtalar joint axis was previously defined as showing a mean, upward orientation of 41° from the transverse plane, and a mean, medial deviation of 23° from the longitudinal reference line of the foot.[11] A wide range of values was also reported for each of these alignments, however, measuring between 20.5 to 68.5° for the upward projection, and between 4 and 47° for the medial deviation. The manner in which the foot functions is dependent on the alignment of the subtalar joint axis and, as demonstrated by the large range, is quite variable. Axis orientation dictates what rotatory motions of the foot are possible based on position of the subtalar axis within the reference coordinate system. The proportion of motion in each plane to the total triplanar motions of pronation/supination are likewise dependent on subtalar axis orientation. A brief review of the cardinal planes and motion around the coordinate axes clearly illustrates this concept. Motion around an axis perpendicular to the sagittal plane, the X axis, can only be the uniplanar rotations of dorsiflexion and plantarflexion occurring in the sagittal plane. Motion around an axis perpendicular to the frontal plane, the Y axis, includes the frontal plane rotations of inversion and eversion. Likewise, motion about the vertical Z axis includes the rotational motions of abduction and adduction in the transverse plane. Because the subtalar axis is not parallel to any of the three coordinate axes, motion around the axis must contain components of motion in each plane. These are, of course, the triplanar motions of pronation and supination. A subtalar axis orientation more closely approximating the alignment of one of the coordinate axes should, however, show a movement that more closely resembles the motion around that coordinate axis. A subtalar axis with a steeper inclination to the transverse plane, closer to the Z axis, would result in greater abduction/adduction motion of the foot around the subtalar axis.[23,33] The triplanar motion of pronation/supination in this high-profile, cavus foot would therefore include a greater transverse plane component. Similarly, a lower inclined subtalar axis with respect to the transverse plane, closer to the Y axis, would permit greater inversion/eversion motion. Pronation/supination in this low-profile, planus foot would then include a greater frontal plane component. This explains the large ranges of calcaneal eversion of those individuals with a low-profile foot. A subtalar axis with a greater medial deviation from the sagittal plane, closer to the X axis, would result in greater dorsiflexion/plantarflexion and a greater sagittal plane component comprising pronation/supination.

Movement of the foot around the subtalar joint is associated with internal

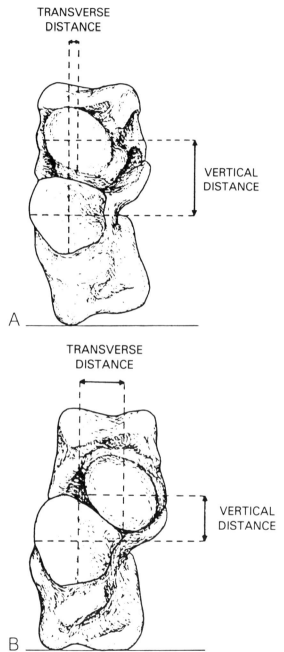

TRANSVERSE
DISTANCE

VERTICAL
DISTANCE

A

TRANSVERSE
DISTANCE

VERTICAL
DISTANCE

B

Fig. 1-11. Change in vertical and transverse distances between the anterior midtarsal joint surfaces of the calcaneus and talus in the (**A**) supinated and (**B**) neutral foot. The height between the supporting surface and the trochlear surface of the talus also changes. (*Figure continues.*)

and external rotation of the lower limb. The primary function of the subtalar joint is to transmit this transverse plane rotation of the leg into the foot. Position of the subtalar axis defines the resultant motion of the foot. This subtalar alignment will likewise dictate the relationship between lower limb rotation and foot pronation/supination. Because the subtalar joint functions as an oblique,

TRANSVERSE
DISTANCE

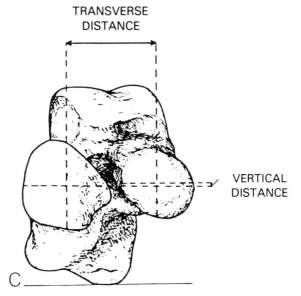

Fig. 1-11 (*Continued*). (**C**) Pronated foot. (Parts A, B, and C adapted from Root ML, Orien WP, Weed JH: Normal and Abnormal Function of the Foot. Clinical Biomechanics, Los Angeles, 1977.)

VERTICAL
DISTANCE

C

mitered hinge, an orientation of 45° from the transverse plane would result in equality in the amount of rotation for each segment.[34] That is, for every 1° of lower limb rotation, there is 1° of calcaneal/foot rotation. The "normal" foot approximates this condition, having a mean orientation of 41°. A subtalar axis showing a greater than normal inclination, 60° for example, would deviate from this 1 : 1 rotational ratio. With this high-profile foot posture, there would be less than 1° of foot rotation for every 1° of lower limb rotation. Correspondingly, excessive lower limb rotation would be required to produce the same amount of foot rotation achieved with the 45° axis. It follows then, that those individuals with a high-profile foot must have greater than normal internal rotation of the lower limb just to achieve medial forefoot contact and the required stability. This is in agreement with the previous discussion that an axis with a steeper inclination would permit greater abduction/adduction rotation but less inversion/eversion. A subtalar axis with a lower than normal inclination, 30° for example, would exhibit a deviation from the 1 : 1 ratio in the opposite direction. This low-profile, or planus foot posture, would show greater than 1° of foot rotation for every 1° of lower limb rotation. Large amounts of calcaneal eversion accompanying lower limb internal rotation would be observed in these individuals due to the more horizontal alignment of the subtalar axis which favors inversion/eversion.

A consequence of foot pronation is a functional shortening of the lower limb secondary to plantarflexion of the talus on the fixed calcaneus.[34] Figure 1-11 shows the relationship between the talus and calcaneus in the supinated, neutral, and pronated positions. The vertical distance between anterior facets of the talus and calcaneus decreases from supination to pronation. Correspondingly, the vertical height between the supporting surface and the superior aspect of the talus is also decreased. Benink[35] reports that variation in subtalar axis orientation results in variability of talar movement and the resultant height change. He examined vertical displacement of the tibia and found that normal subtalar alignment resulted in a height change of almost 4 mm in a specimen that was externally rotated from 0 to 30°. The low-profile foot showed an increase of almost 10 mm in height, whereas the high-profile foot showed no change.

Intraarticular pressure within the subtalar joint was measured by Kyne and Mankin.[36] They report that joint pressure is least in subtalar neutral position and increases as the foot is everted and inverted. The greatest pressure was recorded in inversion, showing a mean value of 75 mm H_2O, whereas the mean pressure in eversion was 29 mm H_2O. They suggest that peroneal muscle spasm that occurs with peroneal spastic flatfoot is initiated through a protective reflex mechanism in response to the elevated pressure within an inflamed subtalar joint during inversion.

Midtarsal Joint

The next distal joint complex, the midtarsal, or transtarsal joint, consists of the articulations between the talus and navicular medially and the calcaneus and cuboid laterally. The talar component has a large, oval, convex joint surface anteriorly, which articulates with the corresponding concave, posterior facet of the navicular.[6,22] Owing to the variable horizontal curvatures of the talar head, Mann[22] and Close et al[30] describe the talonavicular joint as an elliptical paraboloid. The facets comprising the calcaneocuboid joint are somewhat more complex. Bojsen-Møller[37] describes this joint as being concavoconvex, such that the facet of the cuboid presents as a sector of one end of an hourglass-shaped surface of revolution (Fig. 1-12). The corresponding calcaneal facet is similarly shaped, but in the opposite direction. Weston[38] describes the calcaneocuboid joint as being a saddle joint. The cuboid has a bony projection, the calcanean process, directed posteriorly from its medial aspect. It makes contact with the medioplantar aspect of the calcaneus and plays a role in guiding the rotational movement of the cuboid around the calcaneus.[37] Relative position of the talonavicular to the calcaneocuboid joint is variable, depending on the position and degree of mobility at the subtalar joint. This is discussed later in the section. The cuboidnavicular joint contributes little to midtarsal joint mobility and is therefore disregarded.[39]

The midtarsal joint complex contains multiple joint axes. Greenberg[40] states that both the talonavicular and calcaneocuboid joints each have two axes of motion at their respective articulations. Functionally, however, the midtarsal joint can be considered as having two joint axes positioned so that they reflect the combined motion occurring around the previously mentioned four axes. Both of these functional midtarsal axes, the longitudinal and oblique axes, pass medially in the foot near the head of the talus.[41] The average orientation of the oblique joint axis shows a position of 52° upward from the transverse plane and 64° medially from the longitudinal foot reference.[32,42] The longitudinal axis has an average orientation of 15° upward from the transverse plane and 16°

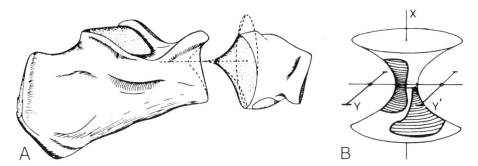

Fig. 1-12. (**A**) Concavoconvex joint surfaces of the calcaneocuboid joint. The main axis at this joint passes longitudinally in the foot through the calcanean process. (**B**) The configuration of these two concavoconvex joint surfaces can be depicted as opposing sectors of an hour glass. (From Calcaneocuboid joint stability of the longitudinal arch of the foot at high and low gear push off, by Bojsen-Møller F. In J Anat 129(1):167. © 1979. Reprinted by permission of Cambridge Univ. Press.)

medially from the longitudinal foot reference. Figure 1-13 shows the position of both axes concurrently.

Because neither axis lies on or is parallel to a principle reference axis, movement around both axes occurs in all three planes and can therefore be defined as triplanar. Each axis does, however, allow one or two primary movements. The primary movements occurring around the longitudinal axis are those of inversion and eversion of the midfoot/forefoot complex,[32,41,42] because its orientation within the reference system is similar to the Y axis around which pure inversion and eversion occur. Because there is a slight deviation from the Y axis, a small degree of dorsiflexion/plantarflexion and abduction/adduction does occur.[41] The opposite motions occur around the oblique midtarsal axis. Root et al[42] state that large amounts of both dorsiflexion/plantarflexion and abduction/adduction are possible, with the magnitude of inversion/eversion being clinically insignificant. This latter statement is easily explained by the degree of deviation from the reference Y axis. The amount of ROM occurring around the oblique axis measured in a cadaver specimen by Hicks[41] was 22°. Rotation around the longitudinal axis is considerably less. Hicks[41] reports a range of 8°, whereas Root et al[42] report that during ambulation, a functional ROM of only 4 to 6° is required. The direction with which this motion occurs is from a neutral forefoot position into inversion and is equal in magnitude to the amount of calcaneal eversion during stance. At maximum midtarsal eversion, position of the forefoot allows the plantar aspect of the forefoot/metatarsal heads to be on the same plane as the plantar aspect of the rearfoot.[29,42] This is the plane perpendicular to the medial to lateral bisection of the posterior tubercle of the calcaneus. It is apparent, then, that it is primarily the function of the midtarsal longitudinal axis to achieve medial contact of the forefoot with the supporting surface during gait. Forefoot posture is determined by the torsion remaining in the talar neck as it derotates from a varus attitude in utero to its final position at 15 to 18 months of age.[43,44] The subtalar joint and the two

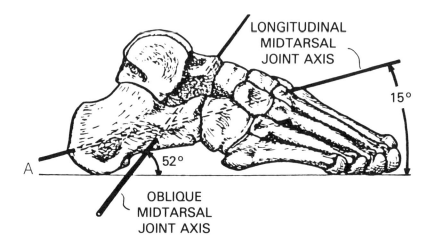

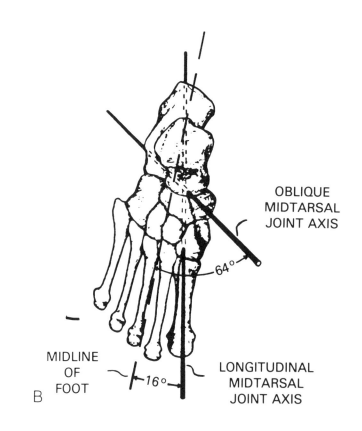

Fig. 1-13. (**A**) Lateral and (**B**) dorsal views of the oblique and longitudinal midtarsal joint axes. (Adapted from Root ML, Orien WP, Weed JH: Normal and Abnormal Function of the Foot. Clinical Biomechanics, Los Angeles, 1977.)

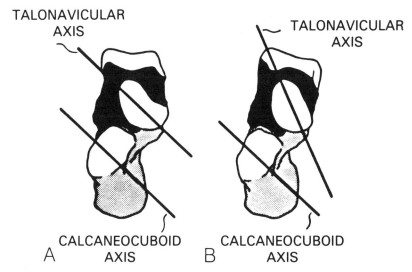

TALONAVICULAR AXIS

TALONAVICULAR AXIS

A CALCANEOCUBOID AXIS

B CALCANEOCUBOID AXIS

Fig. 1-14. Alignment of the oblique axes of the talonavicular and calcaneocuboid joints in the positions of rearfoot (**A**) pronation and (**B**) supination. The parallel alignment during subtalar pronation allows for relatively free midtarsal motion, whereas the divergent alignment when supinated restores midtarsal stability. (Adapted from Mann, RA: Biomechanics of the Foot. p. 257. In American Academy of Orthopedic Surgeons' Atlas of Orthotics; Biomechanical Principles and Application. CV Mosby, St. Louis, 1975.)

functional midtarsal axes during gait are interrelated. The ultimate degree of total ROM at the midtarsal joint is dependent on the position of the subtalar joint. Recalling that there are two axes of motion at the talonavicular joint and two at the calcaneocuboid joint, it is the orientation of these axes that varies with subtalar position and determines the degree of midtarsal motion. Specifically, the orientation of the oblique axes, the major axes at these two joints, is the primary determinant.[25,40] When the foot is pronated at the subtalar joint, the oblique axes of the talonavicular and calcaneocuboid joints assume a parallel alignment. This allows relatively free motion around these parallel axes, resulting in flexibility of the midfoot (Fig. 1-14).[22,25,32,40] Conversely, the effect of subtalar supination alters this parallel alignment, such that the talonavicular and calcaneocuboid oblique axes become divergent. This results in limitation of midtarsal movement and inherent rigidity/stability of the midfoot. This stability is enhanced because the convex joint surface of the talar head is firmly seated into the corresponding convex facet of the navicular.[22]

A complete understanding of midtarsal joint function requires a knowledge of isolated navicular and cuboid movement and the surrounding soft tissues that exert a direct force on them. Huson[39] states that motion between two articulating bones is governed by both the shape of the joint surfaces and surrounding ligaments. He adds that the joint surface actually become incongruent when weightbearing, and the ligamentous structures are necessary to guide joint motion, provided that they are in the proper position and are maintained under tension. Kapandji[19] examined midtarsal joint function and reports that when moving from a position of eversion to inversion over a fixed calcaneus, the navicular moves medially on the talar head when viewed from above and rotates through an arc of 5°. The cuboid moves in similar fashion with the navicular as it is displaced medially with respect to the calcaneus. It is also displaced medially with respect to the navicular as the talar head and consequently the talonavicular joint assume their more superior position above the calcaneocuboid joint (Fig. 1-11) during subtalar supination. Conversely, moving from inversion to eversion would show a lateral displacement of the cuboid with respect to the calcaneus. Greenberg[40] describes a cuboid abduction angle, which measures the acute angle formed by the intersection of the two lines parallel to the lateral borders of the cuboid and calcaneus. He states that this angle is a good measure of midtarsal joint pronation. Values would increase with midtarsal joint pronation and indicates pronation about the oblique midtarsal axis. Kapandji[19] reports that the navicular, when viewed from the side, moves inferiorly under the head of the talus during supination, rotating through an arc of 45°. The cuboid again moves in similar fashion, assuming a position inferior to both the calcaneus and talus and rotating through an arc of 12°. If the midtarsal complex is viewed anteriorly, both the navicular and cuboid are seen to rotate in a relative frontal plane orientation around the longitudinal axes of their respective joints. Observed from the front, this rotational motion for the right foot occurs in a clockwise direction, with the left showing a counterclockwise orientation. Bojsen-Møller[37] states that the calcanean process of the cuboid serves as the pivot around which this rotation occurs. The composite motion of the navicular, then, is a medial and inferior displacement of the navicular over the talar head during supination of the foot and a lateral and superior displacement during pronation (Fig. 1-15). Included in these movements is the clockwise/counterclockwise frontal plane rotation. This lateral movement with its subsequent change of alignment between the medial borders of the navicular and talus explains why the medial aspect of the talar head is easily palpable in full pronation and is obscured with supination. The same rationale holds for the ease of palpation of the lateral talar head in full supination and absence of contact in pronation. The composite motion of the cuboid is similar to that of the navicular.

Metatarsals/MTP Joints

This section concurrently examines the metatarsals as they relate to forefoot function, as well as their distal articulations at the MTP joints. Because it is difficult to disassociate one role from the other completely, a more comprehensive discussion can result from combining these two areas.

The five metatarsal bones share several common features. They each have a wedge-shaped configuration proximally at the base for articulation with the tarsal bones.[6] The first three metatarsals each articulate with a cuneiform bone, the first with the medial, the second with the intermediate, and the third with

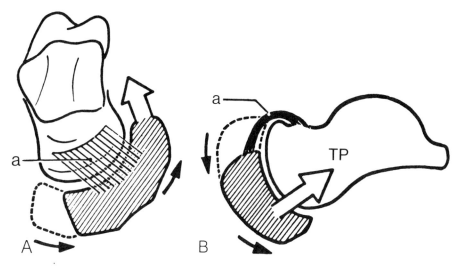

Fig. 1-15. (A) Dorsal and (B) side views show that composite motion of the navicular during supination is (A) medial and (B) inferior, which is assisted by the pull of the tibialis posterior (TP). The dorsal talonavicular ligament (a), helps to check this navicular movement. (Kapandji IA: The Physiology of the Joints. The Lower Limb. 2nd Ed. Vol. 3. Chruchill Livingstone, New York, 1974.)

the lateral cuneiform. Together, the metatarsal with its corresponding cuneiform constitute a ray. The fourth and fifth metatarsals articulate with the cuboid. Each metatarsal also articulates with its neighboring metatarsal, with the second only occasionally articulating medially with the first.[6] Distally, each metatarsal has a convex joint surface for articulation with the corresponding concave facet at the base of the proximal phalanx.[6] The first metatarsal is unique in two respects. First, it has two grooved facets on the plantar aspect of the metatarsal head that allow the two sesamoid bones to glide under it. Each sesamoid is contained within its half of the flexor hallucis brevis tendon and corresponding abductor or adductor tendon at the site of insertion into the proximal phalanx of the great toe. The flexor hallucis brevis divides to allow passage for the flexor hallucis longus tendon.[6] Second, it is the thickest and usually the shortest of the metatarsals. Inman and Mann[34] state that although the first metatarsal is shorter than the second, the sesamoids allow nearly equal functional length by elevating and supporting the first metatarsal head.

The metatarsals normally show a specific orientation with respect to the rearfoot and between themselves. Rowland[45] describes the abduction/adduction position of the forefoot as the forefoot angle, measured between the longitudinal axis of the rearfoot and the longitudinal axis of the second metatarsal. Values reported for normal forefoot posture range between 14 and 16° of adduction, with angles less than 14° representative of a pronated foot. Price[46] examined intermetatarsal angles and reported a normal range of 5 to 9° for the angle formed between the first and second metatarsals and a range of 23 to 29° for the

1-5 intermetatarsal angle. These angles are of clinical significance when considering pathological postures of the forefoot. Price[46] also states that metatarsus primus varus not only can be present when the 1-2 angle exceeds the 9 or 10° upper limit of normal, but can also be present when the 1-5 intermetatarsal angle is greater than normal, even when the 1-2 angle is within normal range. He also examined orientation of the great toe and reported a normal valgus posture between 9 and 17° at the MTP joint and 11 to 19° valgus at the IP joint.

The resultant axes of motion have been identified for three of the five rays, the first, third, and fifth. The first ray axis has a lateral deviation of approximately 45° from the longitudinal reference of the foot, with only a slight upward deviation from the transverse plane (Fig. 1-16).[32,41,42] The axis for the fifth ray, on the other hand, shows a medial deviation from the longitudinal foot reference, measuring 35°. This is similar in alignment to the subtalar and oblique midtarsal joint axis, unlike the first ray axis (Fig. 1-17). The fifth ray axis also shows an orientation of 20° upward from the transverse plane.[32,41,42] The corresponding lateral and medial deviations of the first and fifth ray axes, respectively, result in a near perpendicular orientation between them. The axis for the third ray, as described by Hicks,[41] shows a transverse alignment that runs near the third cuneiform bone and lies nearly perpendicular to the longitudinal reference of the foot.

The resultant motion around the third ray axis is essentially uniplanar owing to its nearly identical alignment with the Y axis of the foot's reference system. The rotational motions occurring are those of plantarflexion and dorsiflexion.[41] Movement around the first and fifth ray axes, however, are triplanar. Rotation around the first ray axis consists of combined dorsiflexion, inversion, and adduction and conversely of the combination of plantarflexion, eversion, and abduction. Root[42] comments that the amount of adduction/abduction in the transverse plane is minimal, due to the near horizontal alignment of the axis; correspondingly, Hicks[41] does not even list these motions as components of first ray mobility.

Total ROM of the first ray around its axis measures 22°.[41] Owing to the near 45° alignment of the axis from the longitudinal reference of the foot, the magnitude of the dorsiflexion-plantarflexion component of motion is nearly equal to the inversion-eversion component.[42] Clinically, normal first ray ROM in dorsiflexion is approximately 10 mm above the plane of the lesser metatarsals; correspondingly, full plantarflexion ROM is 10 mm below the plane. Values for functional ROM around the first ray axis have not been identified, but the following requirements must be achieved. There must be adequate dorsiflexion of the first ray to allow unrestricted movement into this position under the influence of ground reaction forces, particularly if conditions exist leading to excessive pronation and resultant eversion of the foot.[42] Adequate plantarflexion must also be present to ensure attainment of full hallux extension during the propulsive phase of gait. Root[42] reports this functional requirement to be 10°. The mechanical events of first ray plantarflexion and hallux extension are discussed later with the MTP joints.

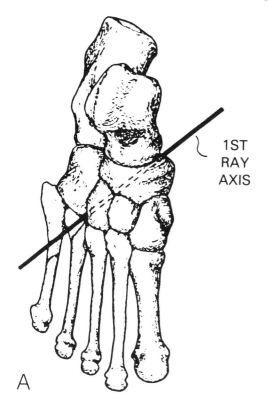

1ST
RAY
AXIS

A

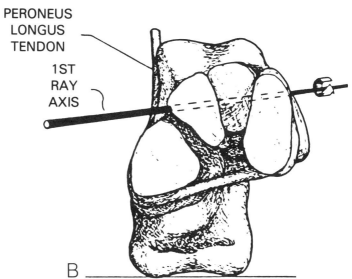

PERONEUS
LONGUS
TENDON

1ST
RAY
AXIS

B

Fig. 1-16. (**A**) Dorsal and (**B**) anterior views of the first ray axis. (Adapted from Root ML, Orien WP, Weed JH. Normal and Abnormal Function of the Foot. Clinical Biomechanics, Los Angeles, 1977.)

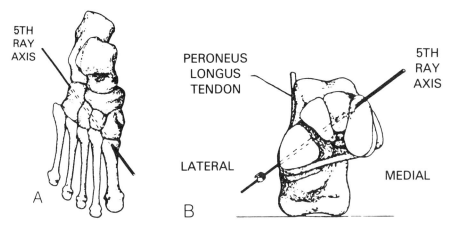

Fig. 1-17. (**A**) Dorsal and (**B**) anterior views of the fifth ray axis. (Adapted from Root ML, Orien WP, Weed JH: Normal and Abnormal Function of the Foot. Clinical Biomechanics, Los Angeles, 1977.)

If the foot is viewed as a whole that rotates into pronation and supination around the subtalar and oblique midtarsal joint axes, alternative first ray motion can be observed. D'Amico[47] and Oldenbrook[48] both describe functional first ray motion as consisting of dorsiflexion occurring with eversion in accordance with forefoot motion. This is shown by the plantar concavity of the first metatarsal pointing laterally with pronation, in contrast to the coupling of dorsiflexion with inversion previously mentioned as occurring around the first ray axis. Oldenbrook[48] also states that this discrepancy between functional and anatomical coupling of motion can be explained by the relatively small degree of motion around the first ray axis when compared with larger magnitudes of the forefoot achieved during pronation of the foot. The degree of forefoot eversion, being one of the component motions of pronation, exceeds the amount of inversion of the first ray, thereby resulting in an apparent net eversion of the first ray coupled with dorsiflexion as pronation occurs about the subtalar and oblique midtarsal joint axes. They report this value to be an average of 3.4° of eversion, as measured on five newly amputated cadavers.

Oldenbrook,[48] in examining motion of the lesser rays, found they showed greater frontal plane ROM than the first ray in all but one case. When sagittal plane mobility was viewed, however, all lesser rays showed less ROM than the first, with the range of dorsiflexion being much less than the plantarflexion range. This is in agreement with Root,[42] who states that on examination, the lesser rays are capable of plantarflexion only from their common position achieved during midstance. Sammarco[32] states that the second ray is the most rigid of the lesser rays.

Motion of the fifth ray is triplanar, consisting of the coupling of dorsiflexion with eversion and abduction, and contrarily, plantarflexion with inversion and adduction. These patterns of movement are similar to those of pronation and supination around the subtalar and oblique midtarsal joints. Because the fifth ray axis deviates from the transverse plane only by 20°, the amount of abduction and adduction is minimal. Hicks[41] reports that the total ROM of the fifth ray is 10°. Functional ROM values are not identified, although there appear to be equal amounts of dorsiflexion and plantarflexion as the foot undergoes pronation and supination.[42]

Functionally, maintaining stability of the first ray in a downward direction is critical. Loss of this plantarflexion stabilization can result in hypermobility of the first ray and lead to development of hallux deformities, particularly hallux valgus and hallux limitus/rigidus.[42] Stability of the first ray is primarily achieved through action of the peroneus longus muscle.[42] An important biomechanical relationship exists between the relative position of the peroneal tendon in the groove of the cuboid and its insertion into the base of the first metatarsal and medial cuneiform. When in the subtalar neutral position, the base of the first metatarsal is at a greater distance from the floor than is the peroneal tendon in the cuboid. When the force generated by the peroneus longus is defined by its component vectors, there is both a laterally directed force and a smaller plantar component (Fig. 1-18). Root[42] therefore states that with this osseous alignment, a plantarflexion stabilizing force is acting on the first ray. When the foot assumes a supinated posture, the talus dorsiflexes over the calcaneus, resulting in a more superior positioning of the talar head in relation to the calcaneus than when in subtalar neutral (Fig. 1-11). The entire medial longitudinal arch is therefore elevated, including not only the talar head, but the navicular, medial cuneiform, and first metatarsal.[35,42] This serves to create an even larger plantarly directed component force of the peroneus longus, thereby increasing its downward stabilization. This is in contrast to the events associated with subtalar pronation. As pronation progresses, the medial arch is lowered, allowing the talar head and calcaneus to lie on almost the same horizontal level. This repositioning effectively eliminates the plantar component of the muscle's force, with the laterally directed component now nearly equivalent to the total force generated by the peroneus longus. The net effect on the first ray is a stronger lateral displacement of its base but, more significantly, a loss of downward stability in response to the dorsally directed ground reaction forces. This renders the first MTP joint hypermobile when the foot assumes a fully pronated position and, in the presence of an everted posture of the hindfoot during pronation, can lead to a dorsiflexed repositioning of the first ray. Root[42] cites the first ray hypermobility as one of the underlying mechanical factors in the development of both hallux valgus and hallux rigidus.

MTP Joints

The MTP joints are composed of the articulations between the distal heads of the five metatarsals with the corresponding bases of the proximal phalanges. The MTP joints are classified as condyloid, being composed of a convex metatarsal surface and a concave phalangeal shape at all five joints.

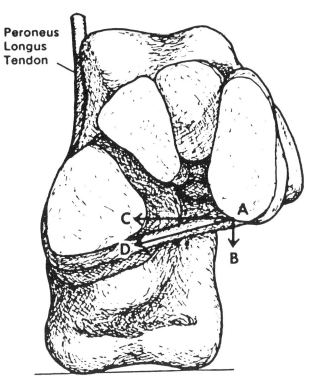

Peroneus Longus Tendon

Fig. 1-18. Relative position between the peroneus longus tendon at the peroneal groove of the cuboid and at the base of the first metatarsal in subtalar neutral position. Vector AB represents the plantar stabilizing force produced by contraction of the peroneus longus muscle. This stabilizing force decreases as the foot pronates due to lowering of the base of the first metatarsal to a level more equal to the groove on the cuboid. This effectively eliminates the plantar stabilizing vector AB and renders the first ray hypermobile. (Root ML, Orien WP, Weed JH: Normal and Abnormal Function of the Foot. Clinical Biomechanics, Los Angeles, 1977.)

Gray[6] describes the articular surface of the metatarsal heads as kidney-shaped, with the plantar portion of the joint surface extending more proximally than the dorsal. The articular cartilage extends over the dorsal aspect of the metatarsal heads to allow full, dorsal motion of the proximal phalanx during MTP extension. Unique to the first MTP joint are two sesamoid bones lying under the plantar aspect of the first metatarsal head and separated by an osseous crest. The medial sesamoid is embedded within the common tendinous insertion of the abductor hallucis brevis and medial portion of the flexor hallucis brevis muscles.[6] The lateral sesamoid is likewise encased within a tendon, now containing the lateral head of the flexor hallucis brevis, oblique head of the adductor hallucis, and transverse head of the adductor hallucis (transversus pedis) muscle.[6,42] The sesamoids have several vital functions, including weightbearing of the first ray, elevating the first metatarsal head to allow subsequent plantarflexion during hallux extension, and enhancing the mechanical lever of those hallux muscles into which they are embedded.

The anatomical relationship allows for motion around two distinct axes at the first MTP joint. Root[42] describes a vertical axis allowing the transverse plane motions of pure adduction/abduction and a transverse axis allowing the pure sagittal plane motions of flexion/extension of the hallux. The vertical axis passes through the first metatarsal at the most proximal aspect of the plantar articulating surface (Fig. 1-19). Sammarco,[32] on the other hand, shows the axis of rotation for transverse plane motion to be near the base of the first metatarsal and subsequently describes the transverse plane motion as translation between the hallux and metatarsal head. The transverse axis lies distally to the vertical axis, being positioned within the metatarsal head.[32,42] Sammarco[32] adds that the position of the transverse axis within the metatarsal head is variable, depending on the position of the hallux in the sagittal plane. The MTP joints of the lesser toes function in the same fashion as the first MTP joint, owing to their similar joint configuration. They each function around a vertical axis for transverse plane abduction/adduction and a transverse axis for sagittal plane flexion/extension.[42] Apparently no frontal plane motion occurs with normal MTP function; therefore, no axis is defined. These motions are clearly apparent in pathological conditions, however, resulting in frontal plane eversion of the great toe in hallux valgus and frontal plane inversion of the fifth toe in digiti quinti varus.

Normal ROM at the first MTP joint measures 30° of flexion and 90° of extension.[32] Values for the lesser MTP joints are similar, showing 90° of extension and slightly greater flexion, now measuring 45 to 50°.[19,32] Functionally, MTP extension rather than flexion is most critical, especially at the first MTP joint, since much larger values are required for proper gait. Reports reflecting the magnitude of functional MTP extension show that the requirements are similar for all MTP joints, but the reported amounts are variable. Bojsen-Møller[49] states that 50 to 60° of maximal MTP extension occurs during push-off; Root[42] reports that a value within the range of 65 to 75° is necessary; Mann[50] cites a slightly larger range of MTP extension, 70 to 90°; whereas Kapandji[19] concurs that magnitudes approaching 90° are observed. The amount of transverse plane abduction/adduction ROM at the MTP joints is small, with no values reported.

An appreciation for normal function at the MTP joints requires a review of the arthrokinematic principles governing the joint. If the toes are passively extended over a stationary metatarsal, the resultant motion is that of a concave joint surface moving on a convex surface (Fig. 1-5a). The arthrokinematics dictate that movement of the concave proximal phalanx will be in the same direction as the osteokinematics of the entire hallux, that being dorsally directed joint motion as the hallux moves dorsally into extension. Conversely, when the toes are stationary and the metatarsals become the moving structure, as occurs following heel-off during normal gait sequence, the direction of motion at the joint surface is now opposite to that of the bony segment (Fig. 1-5). Movement at the articular surface of the convex metatarsal head is plantarly directed as the metatarsal itself moves dorsally. Proper application of these arthrokinematic and osteokinematic concepts becomes clinically relevant when

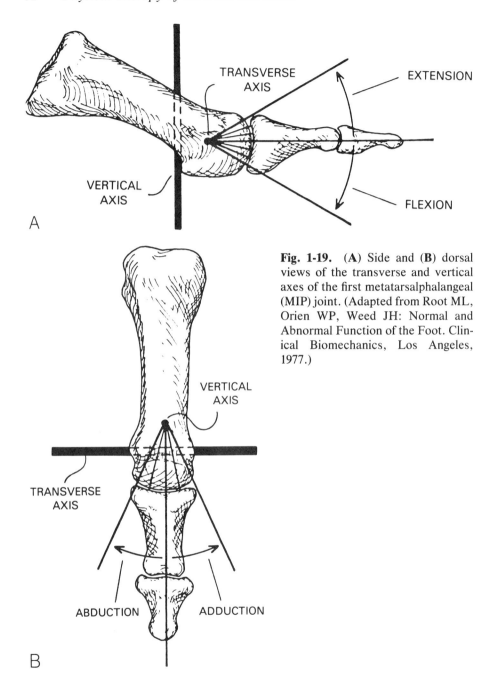

Fig. 1-19. (**A**) Side and (**B**) dorsal views of the transverse and vertical axes of the first metatarsalphalangeal (MIP) joint. (Adapted from Root ML, Orien WP, Weed JH: Normal and Abnormal Function of the Foot. Clinical Biomechanics, Los Angeles, 1977.)

joint mobilization to a hypomobile MTP joint is considered, as would be the case in early stages of hallux limitus.

A closer examination of hallux extension at the first MTP joint reveals that proper function depends on a number of variables, including proper sesamoid function and plantarflexion of the first metatarsal. The degree of hallux exten-

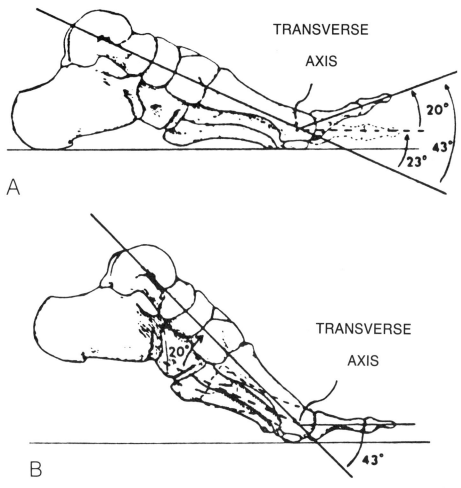

TRANSVERSE

AXIS

20°

43°

23°

A

TRANSVERSE

AXIS

20°

43°

B

Fig. 1-20. (**A**) Maximal hallux extension at the first MTP joint without accompanying plantarflexion of the first ray measures 20° from the supporting surface with the heel on the floor, or (**B**) equivalently, 43° when measured from the long axis of the first ray. (Root ML, Orien WP, Weed JH: Normal and Abnormal Function of the Foot. Clinical Biomechanics, Los Angeles, 1977.)

sion without associated first ray plantarflexion measures 20 to 24° from the floor when standing, or equivalently, 43 to 48° when measured from the shaft of the first metatarsal (Fig. 1-20).[42] If this relationship between the hallux and first metatarsal were maintained throughout the entire propulsive phase of gait, adequate first MTP joint extension would never be achieved and would most likely lead to the development of osteoarthritic changes within the joint. To allow proper MTP motion, the first ray must undergo plantarflexion of approximately 10°.[42] Root[42] adds that this first ray plantarflexion is achieved secondary to proper sesamoid function. The metatarsal head moves posteriorly as the rotating joint surface glides over the fixed sesamoid bones, thereby allowing proper articulation between the proximal phalanx with the dorsal aspect of the metatarsal head joint surface. Although sesamoid bones exist only at the first MTP joint, adequate plantarflexion of the lesser metatarsal heads is likewise necessary to achieve full lesser MTP joint extension.

Proper functioning of the foot requires maintenance of near parallel alignment between the longitudinal axis of all toes with the longitudinal reference of the rearfoot—the position that allows maximum stability of the toes.[42] Price[46] reports a normal range between 9 and 17° of valgus for the hallux at the MTP joint. This transverse plane position of the hallux, and of the lesser toes, in relation to its metatarsal will be properly maintained provided transverse plane alignment of the forefoot remains normal. If forefoot deviations exist in the transverse plane, specifically forefoot adductus, this relationship changes. Root[42] states that the toes will continue to maintain this parallel alignment between the two longitudinal axes by drifting into abduction at the MTP joints, thereby altering the relationship between the toe and its metatarsal. This newly acquired abnormal alignment can lead to development of clinical symptoms and deformity at all joints of the toes, specifically hallux valgus and claw-toes.

An additional anatomical relationship with important biomechanical implications concerns the length of the metatarsals. The second metatarsal is usually the longest[22,34,45,51] followed in length by the first, third, and fourth, with the fifth being the shortest. The outcome of these varying metatarsal lengths is the formation of two functional axes for MTP extension, both of which pass through the second metatarsal, since it is the longest. The first, an oblique MTP axis, passes through the second to fifth MTP joints and is termed the metatarsal break (Fig. 1-21). Mann[22] describes this axis as having a mean deviation of 62° from the longitudinal axis of the foot. The second, the transverse MTP axis, passes between the first and second MTP joints and shows a much more perpendicular alignment to the longitudinal reference. The significance of there being two functional axes is that depending on which is used during the propulsive phase of gait alters significantly the series of levers through which both muscles and ground reaction forces can operate.

During the gait cycle, extension at the MTP joints begins with heel-off, which occurs when the tibia achieves a forward inclination of between 10 and 25° (mean 21°)[49] at approximately 45% of the gait cycle.[52] Initially, this rotation of the rising heel over the stationary toes occurs around the metatarsal break axis. Then, as heel-rise continues, a shift to the transverse axis occurs. Bojsen-Møller[51] states that this shifting between MTP axes results in a 15 to 20% increase in the length of the lever arm. This will correspondingly affect the demands placed on the plantarflexion musculature. He also states that when maximum MTP joint extension is achieved, 55 to 65°, the axis is further displaced anteriorly to the tip of the great toe, providing yet another functional forefoot axis. This effectively increases the lever by an additional 30%.[49] Temporally, rotation around the MTP joint axes continues for 32% of the stance phase (19% of the total gait cycle), with rotation around the tip of the hallux accounting for the remaining 14% of stance phase (8.4% of the total cycle) before swing phase begins.[49] The presence of three distinct levers provides the foot and surrounding musculature with the flexibility to use the lever arm that

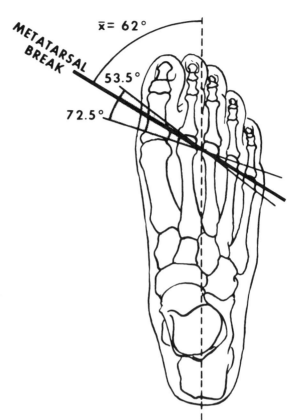

Fig. 1-21. Metatarsal break axis measures an average of 62° from the longitudinal axis of the foot. This axis directs the metatarsal phalangeal (MTP) joint extension at the lesser toes that occurs following heel-off. (Reproduced with permission from Mann RA: Biomechanics of the foot. p. 257. In American Academy of Orthopedic Surgeons' Atlas of Orthotics: Biomechanical Principles and Application. CV Mosby, St. Louis, 1975.)

best meets the requirements imposed by the demands of gait. A fast-paced gait on a level surface requires the longer, transverse MTP axis, whereas uphill walking makes use of the shorter level around the metatarsal break.[49,51]

AUTHOR'S NOTE

This chapter was written in author's private capacity. No official support or endorsement by the United States Department of Health and Human Services is intended or should be inferred.

REFERENCES

1. Kelley DL: Kinesiology: Fundamentals of Motion Description. Prentice-Hall, Englewood Cliffs, NJ, 1971
2. Sgarlato TE. (ed): A Compendium of Podiatric Biomechanics. California College of Podiatric Medicine, San Francisco, 1971
3. Resnick R, Halliday J: Physics. Part I. 3rd Ed. John Wiley & Sons, New York, 1977

4. Maughan RJ, Watson JS, Weir J: Relationships between muscle strength and muscle cross-sectional area in male sprinters and endurance runners. Eur J Appl Physiol 50:309, 1983

5. Perry J: Anatomy and biomechanics of the hindfoot. Clin Orthop Rel Res 177:9, 1983

6. Goss CM (ed): Gray's Anatomy of the Human Body. 29th Ed. Lea & Febiger, Philadelphia, 1973

7. Morris JM: Biomechanics of the foot and ankle. Clin Orthop Rel Res 122:10, 1977

8. Inman VT: The Joints of the Ankle. Williams & Wilkins, Baltimore, 1976

9. Barnett CH, Napier JR: The axis of rotation of the ankle joint in man. Its influence upon the form of the talus and the mobility of the fibula. J Anat 86:1, 1952

10. Frankel VH, Nordin M: Biomechanics of the ankle. p. 179. In Basic Biomechanics of the Skeletal System. Lea & Febiger, Philadelphia, 1980

11. Isman RE, Inman VT: Anthropometric Studies of the Human Foot and Ankle: Technical Report No: 58, University of California, San Francisco, 1968

12. Sammarco GJ, Burnstein AH, Frankel VH: Biomechanics of the ankle: a kinematic study. Orthop Clin North Am 4(1):75, 1973

13. Parlasca R, Shoji H, D'Ambrosia RD: Effects of ligamentous injury on ankle and subtalar joints: a kinematic study. Clin Orthop Rel Res 140:266, 1979

14. Murray MP, Kory RC, Clarkson BH, Sepic SB: Comparison of free and fast speed walking patterns of normal men. Am J Phys Med 45(1):8, 1966

15. Stauffer RN, Chao EYS, Brewster RC: Force and motion analysis of the normal, diseased, and prosthetic ankle joint. Clin Orthop Rel Res 127:189, 1977

16. Jordan RP, Cooper M, Schuster RO: Ankle dorsiflexion at the heel-off phase of gait. J Am Pod Assoc 69(1):40, 1979

17. Ramsey PL, Hamilton W: Changes in tibiotalar area of contact caused by lateral shift. J Bone Joint Surg [Am] 58:356, 1976

18. Eyring EJ, Murray WR: The effect of joint position on the pressure of intra-articular effusion. J Bone Joint Surg [Am] 46:1235, 1964

19. Kapandji IA: The Physiology of the Joints. The Lower Limb. 2nd Ed. Vol. 3. Churchill Livingstone, New York, 1974

20. Bunning PSC, Barnett CH: A comparison of adult and foetal talocalcaneal articulations. J Anat 99(1):71, 1965

21. Isherwood I: A radiological approach to the subtalar joint. J Bone Joint Surg [Br] 43:566, 1961

22. Mann RA: Biomechanics of the foot. p. 257. In American Academy of Orthopedic Surgeons' Atlas of Orthotics: Biomechanical Principles and Application. CV Mosby, St. Louis, 1975

23. Root ML, Weed JH, Sgarlato TE, Bluth DR: Axis of motion of the subtalar joint. J Am Podiatry Assoc 56(4):149, 1966

24. Inman VT, Ralston HJ, Todd F: Human Walking. Williams & Wilkins Company, Baltimore, 1984

25. Kotwick JE: Biomechanics of the foot and ankle. Clin Sports Med 1(1):19, 1982

26. Manter JT: Movements of the subtalar and transtarsal joint. Anat Rec 80(4):397, 1941

27. Green DR, Whitney AK, Walters P: Subtalar joint motion. J Am Podiatry Assoc 69(1):83, 1979

28. Wright DG, Desai SM, Henderson WH: Action of the subtalar and ankle-joint complex during the stance phase of walking. J Bone Joint Surg [Am] 46:361, 1964

29. Subotnick SI: Biomechanics of the subtalar and midtarsal joints. J Am Podiatry Assoc 65(8):756, 1975

30. Close JR, Inman VT, Poor PM, Todd FN: The function of the subtalar joint. Clin Orthop Rel Res 50:159, 1960
31. Imhaeuser G: The constant relationship between forefoot and hindfoot as a basis for treating foot deformities. Arch Orthop Traumatic Surg 94:205, 1979
32. Sammarco GJ: Biomechanics of the foot. p. 193. In Frankel VH, Nordin M (eds): Basic Biomechanics of the Skeletal System. Lea & Febiger, Philadelphia, 1980
33. Levins AS, Inman VT, Blosses JA: Transverse rotation of the lower extremity in locomotion. J Bone Joint Surg [Am] 30:859, 1948
34. Inman VT, Mann RA: Biomechanics of the foot and ankle. p. 3. In Inman VT (ed): Surgery of the Foot. 3rd Ed. CV Mosby, St. Louis, 1973
35. Benink RJ: Biomechanical behavior of the human tarsus related with a new radiological index. p. 191. In Huiskes R, van Campen DH, de Wijn (eds): Biomechanics: principles and Applications. Martinus Nijhoff Publishers, The Hague, 1982
36. Kyne PJ, Mankin HJ: Changes in intra-articular pressure with subtalar joint motion with special reference to the etiology of peroneal spastic flat foot. Bull Hosp Joint Dis 26(2):181, 1965
37. Bojsen-Møller F: Calcaneocuboid joint stability of the longitudinal arch of the foot at high and low gear push off. J Anat 129(1):165, 1979
38. Weston WJ: positive contrast arthrography of the normal midtarsal joints. Aust Radiol 13:365, 1969
39. Huson A: Perspectives in human-joint kinematics. p. 31. In Huiskes R, van Campen DH, de Wijn JR (eds): Biomechanics: principles and Applications. Martinus Nijhoff Publishers, The Hague, 1982
40. Greenberg GS: Relationship of hallux abductus angle and first metatarsal angle to severity of pronation. J Am Podiatry Assoc 69(1):29, 1979
41. Hicks JH: The mechanics of the foot: I. The joints. J Anat 87:345, 1953
42. Root ML, Orien WP, Weed JH: Normal and Abnormal Function of the Foot. Clinical Biomechanics, Los Angeles, 1977
43. Hlavac HF: The Foot Book. World Publications, Mountain View, CA, 1977
44. Hlavac HF: Major considerations in the clinical evaluation of the lower limb. p. 321. In Sgarlato TE (ed): A Compendium of Podiatric Biomechanics. California College of Podiatric Medicine, San Francisco, 1971
45. Rowland RN, Ferris TL, Dobus DC: A study of the metatarsal break. J Am Pod Assoc 69(1):47, 1979
46. Price GFW: Metatarsus primus varus: including various clinicoradiologic features of the female foot. Clin Orthop Rel Res 145:217, 1979
47. D'Amico JC, Schuster RO: Motion of the first ray: clarification through investigation. J Am Podiatry Assoc 69(1):17, 1979
48. Oldenbrook LL, Smith CE: Metatarsal head motion secondary to rearfoot pronation and supination: an anatomical investigation. J Am Podiatry Assoc 69(1):24, 1979
49. Bojsen-Møller F, Lamoreux L: Significance of free dorsiflexion of the toes in walking. Acta Orthop Scand 50:471, 1979
50. Mann RA, Hagy JL: The function of the toes in walking, jogging, and running. Clin Orthop Rel Res, 142:24, 1979
51. Bojsen-Møller F: Anatomy of the forefoot, normal and pathologic. Clin Orthop Rel Res, 142:10, 1979
52. Manley MT: Biomechanics of the foot. p. 21. In Helfet AJ, Gruebel Lee DM (eds): Disorders of the Foot. JB Lippincott, Philadelphia, 1980

2 | Gait and Foot Pathomechanics

Gary C. Hunt
Ronald S. Brocato

GAIT

The average free walking gait cycle is composed of two phases: stance, which constitutes approximately 60 percent, and swing, which constitutes approximately 40 percent of the entire cycle. Stance is composed of a period of single limb support bounded by two periods of double limb support.[1]

As the velocity of ambulation increases to a jog, double limb support is replaced by a floating period, indicating that the body is airborne. The stance phase takes approximately 0.6 second in the average free walking gait cycle and decreases to approximately 0.1 second in a run.[2] Despite this short time frame, a variety of important events occur that enable the efficient transfer of energy, resulting in a smooth gait pattern. The foot plays an important role in allowing the body to use and absorb energy during this process. It is not surprising to encounter a variety of problems when foot dysfunction occurs.

Functions of the Foot

The foot provides primarily four functions: (1) a base of support, (2) shock absorption, (3) mobile adaptation, and (4) a rigid lever. The study of motion (kinematics) and force (kinetics) combine to form the basis for evaluation of human locomotion. A discussion of these two elements will help to explain how the foot is able to satisfy these four functions. Unfortunately, technology has not been able to provide a clear method to study the small intricate motions occurring in the foot; thus, the description of subtalar and midtarsal joint motion is somewhat speculative. The study by Wright et al,[3] which included only a few subjects, has probably been the most widely referenced source on subtalar joint function and despite its limitations, the explanation of foot function is conveniently demonstrated by describing the kinematics of the subtalar joint. Too many variables exist, making absolute values difficult. They include the following:

1. Normal positional variations of the subtalar and midtarsal axes and the fact that they are triplanar
2. Variability of velocity, stride length, and cadence
3. Positional variation of the center of mass affecting standing balance
4. Proximal control and stability of the trunk and pelvis
5. Motor control and neurological maturity

Various studies conducted on the subtalar joint have demonstrated similar patterns of motion, however; therefore, it seems reasonable that discussions of motion patterns rather than magnitudes of motion may be legitimate.[3-6] Therefore, the pattern of subtalar joint motion will be used as the focus to describe how the foot contributes to the functional demands in gait. Figure 2-1 shows the pattern occurring in the subtalar joint. Measurement of subtalar joint motion is not possible owing to its triplanar movement pattern. As a compromise, the frontal plane movement of the calcaneus is measured and is intended to reflect subtalar movement.

A basic requirement of gait is to get from point A to point B with minimal energy expenditure and without falling down. As Perry[7] points out, a smooth forward progression involves (1) shock absorption, (2) momentum control, and (3) forward propulsion. In addition, the individual must have adequate balance, particularly in single limb support.

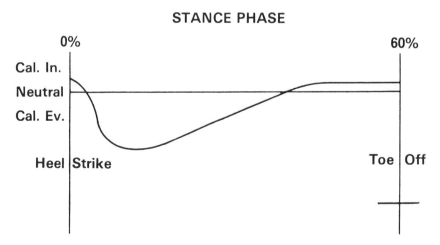

STANCE PHASE

Fig. 2-1. Subtalar joint motion. (Redrawn from Hlavac HF: The Foot Book. p. 92, World Publications, Mountain View, CA, 1977.)

Observational Gait

In observing gait, one may more easily evaluate the foot during gait as its parts relate to the floor. The following discussion identifies the movement in the frontal plane and relates that movement with associated patterns of the remaining limb segments.

Observing the subject from behind offers the best view for calcaneal frontal plane movement as it represents subtalar joint motion. Observation from the anterior view provides better visualization of transverse plane movements of the lower extremity (internal/external rotation) and also movements of the forefoot. Observation from the side provides an assessment of sagittal plane movements (i.e., ankle dorsi/plantarflexion, heel-off, and knee/hip motion patterns). The reader is referred to other references for further gait assessment approaches.[7-9]

Figure 2-2A identifies the movement pattern of the calcaneus during stance and is described as follows. At initial contact during walking, the calcaneus is slightly inverted relative to the floor. As the foot begins to accept weight, rapid calcaneal eversion occurs to a point at which the calcaneus should be perpendicular to the floor. Both the magnitude and velocity of this motion may separately or in combination have a significant impact on the development of overuse syndromes.[6] The first function, base of support, is satisfied merely by the fact that the foot is in contact with the ground. The ability to maintain balance is a prerequisite to efficient motor performance; this is achieved in part as the foot interacts with the supporting surface during stance. The second and third functions, shock absorption and mobile adaptation, respectively, are also achieved early in the stance phase. Shock absorption is achieved in part as the calcaneus everts or rolls in during weight acceptance. As a consequence of calcaneal eversion, the midtarsal region becomes flexible, which adds further to shock absorption but in addition allows the forefoot to adapt or conform to the supporting surface. Maximum calcaneal eversion should be achieved during weight acceptance; therefore, no further eversion should occur in single limb stance.

An important relationship should be emphasized between lower extremity transverse rotation and subtalar motion. As the lower extremity internally rotates on the weightbearing limb, pronation will occur around the subtalar and oblique midtarsal joints. Conversely, as the lower limb externally rotates on the weightbearing limb, the subtalar and oblique midtarsal joint will supinate. This relationship becomes very important because management approaches to control foot pronation will affect transverse rotation of the lower extremity.

During the latter part of stance, the foot must become a stable structure to act as a rigid lever. This is accomplished by supination around the subtalar joint in association with external rotation of the lower extremity relative to the line of progression. Supination around the subtalar axis with the forefoot still in contact with the floor locks the midfoot, thus providing a stable foot. During observational analysis, the heel will be noted to move into inversion (varus) as it leaves the ground and before the forefoot lifts off.

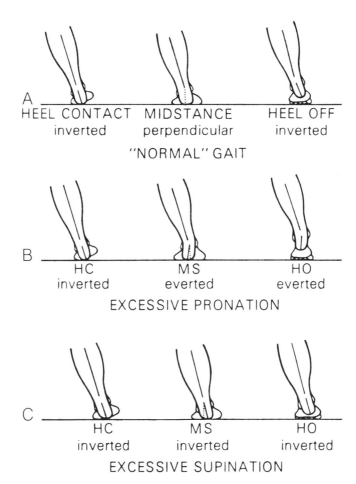

Fig. 2-2. Observational gait analysis. (**A**) ''Normal'' gait, (**B**) Excessive pronation, (**C**) Excessive supination.

The requirements of the foot for jogging and running are the same as walking except that the forces are greater with a shorter time application. Initial contact in jogging may not be heel first for all subjects. Cavanaugh[10] has identified heel strikers, midfoot strikers, and forefoot strikers as normal patterns of running styles. The use of videotape with its slow-motion capabilities is almost essential in studying the athlete in his environment. Movement patterns happen so quickly (stance 0.15 to 0.20 seconds) that foot function is difficult to assess at normal speed.

The timing sequence of these events is important in providing an efficient gait. Repetitive activities associated with excessive or inadequate movement in the foot/ankle seem to result in maldistribution of forces, producing injury. Gait should be evaluated while the patient is barefooted and again while the patient is wearing shoes. Gait abnormalities are often caused by inadequate footwear and not by significant foot dysfunction.

Gait Abnormalities

One of the most common gait abnormalities is excessive subtalar and oblique midtarsal joint pronation. The challenge is to determine the cause of the pronation and then to set up an appropriate management program. Figure 2-2B demonstrates the sequence observed in the excessively pronated gait. Excessive subtalar pronation may occur as a result of the following:[9,11]

1. Sagittal plane deviations
    A compensation for limited ankle joint dorsiflexion
2. Frontal plane deviations
    Excessive tibia vara
    Forefoot varus
    Muscle imbalance between invertors and evertors
3. Transverse plane deviations
    Increased internal lower extremity rotation secondary to
       Femoral anteversion
       Muscle imbalance, with hip internal rotators having greater advantage
4. Miscellaneous
    Short first ray (Morton's foot)

On the other end of the spectrum is excessive supination, which may be caused mainly by frontal plane deviations and include:[9,11]

1. Limited calcaneal eversion
2. Rigid forefoot valgus or plantarflexed first ray
3. Muscle imbalance associated with upper motor neuron deficit (i.e., stronger invertors)

Figure 2.2C illustrates the sequence observed in the excessively supinated gait. It is difficult to determine the primary cause of excessive pronation or supination from the observational gait assessment. Static examination is necessary to identify primary reasons for the gait deviation so that a management scheme can be formulated.

Kinetics: The Influence of Force

Biomechanical assessment is not complete without consideration of how the foot interacts with the forces imposed on it, for it is sandwiched between the pressure of the ground below and the weight and inertional forces of the body above. Investigations have studied these forces through various force or pressure measuring devices,[12] including force plates,[2,13,14] pressure-sensitive crystals,[15] and pressure transducers.[16] Force plate analysis has been one of the more commonly used devices for this assessment. The force plate provides force measurements in the vertical, fore/aft, medial/lateral, and torque movements around the X, Y, and Z axes. By having the individual walk or run over the force plate, therapists can analyze these force parameters.

During walking, the vertical force graph demonstrates an initial maximal force achieved at about 20 percent of the gait cycle which is 115 to 120 percent of body weight. During midstance, the vertical force decreases as the center of body mass is rising; then, during late stance, a second peak force increases again to about 115 to 120 percent of body weight. This second peak force is associated with a maximum contraction of the gastrocnemius and a weight shift to the opposite limb.[2]

The influence of ambulation velocity on force development has been studied and reported.[2,15] Results indicate that as velocity increases so does the vertical force, which approaches 250 to 275 percent of body weight. The cadence and stride length also increases; this is associated with a shorter period of stance phase. Another major difference between walking and jogging/running is that the double limb support phase is replaced by a "floating" or "airborne" phase where at no time are both feet on the ground. This is represented in the vertical force graph by only one maximal peak force in the order of magnitude of about 250 to 275 percent of body weight. When comparing walking with jogging/running, Mann[17] found more variability from step to step in the latter. Figure 2-3 compares the vertical forces produced by walking, jogging, and running.

The other commonly analyzed curves include the fore/aft and medial/lateral forces. In the fore/aft curve, an initial fore force is allowed by an aft force during the end of stance, indicating that the foot is moving in a forward direction when it makes contact with the ground. During stance, as the center of the body mass continues to move over the fixed foot, the force changes to push backward, as indicated in the graph (Fig. 2-4). The pattern is somewhat similar in configuration as the velocity changes except that the magnitude increases approximately 50 percent in running and the rate of rise of the initial peak is sharper.[2]

The medial/lateral force demonstrates that as the foot makes contact with the ground, a rapid rising medial force occurs at all velocities, followed by a more gradual change in the lateral direction during the remainder of stance. This medial directed force is a reflection of foot pronation. The configuration and magnitude of the curve is similar for walking and jogging except that in jogging it occurs in less time. In running, however, the magnitude increases, and there is a double medial force component, the second coming during the latter part of the stance phase.[2] Figures 2-4 and 2-5 illustrate the comparative fore/aft and medial/lateral curves for different ambulation velocities.

The other force curve that has been studied, although less frequently, is the Z axis torque curve, which lies perpendicular to the ground and is illus-

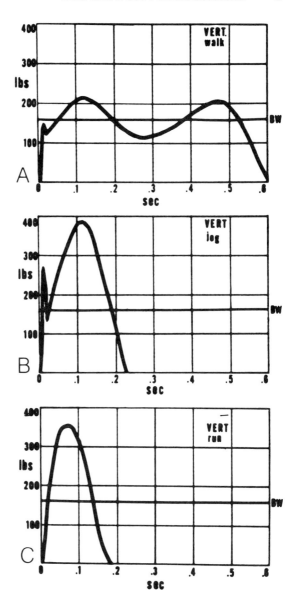

Fig. 2-3. Vertical force curve: (A) walking, (B) jogging, and (C) running. (Reprinted by permission from Mann RA, Hagy JL: Running, jogging, and walking: A comparative electromyographic and biomechanical study. p. 171. In Bateman JE, Trott AW (eds): The Foot and Ankle. New York, Thieme Medical Publishers, Inc., 1980.)

trated in Fig. 2-6. On initial contact, internal torque is demonstrated, followed by external torque. This torque pattern correlates well with the motion patterns of internal and external rotation in the lower extremity during gait.[17] Schoenhaus et al[18] reported increased transverse plane rotatory torque forces in the pronated foot during the stance phase of gait. The subtalar joint complex is the key element in the foot/ankle region in providing absorption and force transfer of this transverse torque. Without its contribution, transverse forces are taken up in other areas that may well fail the task, the result being overuse injuries.

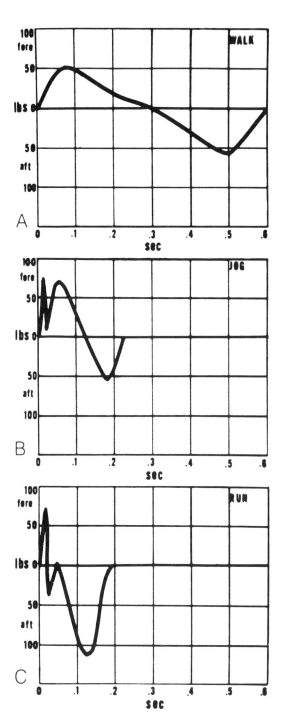

Fig. 2-4. Fore/aft force curve: (**A**) walking, (**B**) jogging, (**C**) running. (Reprinted by permission from Mann RA, Hagy JL: Running, jogging, and walking: A comparative electromyographic and biomechanical study. p. 171. In Bateman JE, Trott AW (eds): The Foot and Ankle. New York, Thieme Medical Publishers, Inc., 1980.)

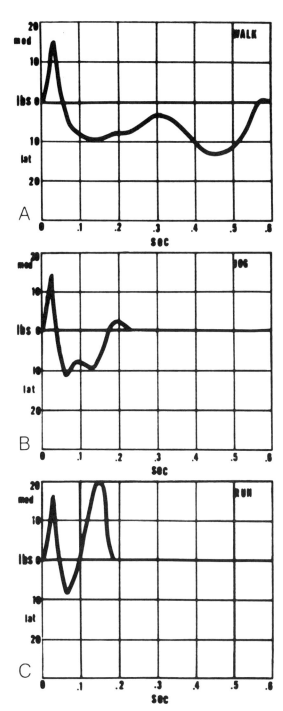

Fig. 2-5. Mediolateral force curve: (**A**) walking, (**B**) jogging, (**C**) running. (Reprinted by permission from Mann RA, Hagy JL: Running, jogging, and walking: A comparative electromyographic and biomechanical study. p. 171. In Bateman JE, Trott AW (eds): The Foot and Ankle. New York, Thieme Medical Publishers, Inc., 1980.)

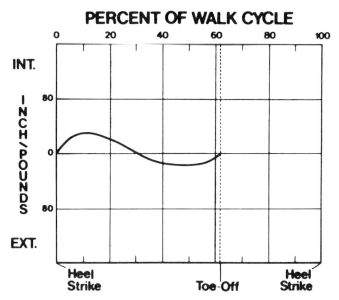

Fig. 2-6.   Force plate analysis of torque during walking. (Reprinted by permission from Mann RA, Hagy JL: Running, jogging, and walking: A comparative electromyographic and Biomechanical Study. p. 171. In Bateman JE, Trott AW (eds): The Foot and Ankle. New York, Thieme Medical Publishers, Inc., 1980.)

Repetitive forces acting on loose articular bodies may cause elongation of the supporting soft tissues, with eventual articular breakdown.[19] Pertinent to the development of this situation is the "windlass" mechanism as described by Hicks[20] and illustrated in Fig. 2-7. This mechanical term has been used to explain how the foot develops stability during stance. During the latter part of stance as the heel lifts off and when midfoot stability is essential, passive dorsiflexion of the metatarsalphalangeal (MTP) joints occurs. This event produces increased tension of the plantar fascia with arch elevation, midfoot stability, and an associated reduction of plantar intersegmental ligament tension. When excessive subtalar joint pronation occurs, the windlass mechanism may be less effective in providing necessary midfoot stability. The result is greater tension development in the midtarsal joint intersegmental ligaments. If this situation persists, it may produce excessive stress, resulting in midfoot pain. Pressure under the first metatarsal head (MTH) can also be greater in the pronated foot because the first metatarsal joint is unable to dorsiflex optimally in late midstance. The net result is pain under the first MTH secondary to increased pressure from inadequate weightbearing of the great toe's distal pad. Indeed, a medial callus on the great toe usually indicates that this reflects the site of greatest pressure. The development of hallux valgus has also been associated with these sequences of pressure distribution. Thus, we can conclude that it is mechanically possible for repeated, excessive pronation to cause hypermobility and eventually lead to joint subluxation.[9,21]

Abnormal pronation can also affect the phasic activity of muscle action

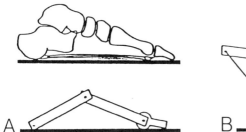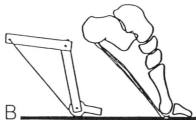

Fig. 2-7. Windlass action: (**A**) plantar fascia during footflat; (**B**) increased tension of plantar fascia during heel off. (Hunt GC, Novick A: Foot Pain: In Echternach JL (ed): Pain. Churchill Livingstone, New York, 1987, as Redrawn from Hicks JH: The foot as a Support. S. Karger AG, Basel. In Acta Anat 25:180, 1955.)

upon the foot. The foot intrinsics are reported to demonstrate increased periods of activity in pronated feet. Stabilization of the midtarsal articulations begin at 35 percent of the gait cycle in the "normal" foot. In the pronated foot, this stabilization begins at zero percent to 26 percent, implying that greater intrinsic muscular activity is required by the midtarsal and subtalar joints in the pronated foot.[22] The same conditions can be postulated for increases in eccentric activity of the anterior tibialis muscle from heel strike to 25 percent of the stance phase as well as the posterior tibialis muscle as it eccentrically contracts to stabilize the medial arch during pronation. The peroneous longus muscle loses its mechanical efficiency as a stabilizer of the first ray when the ray approaches the transverse plane of the cuboid, with pronation occurring within late midstance.[9] This unit may react eccentrically in an attempt to stabilize the medial plantar aspect of the forefoot during abnormal pronation. An inefficient pulley system between the cuboid–tendon interface could create both transverse and longitudinal shearing strains, resulting in tendinitis. It could also result in further destabilization of the cuboid resulting in hypermobility to the fifth ray.[23] This out-of-phase muscular activity as well as mechanical inefficiency secondary to osseous subluxations will alter the musculotendinous unit.

Based on the principle of hypermobility, we can conclude that abnormal compensatory pronation can cause many reported pathologies, including hyperkeratosis,[24] bunions,[9] heel spurs and plantar fasciitis,[25] myofascial pain,[26] anterior tibial syndrome,[27] neuromas,[28,29] postural fatigue and low back pain,[30–32] and chondromalacia patellae.[33,34] In the foot more than in any other body part, variations in the shape of the skeletal articulations and their relationships to one another profoundly modify the stability, shape, and function of the foot.[35]

FOOT PATHOMECHANICS

To describe foot deviations, a frame of reference must be established. The ideal balanced foot is one in which the MTH plane is perpendicular to the longitudinal bisection of the calcaneus with the subtalar joint in neutral position with the midfoot maximally pronated. While in this position, the bisection of the distal one-third of the leg should be contiguous with the calcaneal bisection. Some of the more common deviations from the norm are discussed next. Forefoot and hindfoot assessments are made with the subtalar joint in the neutral position and the midtarsal joints maximally pronated.

Hindfoot

Equinus (Talipes Equinus)

This deviation is a sagittal plane deformity characterized by restricted ankle joint dorsiflexion to less than 10° with the knee completely extended. Its etiology may be secondary to a congenital or an acquired muscle contracture of the gastrocnemius or the soleus muscles. In addition, limited ankle joint dorsiflexion may be secondary to osseous adaptation secondary to congenital talar dome malformation,[36] trauma, or inflammatory disease.

Compensation for this limitation may include excessive pronation of the subtalar and the oblique midtarsal joints during the mid to latter part of stance. The magnitude of the compensation is proportional to the degree of dorsiflexion necessary for a particular gait speed.[37] Studies have reported that these contractures result in increased stress placed on the forefoot.[36–38] Because abnormal pronation must occur about the subtalar joint axis, the midtarsal joints unlock, allowing freedom of movement. Manter[39] and Elftman[40] have reported that the oblique axis of the metatarsal joints will allow dorsiflexion of the forefoot on the rearfoot by as much as 10°. Excessive movement around the longitudinal axis will allow the medial aspect of the foot to flatten as well as place the metatarsals in an abducted position. This abduction results in a medial rolloff during propulsion and hypermobility of the entire first ray complex. The knee joint can also provide compensation by hyperextending to initiate foot flat or flexing, which may cause an early heel rise before 65 to 70 percent of stance. This early heel rise will demonstrate a bounce-type gait characteristic of an equinus deformity.[9,37,38]

Flexible foot structures will demonstrate excessive calcaneal eversion with signs of a rocker-bottom foot.[35] The rocker-bottom foot deformity is secondary to excessive forefoot dorsiflexion on the hindfoot.[41] The forefoot will demonstrate excessive abduction in stance, and the medial talar head will be very prominent. Other deviations may include hallux abducto valgus, hammer toes, and overlapping digits secondary to hypermobility and muscle imbalances. Plantar callus will occur primarily under the second through fourth metatarsal heads as well as along the medial hallux. In addition, some individuals will display limited dorsiflexion of the hallux secondary to a tight plantar aponeurosis. These clinical observations increase or decrease with the severity to the equinus.

Severe postural symptoms,[9,30–32,37,38] talonavicular pain,[9] metatarsalgia,[9] plantar bursitis, fasciitis, and heel spurs[38] have all been associated with this deviation. Equinus deformities in the moderate to severe form can be very difficult foot types to treat conservatively. The least severe acquired muscular imbalances can be treated with stretching and strengthening exercises, heel lifts, or neutral orthotics. All other conservative treatment is accommodative. Indeed, the gastrocnemius or soleus equinus is the greatest symptom producer in the human foot.[38]

Rearfoot Varus (Subtalar Varus)

The frontal plane deviation known as rearfoot or subtalar varus causes the calcaneus to be inverted to the ground when the subtalar joint is in the neutral position.[41] It occurs as a result of a developmental longitudinal varus torsion of the calcaneus or a structural tibia vara.[42] Compensation for this deviation is pronation of the subtalar joint during the initial part of stance, which may prevent normal supination during early propulsion.[9] Calcaneal eversion is generally limited, and the total range of motion (ROM) is reduced to between 17 and 21°.[42] The neutral subtalar joint position is 3 to 5° of varus. Because of the range limitations, the foot is moderately to severely rigid depending on the occurrence of other related pathology. Shearing keratomas may be noted under the second, fourth, and fifth MTHs as well as a retrocalcaneal prominence (pump bump).[41] Sometimes the first ray will plantarflex to reach foot flat. In addition, the tibia will internally rotate and adduct as another means of compensation.[43]

Generally, during gait, the calcaneus will stay in an inverted or varus position relative to the ground (see Fig. 2-2C).[9] As a result, the duration of pronatory compensation is minimal and does not extend into the propulsive periods. Signs of hypermobility are few. Symptomatology related to the abnormality is mild when associated with activities of daily living (ADL). Increased recreational endeavors could aggravate knee and ankle pathology.[34,44] This rearfoot abnormality is often associated with other structural deformities such as tibia vara and forefoot valgus. As the amount of tibia vara increases, so does the need for calcaneal eversion. Large amounts of subtalar vara combined with any of the above will augment symptoms in both the proximal and distal articulations.

Forefoot

Inverted Forefoot

Forefoot varus is considered a frontal plane structural deviation of the midtarsal joint in which the forefoot is inverted to the rearfoot when the subtalar joint is in its neutral position and the midtarsal joint is completely pronated (Fig. 2-8).[9]

The etiology is perceived to be a delay in the normal ontogeny of the

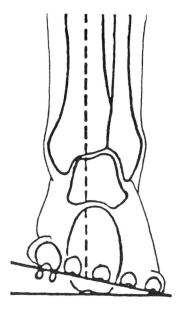

Fig. 2-8. Forefoot varus. (Hunt GC, Novick A: Foot Pain: In Echternach JL (ed): Pain. Churchill Livingstone, New York, 1987.)

midtarsal joint in which the head and the neck of the talus fail to complete the necessary valgus torsion.[45] In adult life, this equals approximately a valgus tilt of 35 to 40° of the head and neck of the talus to its trochlea.[46]

For the medial aspect of the foot to make contact with the ground during the first part of the stance phase, excessive pronation occurs around the subtalar and oblique midtarsal joints axes.[43,45,47] As subtalar pronation occurs, the planes of the midtarsal axes become parallel, allowing the midfoot to evert around the longitudinal axis.[40] This pronatory cycle is continued into the latter part of stance. Root et al[9] reported that continued pronation through the end of the stance phase is the most destructive cause of forefoot structures.

In static stance, the calcaneus will rest in an everted posture, and the forefoot may abduct if sufficient motion exists in the subtalar joint. The medial talar head will also be prominent as the medial arch collapses. A hallux valgus with a callus over the medial aspect of the great toe pad often exists due to shearing forces and pressure. As a consequence of forefoot hypermobility, keratomas develop under the second, third, and sometimes the fourth MTHs.[21] When limited subtalar joint motion is available, the calcaneus will not assume a valgus position and indeed may be inverted. Weightbearing is shifted to the lateral side of the foot; as a result, callus is located under the fourth and fifth MTHs. Keratomas that develop secondary to abnormal pronation are likely to be located distal and lateral to the MTHs.[48]

Symptoms associated with forefoot varus include postural fatigue,[43] chondromalacia patella,[33,34] Morton's neuroma,[28] plantar fasciitis, tendinitis, and shin splints.[9]

Everted Forefoot

The frontal plane position of the forefoot is everted relative to the calcaneal bisection while the subtalar joint is held in neutral position with the midfoot completely pronated.[9] Terminology regarding acquired and congenital foot types can become confusing. The terms pes cavus and pes planus are frequently used. The former has multiple classifications depending on the etiology and is often associated with everted forefoot postures.[49,50] Two main variations illustrated in Figs. 2-9 and 2-10 have been described and include the following:[51]:

1. Forefoot valgus—This deviation exists when the head and neck of the talus exceeds the necessary valgus torsion of 35 to 40° relative to the trochlear of the talus.[43] All five MTHs are everted relative to the calcaneal bisection.

2. Plantarflexed first ray—The first ray lies below the level of the remaining MTHs and produces an everted forefoot when the forefoot alignment includes the first through the fifth MTH. If congenital, this abnormality describes a pure cavus foot.[9] It is the most common form of an everted forefoot and is generally acquired as a compensation from excessive tibia vara with limited calcaneal eversion. The first ray plantarflexes in order for the medial side of the foot to make contact with the supporting surface. The plantarflexion results from a strong pull of the peroneus longus tendon in an effort to arrive at foot flat to provide stance stability.

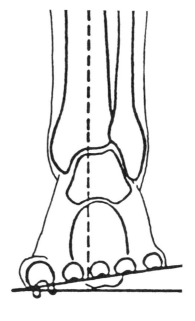

Fig. 2-9.   Forefoot valgus. (Hunt GC, Novick A: Foot Pain: In Echternach JL (ed): Pain. Churchill Livingstone, New York, 1987.)

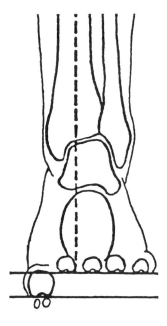

Fig. 2-10. Plantarflexed flexed first ray. (Hunt GC, Novick A: Foot Pain: In Echternach JL (ed): Pain. Churchill Livingstone, New York, 1987.)

Gait deviations largely depend on the degree of abnormality and whether the forefoot is rigid or flexible. If the foot posture is rigid and greater than 6°, lateral instability during stance will occur and the calcaneus will remain in varus throughout stance.[9] Keratomas under the first and fifth MTHs are very common. In the latter stages of deformity, digital contractures are common, especially of the fourth and fifth toes.[52,53] Chronic ankle sprains[44,54] occur due to the lateral weightbearing tendency and can pose a management problem. Other associated problems include iliotibial band syndrome,[55] anterior tarsal tunnel syndrome,[56] sesamoidities,[9] plantar fasciitis,[42] and leg and thigh pain.[9,44]

Schoenhaus and Jay[52] described a flexible forefoot valgus deviation. This foot resembles a true forefoot valgus in a nonweightbearing position. The flexibility of the first and fifth rays, however, allows the midtarsal articulations to remain unlocked, assuming a pes planus attitude during midstance. During gait, the unstable hindfoot may produce calcaneal inversion through the longitudinal axis of the midtarsal joint. Because of this supinatory instability during the first part of stance, the subtalar joint may respond by pronating during the latter part of stance in an attempt to improve balance. As a consequence to this subtalar joint pronation, the midfoot will unlock, producing forefoot instability during pushoff. This instability as described will result in significant forefoot deviations such as hallux abducto valgus and a variety of submetatarsal lesions.

A number of other anatomic factors can contribute to the development of abnormal gait patterns. These include internal or external malleolar torsion,[42,57] femoral anteversion[58] or retroversion, and medial or lateral hamstring contractures.[37] Interestingly enough, gait deviations such as excessive pronation can be caused by limited ankle dorsiflexion, forefoot varus, or excessive internal rotation of the lower limb. The key to a successful resolution is to note the gait abnormality first and then to conduct a clinical examination systematically to identify the primary cause(s). Only then can an appropriate management program be developed.

AUTHORS' NOTE

This chapter was written in authors' private capacity. No official support or endorsement by the United States Department of Health and Human Services is intended or should be inferred.

REFERENCES

1. Murray MP: Gait as a total pattern of movement. Am J Phys Med 46:290, 1967
2. Mann RA, Hagy JL: Running, jogging, and walking: A comparative electromyographic and biomechanical study. p. 167. In Bateman JE, Trott AW (eds): The Foot and Ankle. Brian C. Decker, Thieme-Stratton, New York, 1980
3. Wright DG, Desai SM, Henderson WH: Action on the subtalar and ankle-joint complex during the stance phase of walking. J Bone Joint Surg [Am] 46:361, 1964
4. Bates BT, Osternig LR, Mason B: Lower extremity function during the support phase of running. Biomechanics VI Baltimore: University Park Press, VI-B:31, 1978
5. Cavanaugh PR, Clarke TE, Williams KR, Kalenak A: An evaluation of the effects of orthotics on pressure distribution and rearfoot movement during running. Paper presented at the meeting of the American Orthopaedic Society for Sports Medicine, Lake Placid NY, June 1978
6. Clarke TE, Frederick EC, Hamill C: The study of rearfoot movement in running. p. 166. In Frederick EC (ed): Sport Shoes and Playing Surfaces. Human Kinetics Publishers, Champaign, IL, 1984
7. Perry J: The mechanics of walking. J Am Phys Assoc 47:9, 1967
8. Inman VT, Ralston HJ, Todd F: Human Walking. Baltimore, Williams & Wilkins, 1981
9. Root ML, Orien WP, Weed JH: Normal and Abnormal Function of the Foot: clinical Biomechanics. Vol. 2, Clinical Biomechanics, Los Angeles, 1977
10. Cavanaugh PR: The Running Shoe Book. World Publications, Mountain View, CA, 1981
11. Hlavac HF: The Foot Book. World Publications, Mountain View, CA, 1977
12. Lord M: Foot pressure measurement: a review of methodology. J Biomed Eng 3:91, 1981
13. Cavanaugh PR, LaFortune MA: Ground reaction forces in distance running. J Biomech 13:397, 1980
14. Katoh Y, Chao EYS, Morrey BF, Laughman RK: Objective technique for evaluating painful heel syndrome and its treatment. Foot Ankle 3:227, 1983
15. Scranton PE, Hootman BD, McMaster JH: Forces under the foot: A study of walking, jogging, and sprinting force distribution under normal and abnormal feet. p. 186. In Bateman JE, Trott AW (eds): The Foot and Ankle. Thieme Medical Publishers Inc., New York, 1980

16. Bauman JH, Brand PW: Measurement of pressure between foot and shoe. Lancet 1:629, 1963
17. Mann RA: Biomechanics of running. p. 1. In Mack RP (ed): The Foot and Leg in Running Sports. CV Mosby, St. Louis, 1982
18. Schoenhaus HD, Gold M, Hylinski J, et al: Computerized analysis of gait: clinical examples relating to torque. J Am Podiatry Assoc 65:953, 1975
19. Jaworek TE: The Histologic patterns in functional bony adaption as applied to congruous and subluxed joints. J Am Podiatry Assoc 65:953, 1975
20. Hicks JH: The three weight bearing mechanisms of the foot. p. 161. In Evans EG (ed): Biomechanical Studies of the Musculoskeletal System. Charles C. Thomas, Springfield, IL, 1961
21. Hutton WC, Dhanendran M: The mechanics of normal and hallux valgus feet: a quantitative study. Clin Orthop 157:7, 1981
22. Mann RA, Inman VT: Plasic activity of intrinsic muscles of the foot. J Bone Joint Surg [Am] 46:469, 1964
23. Viel ER, Desmarets JJ; Mechanical pull of the peroneal tendons on the fifth ray of the foot. J Orthop Sports Phys Ther 7:102, 1985
24. Gibbs RC, Boxer MC: Abnormal biomechanics of the feet and their cause of hyperkaratoses. J Am Acad Dermatol 6:1061, 1982
25. Schuster RO: Podiatry and the foot of the athlete. J Am Podiatry Assoc 62:465, 1972
26. Louis JM, Naftolin WH: Myofascial pain syndrome in the foot. J Am Podiatry Assoc 70:89, 1980
27. Bresnahan TP, Redmond CT: Injuries to the leg. J Am Podiatry Assoc 69:577, 1979
28. Tate RO, Rusin J: Morton's neuroma—its ultra-structural anatomy and biomechanical etiology. J Am Podiatry Assoc 68:797, 1978
29. Carrier PA, Janigan JD, Smith SD, et al: Morton's neuralgia: a possible contributing etiology. J Am Podiatry Assoc 65:315, 1975
30. Kendall H, Kendall F: Posture and Pain. Williams & Wilkins, Baltimore, 1952
31. Bottee RR: An Interpretation of the pronation syndrome and foot types of patients with low back pain. J Am Podiatry Assoc 71:243, 1981
32. Sanner WH, Page JC, Tolkol HR, et al: Ankle joint height changes with subtalar joint motion. J Am Podiatry Assoc 71:158, 1981
33. Bogden RJ, Jenkins D, Hyland T: The runner's knee syndrome. p. 159. In Rinaldi RR, Sabia M (eds): Sports Medicine. Futura, New York, 1978
34. Olerud C, Berg P: The variation of the Q angle with different positions of the foot. Clin Orthop 191:162, 1984
35. Harris RI, Beam T: Hypermobile flat foot with short tendo achilles. J Bone Joint Surg [Am] 30:116, 1948
36. Melillo TV: Gastronemius equinus—its diagnosis and treatment. Arch Pod Med and Foot Surgery 2:159, 1975
37. Sgarlato TE: Tendo achilles lengthening and its effect on foot disorders. J Am Podiatry Assoc 65:849, 1975
38. Subotnick SI: Equinus deformity as it affects the forefoot. J Am Podiatry Assoc 61:423, 1971
39. Manter JT: Movements of the subtalar and transverse talar joints. Clin Orthop 30:20, 1941
40. Elftman H: The transverse tarsal joint and its control. Clin Orthop 16:41, 1960
41. Subotnick SI: Rearfoot Varus Biomechanical Compendium. PAL Biomechanical Research and Education Laboratory, Perkin, IL, 1985

42. Subotnick SI: Podiatric Sports Medicine. Futura, Mount Kisco, NY 1975
43. Subotnick SI: Biomechanics of the subtalar and midtarsal joints. J Am Podiatry Assoc 65:756, 1975
44. Weil LS, Moore JW: A Biomechanical study of lateral ankle sprains in basketball. J Am Podiatry Assoc 69:687, 1979
45. Hlavac H: Compensated forefoot varus. J Am Podiatry Assoc 60:229, 1970
46. Strauss WL: Growth of the human foot and its evolutionary significance. Contrib Embry, Carnegie Institute 19:93, 1927
47. Root ML, et al: Axis of motion of the subtalar joint. J Am Podiatry Assoc 56:149, 1966
48. Moeller FA: Biomechanics and its relationship to foot surgery. J Am Podiatry Assoc 63:383, 1973
49. Samilson RL, Dillin W: Cavus, cavovarus, and calcaneovarus: an update. Clin Orthop 177:125, 1983
50. Jahss MH: Evaluation of the cavus foot for orthopedic treatment. Clin Orthop 181:52, 1983
51. Sgarlato TE: A Compendium of Podiatric Biomechanics. California College of Podiatric Medicine, San Francisco, 1971
52. Schoenhaus HD, Jay RM: Cavus deformities: conservative management. J Am Podiatry Assoc 70:235, 1980
53. Haber L, Winthrop L, Weiner S: Biomechanical findings in a random survey of fifth toe abnormalities. J Am Podiatry Assoc 65:206, 1975
54. Steindler A: Kinesiology of the Human Body Under Normal and Pathological Conditions. Charles C Thomas, IL, 1970
55. Cangialosi CP, Schnall SJ: The biomechanical aspects of anterior tarsal tunnel syndrome. J Am Podiatry Assoc 70:291, 1980
56. Weiner DS, Weiner SD: The natural evolution of internal tibial torsion. Orthophedics 2:583, 1979
57. Mittleman G: Transverse plane abnormalities of the lower extremities: intoe and outtoe gait. J Am Podiatry Assoc 61:1, 1971

3 | Examination

William A. Fromherz

The examination procedure presented in this chapter is designed to serve as a guide to the physical therapist involved in the treatment of the foot and ankle. Regional examinations of related structures such as the knee are based on the principles outlined in the chapters on biomechanics and pathomechanics. Physical therapists must exercise good clinical judgment to determine if a more detailed examination of related structures is indicated, (e.g., accessory movement testing of the lumbar spine and stability testing of the knee).[1-10]

Standardization of the examination procedure and the recording of valid and reliable data serve as the basis for assessment of the client's problem, establishment of goals, and development of a realistic and effective treatment program. Without these data, a valid assessment of the client's progress cannot be made, and the treatment program cannot be justified.

Standardization of the tests and measurements used in the examination procedure provides a means for the clinician to analyze data and, in effect, carry out research projects in a clinical setting.

A modified problem-oriented format is used in presenting the material in this chapter. The information is sequenced in such a manner that the therapist may easily refer to the material when questions arise concerning certain examination procedures.

An examination worksheet that follows the sequence in which information is presented has been developed (Fig. 3-1). Readers are encouraged to use this format or to develop their own format for recording the examination data. In some clinical settings, this type of form may be included as part of the client's official record. In other settings, such a form may not be approved; however, the data are recorded in a manner that may be easily consolidated to meet any required progress note format.

The examination procedures presented in this chapter are primarily based on the principles outlined in the chapters on biomechanics and pathome-

LOWER EXTREMITY EXAMINATION WORKSHEET

Date ______________ **FOOT AND ANKLE** Weight _____ Height _____ Age _____
Name ____________________ Sex ______ Occupation __________
No. ______________ ______________________________

I. Problem:

II. History:

III. Subjective:

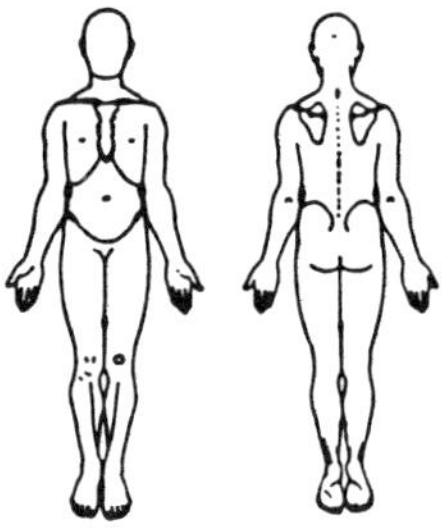

IV. Objective:

A. Posture

B. Sensation - Stress Patterns

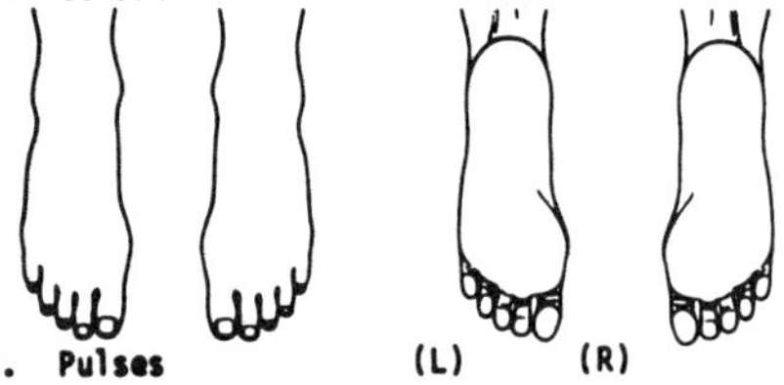

D. Footwear

(L) (R) (L) (R)

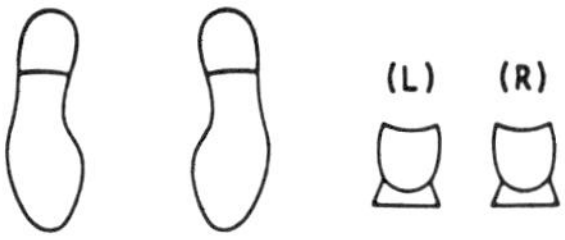

C. Pulses

	(L)	(R)
Dorsalis Pedis	____	____
Post Tibialis	____	____

E. Gait Assessment

1. Initial Contact

	(L)	(R)
Forefoot	____	____
Heel:		
Inverted	____	____
Neutral	____	____
Everted	____	____

2. Mid-stance

	(L)	(R)
Neutral	____	____
Everted	____	____
Inverted	____	____
Early Heel-Off	____	____

3. Heel Off

	(L)	(R)
Inverted	____	____
Neutral	____	____
Everted	____	____
Medial Heel Whip	____	____

F. Range of Motion/Position

1. Prone

	(L)	(R)
Dorsiflexion (knee extended)	______	______
Dorsiflexion (knee flexed)	______	______
Plantarflexion	______	______
Calcaneal inversion	______	______
Calcaneal eversion	______	______
Tibial Varum (stance)	______	______
[Hindfoot] in subtalar neutral	______	______
[Forefoot]	______	______
Plantar flexed 1st Ray	______	______

Fig. 3-1. Lower extremity examination worksheet (PAGE 1 and 2).

2. Modified Supine   (L)   (R)   COMMENTS:

       Tibial Torsion (sitting)
       Hip: Int. rotation
             Ext. rotation
       Straight leg raise
       Medial Hamstring
       Hip Flexors
       Rectus Femoris
       Tensor Fascia Lata
       (also in side lying)

3. Supine

       Limb Length - Real
                  Apparent
       Knee -   Flexion
                 Extension

4. Stance

       Great Toe Extension
       Resting Calcaneal Position
       Neutral Calcaneal Position
       Tibial Varum (see above)
       Limb Length (board width)
       "Q" Angle

G. Strength Assessment (Tone)   (L)   (R)

Hip:
     Gastroc/Soleus   Flexion
     Anterior tibialis   Extension
     Posterior tibialis   Abduction
     Peroneal   Adduction
     Extensor hallucis longus   Ext. rotation
     Extensor digitorum longus   Int. rotation
     Flexor hallucis longus
     Flexor digitorum longus   H. Podoscope
     Intrinsics

     Quadriceps
     Hamstrings

   I. Other

V. <u>Assessment</u>

VI. <u>Plan</u>

Fig. 3-1. (*Continued*).

chanics. Examination procedures are presented in other chapters to meet specific needs, (e.g., Doppler examination if vascular insufficiency is suspected). These additional procedures may easily be incorporated into the plan for the objective examination.

IDENTIFICATION OF THE PROBLEM

The "problem" is the first item listed in a note using the problem-oriented format.[11,12] It will be discussed in sequence for the purposes of this chapter; however, the problem for which the examiner will eventually institute treatment cannot be accurately identified until an assessment of all subjective and objective data has been completed.

Rothstein suggests that development of a problem statement should begin after completion of the history and subjective examinations to guide the therapist in the development of goals and a plan for the objective examination.[13] Problems should be stated in terms that express why the client is seeking treatment. When possible, the problem is expressed as a functional loss (e.g., unable to bear full weight on foot). "Anticipated" problems such as development of knee dysfunction are often identified when dealing with problems related to the foot and ankle.

When clients are unable to communicate, as in central nervous system involvement, it may be necessary to express the problem as "inferred" as well as "functional" or "anticipated."

HISTORY

For the purposes of clarity and ease of data retrieval, the history is not included in the "subjective examination" as presented in most versions of the problem-oriented format.[11,12] If a thorough history is obtained, it will not change unless the data are inaccurate or incomplete. Subjective data is expected to change with the institution of treatment. *History is not affected by treatment.* Although the history is taken into consideration during reassessment of the problem, only the change or lack of change in subjective and objective data is recorded.

The history includes information that may or may not be verified by the medical record. The source of the information should be identified (e.g., "client states . . .", "medical records states . . .").

Personal data including (1) age, (2) sex, (3) weight, and (4) height are conveniently recorded in the history portion of the initial note. Activities that may be directly or indirectly related to the problem should be noted (e.g., jogging 5 miles a day, tennis three times a week). Related occupational activities should also be documented (e.g., standing 2 hours at a time, climbing stairs).

The history includes information related to events that took place prior to the initial visit. The therapist documents the circumstances related to the onset of the problem and follows through up to the day of the initial visit.

Maitland[8] has developed a scheme of asking questions that assists in collection of historical data. A modification of Maitland's original scheme is presented in Figure 3-2. Readers are encouraged to follow this sequence of questioning or to develop their own so that the data are collected in an organized and thorough manner.

If not included in the initial questioning, relevant previous history is recorded. The first incident is reviewed in detail. The frequency and ease with which the symptoms and signs have recurred is also reviewed and recorded. The history of referred and/or associated symptoms as well as the local symptoms should be considered (e.g., ankle pain is decreasing; however, medial knee pain is increasing).

Current and/or past treatment(s) related to the problem are reviewed in detail (e.g., surgical procedures, bracing, casting, exercises, orthotics, etc.). Approximate dates on which the treatment(s) were received and the client's estimation of benefit should be noted.

Information obtained in the history will be used to guide the therapist in conducting the subjective and objective examinations. This information is also to be considered during treatment planning and goal setting as well as during program implementation and assessment of the effects of treatment.

SUBJECTIVE EXAMINATION

The subjective portion of the examination includes the client's description or interpretation of the "current" symptoms. It also includes responses to specific questions, which improves understanding of the problem. (see special questions) The subjective data is used in: (1) planning for the objective examination, (2) assessing the problem, (3) goal setting, and (4) treatment program planning. Most important, the subjective data are reassessed throughout the treatment process to guide the therapist and to assist in determining the efficacy of each procedure.

Area of Symptoms

The client is requested to point out the specific area(s) of symptoms (e.g., discomfort, "pain," paresthesia, anesthesia, etc.). If pain is experienced, terms that describe its quality should be used (e.g., ache, burning, etc.). A pain scale may also be used and is an effective tool in the assessment and reassessment process.[14-16] Symptoms involving associated areas should also be documented in detail (e.g., knee, hip, back, etc.).

The examiner may use light finger touch to assist the client in defining the

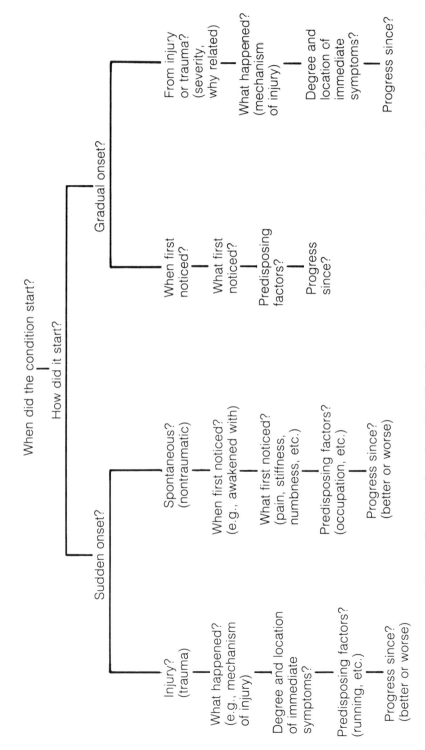

Fig. 3-2.   Scheme for history interview. (Modified from Maitland GD: Peripheral Manipulation. 5th Ed. Butterworth, London, 1977.)

anatomic boundaries of the symptoms. Care must be taken not to elicit symptoms through palpation during the "subjective examination."

The area of symptoms may be recorded on the diagrams of the body and/or feet as indicated. (Fig. 3-1) A key of symbols representing various symptoms may be incorporated into the diagrams.[17]

Behavior of Symptoms

The therapist attempts to obtain a clear picture of how each symptom behaves during static position and activity (e.g., ankle pain when descending stairs; no pain on walking, standing, or ascending stairs.). Maitland[8] has developed a questioning scheme to assist the examiner when interviewing relative to the behavior of symptoms. A modification of Maitland's interview scheme is presented in Figure 3-3.

If a patient states that there is not a position, movement, and/or activity that either relieves or intensifies the symptoms, a nonmechanical problem must be considered (e.g., tumor, inflammation, etc.).

The therapist should have a clear understanding of how the symptoms behave with rest vs activity: If pain awakens the client at night, is it because of mechanical dysfunction and/or inflammation? What are the symptoms like when the patient first arises vs during the day with activity? Do the symptoms increase with activity, indicating the possibility of inflammation?

Symptoms referred from distant anatomic structures should be carefully considered. Nerve root and peripheral nerve involvement frequently result in symptoms experienced in the lower leg and foot.

Clarifying (Special) Questions

Special questions are asked to assist the therapist in ruling out possible complicating factors that may need further investigation and/or may suggest contraindications to further objective examination or treatment.

General health? Seemingly unrelated health problems may have an indirect as well as a direct influence on the problem for which the client is being seen (e.g., diabetes mellitus often leads to sensory and motor changes is the extremities).

Significant weight loss? In a client who is not on a diet, weight loss may be indicative of serious pathology unrelated to the problem for which the therapist is seeing the client.

Have x-ray films been taken? In most cases, radiographs are reviewed following the examination since they may tend to bias the objective examination. Radiographs should be reviewed prior to the objective examination in the case of moderate to severe trauma.

Medications taken for this problem or other problem? Medications may

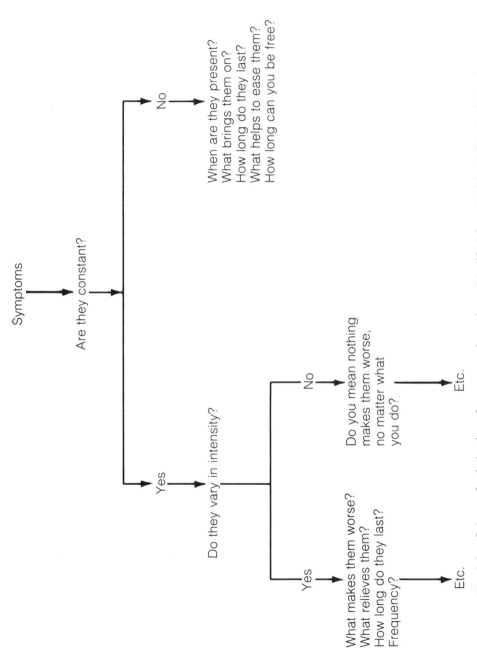

Fig. 3-3. Scheme for behavior of symptoms interview. (Modified from Maitland GD: Peripheral Manipulation. 5th Ed. Butterworth, London, 1977.)

mask symptoms or have side effects. When the medications were first taken is an important factor to be considered in the assessment process. If medications were first taken following treatment, it becomes difficult to assess whether a change or lack of change in symptoms and signs are due to the medications and/or treatment.

Which is the dominant hand/foot?

Patient and/or family history of the following conditions should be clarified and documented:

Rheumatoid arthritis
Osteoarthritis
Diabetes mellitus
Neurological disorders
Weakness in lower extremities
Circulatory problems (type)
    Frequent or unhealed ulcers
    Cold feet
    Burning feet (irritation from shoes or socks)
    Sweaty feet
    Nail problems
    Conditions requiring lower extremity or back surgery (type of surgery and when)
"Flat feet"
Special shoes
Orthotic devices ("arch supports"—bracing)
Sprained ankle(s)
Osteoporosis

McPoil has developed a list of *special questions* for runners/joggers (T. McPoil, personal communication, 1986).

Type of workout: distance, interval etc.?
Terrain (e.g., hill, level, track?)
Surface (e.g., paved road, sidewalk, packed sand etc.?)
Time of day?
Shoe style (e.g., tennis, long distance etc.?)
Type of shoe (name brand)?
Socks vs no socks, how many pair?
Workouts per week?
Miles per week, miles per workout?
How long has the client been running (jogging)?
Participation in races: 5 k, 10 k, marathon etc.?
Warm-up time, warm-down time, stretching included?
How does the client classify his/her foot structure?
Have orthotics been used, currently using, type (rigid vs flexible), for what purpose, do they help?

Additional special questions should be asked of the client if associated areas of the body are involved (e.g., Bowel and/or bladder involvement?) if the client complains of significant back pain.

On completion of the subjective examination, the therapist is ready to develop a plan for carrying out the objective examination.

OBJECTIVE EXAMINATION

The objective examination is approached in an organized manner and planned based on the history and subjective examination findings. the plan may be written; however, it is not included in the client's record. The objective examination section of the worksheet may be reviewed to assist the therapist in selecting the appropriate tests and measurements (Fig. 3-1). The worksheet is to be used as a *guide* and is not intended to be all-inclusive. As the examiner progresses through the objective plan, it may be revised as indicated by the preceding test and measurement findings. Items are to be deleted or added to those listed on the worksheet based on the clinical judgment of the examiner.

After reviewing the history and subjective examination findings the therapist should consider, *but not be limited to, the following questions:*

Which muscles, joints or other structures must be examined as a possible cause of the symptoms? How does the foot and ankle relate to the knee, hip, and spine?

What structural, dynamic, and static relationships need to be examined (e.g., tibia vara, hindfoot, forefoot, free walking vs running)?

What other contributing factors need to be examined (e.g., posture, muscle length, weakness, sensation, reflexes)?

What equipment is required to perform the tests and measurements?

Would videotaped gait, postural, and movement analysis be helpful?

What is the assessment of the client's history and subjective examination findings in regards to the *severity, irritability, and nature* of the condition?

Severity: "Harsh," "Intense"

Irritability: How easily are the symptoms brought on and how long does it take for them to ease?

Nature: Based on the history and subjective examination findings, does the condition appear to be one in which caution must be taken in performing the objective examination (e.g., neurologic involvement, rheumatoid arthritis, recent trauma or fracture, steroid therapy)?

The therapist's subjective impression of the Severity, Irritability, and Nature (SIN) of the condition will serve as a guide as to how vigorous the examination procedures are to be performed and if extreme caution is indicated. The subjective SIN when compared with the assessment of the objective SIN following completion of the objective examination is an essential element in the total *assessment* of the client's condition.

Example: A client states that he is unable to dorsiflex his foot actively due to a direct blow to the dorsum of the foot while working. It is noted during ambulation that the client exhibits a normal loading response at the ankle and there are no other objective findings except that he refuses or is unable to dorsiflex on request.

Assessment: The subjective and objective findings do not correlate, indicating that further testing may be indicated and/or that the possibility of secondary gain must be considered.

Before making the objective examination, the therapist should consider whether to review the client's record, if available. If review of the record is not warranted by the history, subjective examination, or SIN, the therapist should proceed with the objective examination. Reviewing another examiner's findings may bias the examination. If there is any question concerning client safety, the record should be reviewed prior to initiating the objective examination.

If the client's medical record is available, it should always be reviewed immediately following the objective examination. This review is performed to confirm or rule out complicating factors as well as to review: (1) notes written by other health care professionals, (2) laboratory results, and (3) results of diagnostic tests (e.g., Doppler studies, radiographs, computed tomography (CT) scans, lab results.

The tests and measurements to be discussed correspond to those listed on the lower extremity examination worksheet (Fig. 3-1). The worksheet is to serve only as a guide and a mechanism for recording the test and measurement results. The objective examination plan earmarks those tests and measurements to be performed. The objective plan may be modified at any time depending on the findings obtained as the therapist progresses through the examination.

Posture

Kendall and others[9,18] have described methods by which a complete postural examination may be conducted. For the purposes of the lower extremity examination, emphasis should be placed on determining the relative height of the iliac crests, posterior superior iliac spines, anterior superior iliac spines, patellae, gluteal folds, posterior knee creases, and medial malleoli. If asymmetry is noted, an examination of the sacroiliac joints and spine may be indicated. Foot posture and stance width should be observed. Excessive pronation or supination may decrease or increase the functional limb length.

Abnormal knee posture in frontal plane (genu varum, genu valgum), saggital plane (flexion, hyperextension), and transverse plane (internal or external) femoral rotation should be observed. Saggital, frontal, and transverse plane posture should be examined above the level of the pelvis if the client complains of spinal-related symptoms or if assymetry is detected at or below the pelvis. Postural deviation may be recorded on the body chart (Fig. 3-1).

Sensation

Sensation testing, including pain, light touch, two-point discrimination, vibration, etc., are to be tested as indicated. Areas of decreased or absent sensation as well as areas of hypersensitivity are recorded on the body chart or diagrams of the foot and ankle (Fig. 3-1).

Trophic Changes and Stress Patterns

Skin color, texture, ulcers, calluses, and corns, are noted on the body chart or diagrams of the foot and ankle.

Peripheral Pulses

If there is any suggestion of sensory and/or trophic changes, the dorsalis pedis and posterior tibialis pulses should be examined. Pulses proximal to the foot and ankle should be examined if the distal pulses are absent. Appropriate referral should be made when a primary vascular problem that is not being managed is suspected.[19]

Footwear Diagrams

Abnormal wear patterns on the sole of the shoe and breakdown of the heel counter should be carefully observed and noted on the footwear diagrams. (Fig. 3-4) Wear patterns may be correlated with other objective findings such as gait deviations and imbalances in strength and/or range of motion (ROM).

The type of preferred footwear should be noted. Many clients select footwear based strictly on cosmetic considerations without regard to function. If a client states that function and comfort are not the primary factors considered, an explanation of the criteria for appropriate selection of footwear should be considered.

Gait Assessment

A gait screening examination should be performed to identify abnormalities that may be accounted for in the tests and measurements to be carried out later in the examination. A complete observational gait examination such as that developed by Perry and others may be considered when gross abnormalities are noted.[20]

The gait screening examination is limited to observation of the position of the calcaneus in relation to the supporting surface during the stance phase. As noted in Chapter 2, the calcaneus is slightly inverted at initial contact, everts

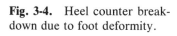
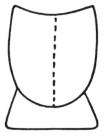
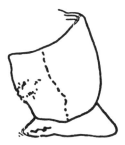

Fig. 3-4. Heel counter break-down due to foot deformity.

toward the perpendicular position at midstance, and is inverted at heel-off. The evidence of forefoot contact at heel contact, early heel-off at midstance, and medial heel whip at heel-off should also be noted. (Fig. 3-1)

Slow-motion videotape analysis of the client's gait is often useful in performing the screening examination. (Fig. 3-5) Slow-motion analysis is helpful in performing a full observational gait analysis when it is indicated. Hard-copy video recordings may be used to document gait deviation for the record. Computerized motion analysis is useful in an attempt to document gait deviation objectively; however, these systems are not readily available in most clinical settings.

Range of Motion/Position

Range of motion and static structural position measurements are taken to assist the therapist in assessing the biomechanical components of the client's symptoms, signs and/or gait deviations. Measurements are taken in the (1) prone, (2) sitting, (3) modified supine, (4) supine, and (5) stance positions (Fig. 3-1). Other positions may be used as indicated or required by the patient's condition.

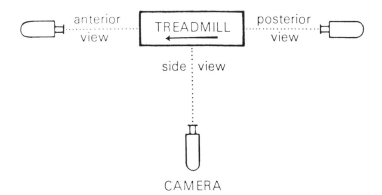

Fig. 3-5. Camera position for videotaping with treadmill.

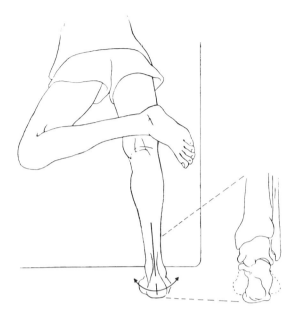

Fig. 3-6. Positioning in preparation for subtalar joint measurements and static alignment of the hindfoot and forefoot.

Subtalar Neutral Position

The subtalar neutral position serves as a reference from which many structural, and ROM measurements are taken.[21,22] The subject is placed in the prone position with the foot and ankle to be measured extending well over the end of the examination table. The opposite hip may be flexed to align the sagittal plane of the distal leg perpendicular to the floor (Fig. 3-6). The thumb is used to palpate the medial aspect of the talar head, which is slightly inferior and anterior to the medial malleolus and proximal to the navicular (Fig. 3-7). The index finger is used to palpate the lateral aspect of the talar head, which is anterior to

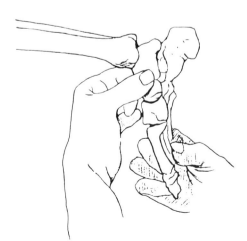

Fig. 3-7. Thumb palpates medial aspect of the talar head.

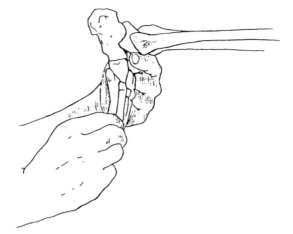

Fig. 3-8. Index finger palpates the lateral aspect of the talar head.

the lateral malleolus and toward the midline of the foot. A sulcus that represents the sinus tarsi and the location of the lateral aspect of the talar head during supination should be palpated (Fig. 3-8).

By grasping the fourth and fifth metatarsal heads (MTHs) with the thumb and index finger, the therapist takes up the slack in the midtarsal joints, and the hindfoot is pronated and supinated through an arch of motion around the axis of the subtalar joint. During pronation and supination, the medial and lateral aspect of the head of the talus become prominent, respectively. Care is taken not to push the metatarsals in a single plane motion as may occur with a straight dorsiflexion movement. Subtalar neutral is defined for clinical purposes as the position at which the medial and lateral aspects of the talar head are palpated equally.

Dorsiflexion
(Talofibular-Tibial Joint) (Talocrural Joint)

The literature indicates that 10° of dorsiflexion at the talofibular-tibial joint is required during the stance phase of gait.[20,21,23] The dorsiflexion component of pronation occurring at the subtalar joint and the oblique metatarsal joint also increases the functional ROM and may become excessive if dorsiflexion of the talocrural joint is restricted.

To eliminate the subtalar joint's contribution to total dorsiflexion ROM and to obtain a more accurate measurement of motion occurring at the talocrural joint, pronation is passively controlled. The subtalar neutral position is attained as described. The distal arm of a small goniometer is aligned parallel to an imaginary line from the plantar aspect of the calcaneus to the plantar surface of the fifth MTH. Palpation of anatomic landmarks is required especially when excessive soft tissue exists. The proximal arm of the goniometer is aligned parallel to the lateral bisection of the lower leg, which usually runs through the lateral malleolus (Fig. 3-9).

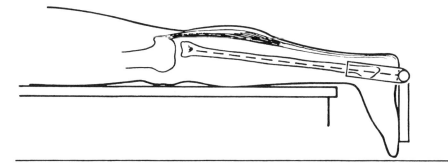

Fig. 3-9. Limited dorsiflexion measured while pronation is controlled.

The talocrural joint is passively dorsiflexed to the point of resistance and is then actively dorsiflexed by the client while the examiner passively controls any pronation occurring at the subtalar joint.

If maximum dorsiflexion is less than 10°, the knee is flexed to 90° and the dorsiflexion is measured again (Fig. 3-10).[23,24] If the dorsiflexion range is greater with the knee flexed than extended, the two-joint relationship of gastrocnemius is implicated. If limitation of motion is unchanged in the knee-flexed position, the soleus and/or articular structures are implicated.

The lateral border of the calcaneus may serve as the landmark for placement of the distal arm of the goniometer when a foot that appears to have a high inclined subtalar joint axis is measured. An increase in functional dorsiflexion range results if pronation at the subtalar joint is allowed to occur.

Plantar Flexion (Talofibular-Tibial Joint)

Plantar flexion is measured with essentially the same goniometric techniques as those noted in the measurement of dorsiflexion. Twenty degrees of plantarflexion is required for normal gait.[21]

Calcaneal Inversion/Eversion (Subtalar Joint)

Clinically, the best estimate of subtalar joint motion is calcaneal inversion and eversion. This measurement is taken in the frontal plane.[25] Associated component motions of subtalar plantar flexion, adduction, dorsiflexion, and abduction may be estimated indirectly (e.g., observation, the type of foot structure, radiograph, etc.). When frontal plane measurements are taken, approximately one-third of the motion is believed to occur in calcaneal eversion representing pronation and two-thirds in inversion representing the best estimate of subtalar joint supination.[21]

Reference landmarks for measuring calcaneal inversion and eversion in the frontal plane are the frontal plane bisection of the posterior calcaneus as it

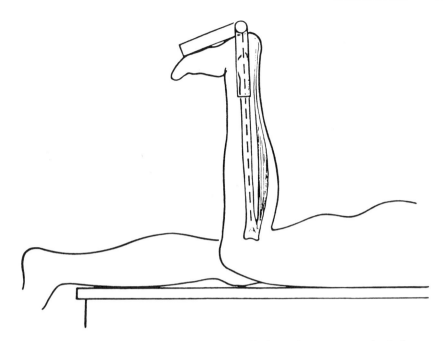

Fig. 3-10. Dorsiflexion with the knee flexed to eliminate the gastrocnemius influence as a two-joint muscle.

relates to the frontal plane bisection of the posterior aspect of the distal one-third of the lower leg (Fig. 3-11).

Dots representing the axis of motion, as well as distal points of the bisections may be drawn with a pen to assist in aligning the goniometer. Skin lines connecting the dots may also be drawn.[23,25] It must be remembered that the relationship between osseous structures is being measured. Extreme care must be taken to account for Achilles tendon and other soft tissue deformation that occurs during inversion and eversion. Skin markings must be redrawn when measuring from maximum inversion to maximum eversion due to this soft tissue deformation. The decision to use skin markings in a clinical setting is based on preference of the examiner.

Calcaneal Inversion

The client is placed in the same position as that for determining the subtalar neutral position with the calcaneus perpendicular to the floor. When the midfoot is grasped, the subtalar joint is inverted and then everted while the perpendicular relationship of the calcaneus is maintained without allowing the leg to rotate internally or externally. The axis of the frontal plane motion is visually identified slightly superior to the calcaneus.

The calcaneus is visually bisected following careful palpation of its medial

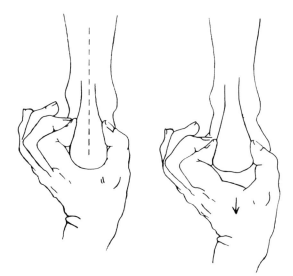

Fig. 3-11. Palpation and visual bisection of the calaneus and distal one-third of the lower leg.

and lateral borders. Care is taken to disregard the soft tissue that may be deformed during the palpation of the calcaneus (Fig. 3-11).

The calcaneus is maximally inverted, and palpation is repeated. Manual overpressure may be applied by grasping the calcaneus directly to assure that maximum motion has been attained. When full inversion has been attained, the hand placement should be adjusted distally to grasp the midfoot while maintaining the end-range position. The proximal and distal arms of a small goniometer are aligned with the bisections of the distal one-third of the lower leg and calcaneus, respectively. (Fig. 3-12). It is important to disregard the influences of the change in Achilles tendon position and deformation of the soft tissue overlying the cancaneus during the palpation and visual bisection.

Calcaneal Eversion

Maximum eversion is measured using the same technique as described for measuring inversion (Fig. 3-13). Care is again taken to disregard the visual influence of Achilles tendon movement and deformation of the soft tissue surrounding the calcaneus.

Hindfoot Position

Static calcaneal position is determined by the relationship of the bisection of the distal one-third of the lower leg to the bisection of the calcaneus when the subtalar joint is in the neutral position.[21-24]

The client is placed in the prone position, and the subtalar neutral position is attained. The distal one-third of the lower leg and calcaneus are visually bisected as previously described.

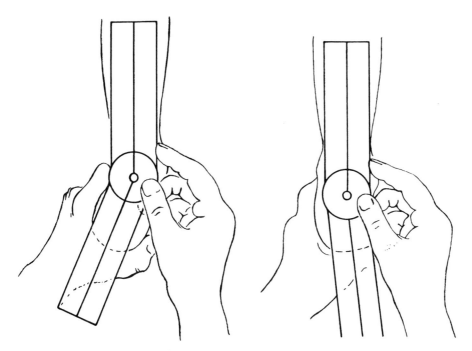

Fig. 3-12. Goniometric measurement of inversion.

Fig. 3-13. Goniometric measurement of eversion.

A hindfoot deformity is not suspected if the bisection of the distal one-third of the lower leg is parallel to the bisection of the calcaneus. A *hindfoot varus* is suspected if the bisection of the calcaneus angles medially from the bisection of the distal one-third of the lower leg (Fig. 3-14). A *hindfoot valgus* is suspected if the bisection of the calcaneus angles laterally from the bisection of the distal one-third of the lower leg. Goniometric measurement of the hindfoot relationship to the distal one-third of the lower leg may be made by using the previously described technique.

Forefoot Position

Static forefoot position is determined by the relationship between the longitudinal bisection of the calcaneus and the transverse plane alignment of the second through the fifth MTHs.[23,26]

The subtalar neutral position is attained and the calcaneus is visually bisected as prevously described. The clinician is careful to take the slack out of the midtarsal joints only and not to dorsiflex the fourth and fifth metatarsal excessively, because that may give the false impression of a forefoot deformity.

The plantar surface of the metatarsal heads are palpated to determine their plane of alignment and to identify any prominences. With the exception of ruling out rotation of the lower extremity, the position of the lower leg is ignored. The examiner must visualize the forefoot to hindfoot relationship and not be influenced by any deformity existing between the calcaneus and the lower leg (i.e., hindfoot varus or valgus). Chapter 2 describes some of the possible relationships of the forefoot to the hindfoot.

A forefoot deformity is not suspected if the calcaneal bisection is perpendicular to the plane of the MTHs (Fig. 3-14). A *forefoot varus* deformity is suspected if the plane of the MTHs is inverted (i.e., angled medially upward in relation to the calcaneal bisection). A *forefoot valgus* is suspected if the plane of the MTHs is everted (i.e., angled laterally upward in relation to the calcaneal bisection).

Quantifiable forefoot measurements are clinically difficult to obtain and may be unreliable although both goniometric and protractor techniques have been described.[24] It is often possible to determine the degree of forefoot deformity from a model of the foot if orthotics are to be constructed.[23] If a forefoot measurement is taken with a goniometer, the subtalar neutral position is attained as previously described. One arm of a goniometer is aligned parallel to the calcaneal bisection and the other arm is visually aligned with the best estimate of the plane of MTHs two through five. Care is taken not to be influenced by the presence of a plantarflexed first ray, which may give the appearance of a forefoot valgus.

Plantarflexed First Ray

The first ray may plantarflex below the plane of the second through the fifth metatarsal heads in an attempt to balance the foot in the presence of a hindfoot and/or forefoot varus deformity. A "rigid" plantarflexed first ray is one that cannot be passively dorsiflexed to the plane of the remaining MTHs. A "flexible" or mobile plantarflexed first ray may be passively dorsiflexed to or beyond the plane of the remaining MTHs.[22]

A plantarflexed first ray is detected in the subtalar neutral position and through careful palpation of the first MTH as it relates to the plane of the second through the fifth MTHs. The magnitude of the first ray mobility is examined during this palpation procedure. The length of the metatarsals as noted in a "Morton's toe" and the prominence of the second and/or other MTH may also be detected during the palpation procedure.[19,24]

Tibial Torsion (Malleolar Torsion)

Tibial torsion describes the ankle axis in the frontal plane as it relates to the tranverse axis of the knee. It has been measured with an approximate 15° external rotation orientation.[21]

The client is placed in the sitting position with the knee axis parallel to the examination table. The transverse plane relationship of the lateral to medial malleoli is observed with the examiner placing one thumb just anterior to the

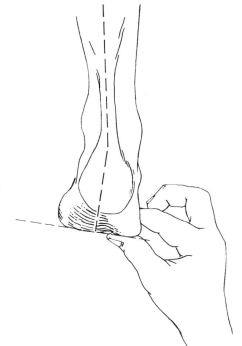

Fig. 3-14. Hindfoot varus measured in subtalar neutral. Neutral forefoot in relation to the hindfoot.

lateral malleolus and the index finger on the apex of the medial malleolus.[27] The examiner then visually determines the relationship of a line connecting the thumb and index finger to a line representing the axis of the knee (Fig. 3-15). A qualitative estimate of "normal" is determined if these lines are parallel. Although the procedure is not quantitative, it does allow the examiner to gain a feel for the presence of internal or external tibial (malleolar) torsion.

Hamstring Length

Many methods have been described for determining the length of the hamstrings.[18,19] Passive straight leg raising has been used traditionally; however, the influence of medial hamstrings on gait has frequently been overlooked. To identify the presence of medial hamstring tightness, the hip is flexed to 90° and passively externally rotated to the end of range. The medial hamstrings are placed on stretch by passively extending the knee while maintaining the hip position. The hip is then passively internally rotated while maintaining flexion at 90°. Any increase in the degree of passive knee extension that would implicate medial hamstring tightness is carefully noted.[28] If knee extension range does not increase, selective medial hamstring tightness is not suspected. The reverse maneuver with hip being moved from internal rotation to neutral while any increase in passive knee extension may be noted may be indicative of lateral hamstring tightness.

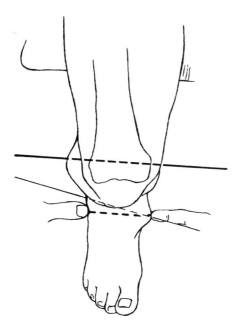

Fig. 3-15.   Visualization of tibal torsion.

Hip Rotation (Transverse Rotation) ROM

ROM imbalances may effect hip muscular function; this also requires careful assessment. Forty-five degrees of hip internal and external rotation is considered to be within normal limits.[24,29] Measurements should initially be taken with the client relaxed in the supine position and the knees flexed freely over the end of the examination table (modified supine position). A standard goniometer or angle-finder attached to a shaft may be used to measure the angle at which maximum passive range is attained. End range is determined with the initiation of pelvic movement. Figure 3-16 demonstrates the use of an angle finder. The modified supine position closely approximates the functional position of the hip through much of the gait cycle.[20,28]

Measurements may also be taken with the client in the sitting position in an attempt to determine if restricted motion is due to position and soft tissue tightness or due to structural abnormalities as seen in femoral anteversion and retroversion. An increase in range in the sitting (hip flexed) position over the extended (modified supine) position may implicate soft tissue rather than osseous structures. Increases in ROM through exercise would not be expected if limitations were due to abnormalities in the alignment of bone.

Hip Flexor Tightness

Hip flexor tightness may be determined through use of the Thomas test position. With the hips maximally flexed and the pelvis posteriorly rotated so that the lumbar spine is parallel to the examination table, the test leg is slowly

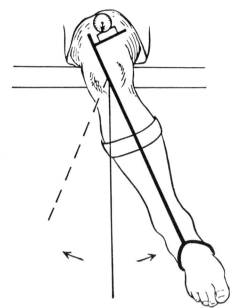

Fig. 3-16. Hip rotation measured with an "angle finder."

lowered into extension until pelvic and lumbar spine movement is noted (Fig. 3-17). If the thigh extends to a position that is parallel to the examination table, normal range has been attained.[18]

If tightness exists in the primary single joint hip flexors (psoas and iliacus), external rotation of the thigh may be noted, since their line of pull is medial to the axis of hip rotation. Increase in hip internal rotation in sitting vs the modified supine position may also be noted since the flexors are on slack in the flexed position.

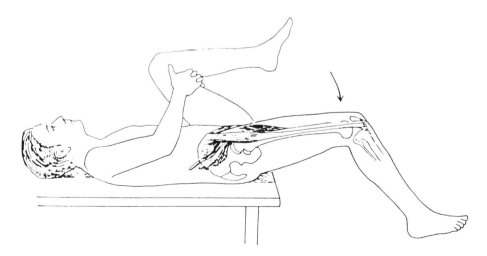

Fig. 3-17. Thomas test position to identify hip flexor tightness.

The tensor fasciae latae is a hip flexor, abductor, and internal rotator. If the thigh abducts as it is lowered towards extension, tensor and/or IT band tightness is suspected.

Rectus femoris, tensor fasciae latae and sartorius function as hip flexors. They also cross the knee and are considered two-joint muscles. The rectus femoris and, to some extent, the tensor fasciae latae act as knee extensors while the sartoris acts as a knee flexor. The two-joint knee extensors are considered to have normal length if the knee is able to flex at least 80° during the final manuever of the Thomas test.[16] Frontal plane (abduction/adduction) and transverse plane (internal/external rotation) motion as well as sagittal plane flexion at the hip should be noted and/or eliminated through passive stabilization by the examiner (Fig. 3-18).

Tensor fasciae latae and IT band tightness may also be identified with the client in the sidelying position, the thigh in neutral in the transverse plane, and the hip slightly extended. As the thigh is passively guided into adduction, care is taken to stabilize the pelvis so that frontal plane side bending does not occur. The toes should drop below the level of the examination table top.[18,19] An increased stretching sensation experienced by the client with active and passive knee flexion during the final test maneuver may implicate the knee extensor portion of the tensor and IT band (Fig. 3-19).

Limb Length

Assessment of limb length has long been studied, discussed, and disagreed on, and in many cases has confused the clinician. Structural, muscle, and ROM imbalances around the pelvis, hip, knee, foot and ankle may all influence the functional length of the lower extremity[19]:

Unilateral anterior or posterior rotation of the illium vs displacement of the sacrum

Hip and pelvis ROM and muscular imbalances

Structural deformities of the proximal femur (e.g., coxa vara, coxa valga, coxa plana, etc.)

Structural, muscular, and ROM imbalances at the knee (e.g., flexion contractures, genu recurvatum, genu vara, genu valga, rotatory and straight instabilities, etc.)

Structural, muscular, and ROM imbalance of the lower leg, ankle and foot (e.g., tibia vara, tibial torsion, excessive pronation or supination, etc.)

Clinically, the functional limb length may be determined by placing the client in the standing position and carefully palpating just inferior to the posterior superior iliac spines (PSIS) illustrated in Figure 3-20 and anterior superior iliac spines (ASIS). A line is visualized connecting the PSIS and another line is visualized connecting the ASIS. If both lines are parallel to the floor, a limb length discrepancy is not suspected. If both the ASIS and the PSIS appear low,

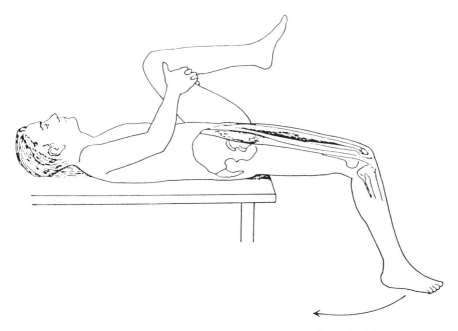

Fig. 3-18. Thomas test position to identify rectus femoris tightness.

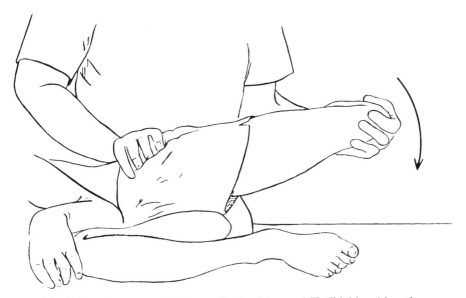

Fig. 3-19. Assessment of tensor fasciae latae and iliotibial band length.

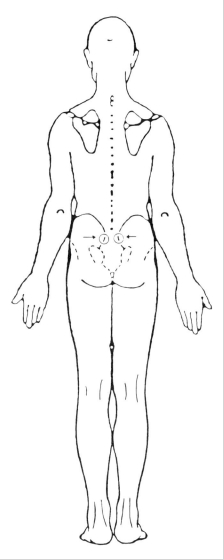

Fig. 3-20. Assessment of limb length in standing. Location of posterior superior iliac spine (PSIS) palpation landmarks.

careful observation is required to determine if the center of gravity is shifted away from that side. If the ASIS and PSIS continue to appear low following the shift back to the midline, a leg length discrepancy is suspected. The degree of shortening may be determined by the use of graduated boards that are placed under the foot. If the PSIS appears low and the ASIS appears high on the ipsilateral side, a possible rotated ilium may be suspected. This may be confirmed if the same PSIS alignment is observed with the client sitting on a firm surface.

Other methods of determining limb length vs pelvic rotational abnormalities (including the use of a tape measure and x-ray films) have been described in

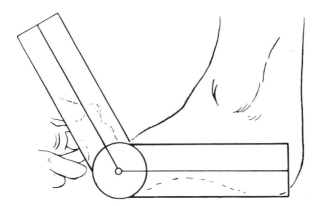

Fig. 3-21.   Great toe metarsalphalangeal joint extension measured in stance.

detail.[2,16,18,19] Use of these methods should be considered if the indications for a shoe lift in the case of a true leg length discrepancy vs exercise in the case of positional, muscular, or ROM imbalances are not clearly identified.

Great Toe Extension

Although minimum requirements vary with specific activities, 45° of great toe extension are adequate for general ambulation.[30] Limited range may result from restriction of the joint proper or may result from a combination of biomechanical factors such a short tendons, excessive pronation, etc. To determine functional range, great toe extension should be measured in the standing position with one arm of the goniometer parallel to the floor and the other arm parallel to the bisection of the proximal and distal phalanges. Evidence of supination with associated external rotation of the tibia should be noted upon passive overpressure (Fig. 3-21). If limited range is suspected, the measurement is taken nonweightbearing with the foot in plantarflexion to rule out restriction of the metatarsalphalangeal (MTP) joint.

Tibia Vara

The degree of calcaneal eversion must match the degree of tibia vara for the calcaneus to rest flat on the supporting surface without compensatory motion occurring at other joints in the lower extremity. The degree of tibia vara is determined by the goniometric measurement of the frontal plane bisection of the distal one-third of the lower leg in reference to the transverse plane of the supporting surface. To simulate a functional position seen during gait, the measurement is taken in single limb stance using contralateral toe contact to assist balance (Fig. 3-22).

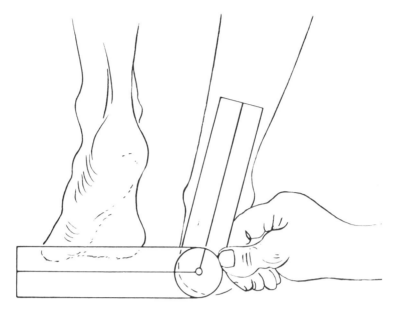

Fig. 3-22.   Tibia vara measured in single limb stance.

Neutral Calcaneal Position (Single Limb Stance)

Neutral calcaneal position is determined by goniometric measurement of the frontal plane angle of the calcaneal bisection in reference to the transverse plane of the supporting surface (floor). The measurement is taken in single limb stance using the contralateral toe contact to assist balance. The client carefully internally and externally rotates the lower limb which results in pronation and supination at the subtalar joint. The medial and lateral aspects of the talar head are palpated until they are equally prominent (see subtalar neutral position). The calcaneus is then palpated and visually bisected with care to disregard the displacement of the calcaneal fat pad and Achilles tendon. The client must hold the position while the goniometric measurement is taken (Fig. 3-23).

Resting Calcaneal Position (Single Limb Stance)

After the neutral calcaneal position has been determined, the client is allowed to return to the single limb stance position without regard to transverse plane rotation position of the tibia. Calcaneal motion is carefully observed. If any change in calcaneal angulation is noted, the angle of the frontal plane

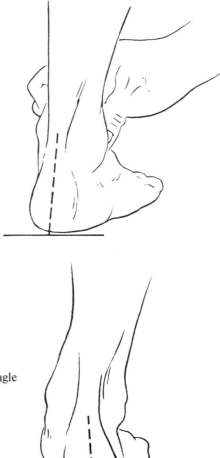

Fig. 3-23. Neutral calcaneal position in single limb stance.

Fig. 3-24. Resting calcaneal position in single limb stance.

bisection of the calcaneus in relation to the floor is remeasured (Fig. 3-24). The calcaneal resting position may be determined prior to positioning the lower extremity in the calcaneal neutral position.

Q Angle

The Q angle is the angle formed by lines from the anterior superior iliac spine and the tibial tubercle as they pass through the mediolateral, superior-inferior bisection of the patella. This angle influences direction of the quadriceps pull and tracking of the patella. In an effort to determine the functional angle, the measurement is taken with the client standing and simulating the angle and base of gait (Fig. 3-25).

•ASIS

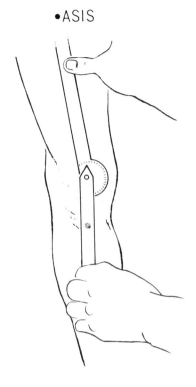

Fig. 3-25. Q angle measured in stance.

Knee ROM

ROM of the knee should be examined and measured with a goniometer if hyper- or hypomobility is suspected. Evidence of hyperextensibility is examined with the client in the supine position by lifting the client's lower leg by the toes. If the lateral plateau of the tibia moves posteriorly with apparent external rotation of the tibia and hyperextension of the knee, a posterior-lateral rotatory

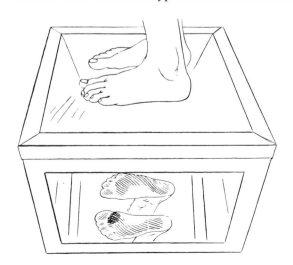

Fig. 3-26. Plantar surface contact and high-pressure areas noted with the podoscope.

instability is suspected. If alignment abnormalities or complaints of knee instability or pain exist, a thorough knee examination should be conducted.[4,5,6,7,31]

Muscle Testing (Tone)

Kendall and McCreary[18] and Daniels and Worthingham[29] are excellent references for muscle testing procedures for the trunk and lower extremities. The concepts of "stretch weakness" and "handedness patterns" should be kept in mind when structural and ROM imbalances are noted. Palpation and stabilization skills are critical, especially in the presence of neuromuscular involvement.

Podoscope

A podoscope is a device designed to provide a visual image of the pressure distribution over the plantar surface of the foot during standing and single limb stance. Patterns of pressure distribution may be photographed, videotaped, or drawn on foot diagrams of the worksheet (Fig. 3-26).

Other

On completion of the objective examination, the therapist is ready to assess the examination in total, to identify the problem, and to plan a treatment program.

AUTHOR'S NOTE

This chapter was written in author's private capacity. No official support or endorsement by the United States Department of Health and Human Services is intended or should be inferred.

REFERENCES

1. Gould III JA, Davies GJ (eds): Orthopaedic and Sports Physical Therapy. CV Mosby, St. Louis, 1985
2. Edmonson AS, Crenshaw AH (eds): Campbell's Operative Orthopaedics. 6th Ed. Vol. 1. CV Mosby, St. Louis, 1980
3. Kessler M, Hertling: Management of Common Musculoskeletal Disorders Physical Therapy Principles and Methods. Harper & Row, Philadelphia, 1983
4. Malone T, Blackburn TA (eds): The knee athletic injuries. Phys Ther 60:12, 1980
5. Cyriax J: Textbook of Orthopaedic Medicine. 8th Ed. Vol. 1. Diagnosis of Soft Tissue Lesions. Balliere Tindall, London, 1982
6. Hughston JC, Andrews JR, Cross MJ, et al: Classification of knee ligament instabilities: 1. The medial compartment and cruciate ligament. J Bone Joint Surg [Am] 58:000, 1976

7. Hughston JC, Andrews JR, Cross MJ, et al: Classification of knee ligament: 2. The lateral compartment. J Bone Joint Surg [Am] 58:000, 1976
8. Maitland GD: Vertebral Manipulation. 5th Ed. Butterworth, London, 1986
9. Corrigan B, Maitland GD: Practical Orthopedic Medicine. Butterworth, London, 1983
10. Maitland GD: Peripheral Manipulation. 2nd Ed. Butterworth, London, 1977
11. Weed LL: Medical Records, Medical Education and Patient Care. Yearbook Medical Publishers, Chicago, 1970
12. Echternach J: Use of the problem oriented clinical note in physical therapy department. Phys Ther 54:19, 1974
13. Rothstein JM, Ecternach J: Hypothesis oriented alogorithm for clinicians: A method for evaluation and treatment planning. (in press)
14. Gracely RH: Psychophysical assessment of human pain. Adv Pain Res Ther 3:000, 1979
15. Melzack R (ed): Pain Measurement and Assessment. Raven Press, New York, 1983
16. Wall PD, Melzack R (eds): Textbook of Pain. Churchill Livingstone, Edinburgh, 1984
17. Grieve GP: Common Vertebral Joint Problems. Churchill Livingston, Edinburgh, 1980
18. Kendall FP, McCreary EK: Muscles Testing and Function. 3rd Ed. Williams & Wilkins, Baltimore, 1983; (Appleton-Century-Crofts, Norwalk, CN, 1976)
19. Hopenfield S: Physical Examination of the Spine and Extremities. Appleton-Century-Crofts, Norwalk, 1976
20. Pathokinesiology service and physical therapy department Ranch Los Amigos Hospital: Normal and pathological gait syllabus. Professional staff association of Rancho Los Amigos Hospital, Downey, CA 1981
21. Root ML, et al: Biomechanical Examination of the Foot. Vol. 1. Clinical Biomechanics, Los Angeles, 1971
22. Wernick J, Langer S: A Practical Manual for a Basic Approach to Biomechanics. Langer Laboratories, Deer Park, NY, 1973
23. Mcpoil TG, Brocato RS: The foot and the ankle: Biomechanical evaluation and treatment. In Gould III JA, Davies GJ (eds): Orthopaedic and Sports. Vol. 2. CV Mosby, St. Louis, 1985
24. Hlavac HF: The Foot Book. World Publications Inc., Mountain View, CA, 1977
25. Sgarlato TE: A Compendium of Podiatric Biomechanics. California College of Podiatric Medicine Press, San Francisco, 1971
26. Root ML: Axis of Motion of the Subtalar Joint. J Am Podiatry Assoc 56:149, 1966
27. Hunt GC: Examination of lower extremity disfunction. In Gould III JA, Davies GJ (eds): Orthopaedic and Sports. Vol. 2. CV Mosby, St. Louis, 1985
28. Root ML, Orien WP, Weed JH: Clinical Biomechanics. Vol. 2. Normal and Abnormal Junction of the Foot. Clinical Biomechanics, Los Angeles, 1977
29. Daniels, Worthingham: Muscle Testing Techniques of Manual Examination. WB Saunders, Philadelphia, 1972
30. Mann RA, Hagy JL: Running, jogging, and walking: A comparative electromyographic and biomechanical study. In Bateman JE, Trott AW (eds): The Foot and Ankle. Brian C. Decker, Thieme-Stratton, New York, 1980
31. Wallace LA, Mangine RE, Malone T: The Knee: In Bateman JE, Trott AW (eds): The Foot and Ankle. Brian C. Decker, Thieme-Stratton, New York, 1980

4 | The Foot in Arthritic Diseases

Lynn H. Gerber

The term *arthritis* means inflammation of the joint, and most arthritic conditions are characterized by the hallmarks of inflammation: pain and swelling. In several arthritic conditions, however, there is little if any evidence for inflammation. It is useful to distinguish between the two types because the inflammatory types are more often progressive, involve more joints, and are generally associated with more disability. Arthritis of the noninflammatory type usually involves one or only a few joints, is rarely associated with systemic symptoms, and produces less disability. Examples of each type of arthritis are listed in Table 4-1. In inflammatory arthritis, the joints usually appear swollen, red, and warm; in noninflammatory arthritis, the joints often appear swollen, but lack redness and warmth. In osteoarthritis (OA) the joints may be enlarged, with extra bony growth, but are rarely swollen with fluid. The two general types of arthritis are further distinguished by the composition of the synovial fluid. Inflammatory fluid is usually high in WBC and has less viscosity and more degradative enzyme activity than does noninflammatory fluid. The WBCs themselves are believed to contribute to perpetuation of inflammation and joint destruction by releasing enzymes and chemotactic factors that attract more WBCs to the area.

Other schema are used to classify arthritis. These include the division into polyarthritis vs oligoarthritis or monoarthritis—differentiating between arthritides involving many joints vs those involving a few or one. This distinction helps to establish a diagnosis and predict the course or prognosis. Two other classifications include the symmetry of the arthritis and its distribution (peripheral or axial). A classification is given in Table 4-1.

Inflammation, pain, or swelling of the small joints of the foot and ankle is a frequent finding in arthritis. Indeed, foot pain, particularly metatarsalgia, is

TABLE 4-1. Classification of Arthritis

Arthritis	Inflammatory (I) vs Noninflammatory (N)	Polyarticular (P) vs Oligo- or Monoarticular (O,M)	Symmetrical (S) vs Asymmetrical (A)
Rheumatoid arthritis	I	P	S
Juvenile rheumatoid arthritis	I	P,O,M	S
Psoriatic rheumatoid arthritis	I	P,O,M	A
Reiter's syndrome	I	O	A
Gout	I	O,M	A
Pseudo-gout	I	O,M	A
Septic	I	M	M
Osteoarthritis	N	O,M	A,S
Traumatic	N	O,M	A
Reactive	N	O,M	A

often an initial symptom of arthritis patients. It is estimated that 85 percent of persons with rheumatoid arthritis (RA) will have foot problems at some time during the course of the disease.[1] Among patients with arthritis in which the spine is involved and the rheumatoid factor is absent, the likelihood of having either foot or ankle involvement is almost certain.[2]

Foot involvement clearly is common in arthritis, and its management will vary depending on the nature of the underlying disease process and the extent of inflammation as well as its anatomic location. The remainder of the chapter lists the arthritic processes and the associated foot problems.

OSTEOARTHRITIS

OA is the most common of the various forms of arthritis affecting humans. It occurs more frequently in old people, but it is not exclusively found in the aged. Those in younger age groups are often asymptomatic, suggesting that the process begins earlier in life and continues throughout later years, at which time it is almost universal.[3] OA can be classified as primary (having no known cause) or as secondary (in which anatomic or pathophysiologic causes for the arthritis can be shown). Primary OA of the foot usually involves the first metatarsophalangeal (MTP) joint. Secondary OA may result from trauma, RA, diabetes, and many other processes; when it does, any joint may be affected.

OA is a process that involves articular cartilage and subchondral bone. A structural breakdown of cartilage occurs leading to fissuring, pitting, and erosion of the cartilagenous surface. The body responds to this with a proliferation of cartilage and bone at the joint periphery, leading to bony spurs at the joint margins. The process is primarily a reparative one, but when repairs fail, the release of enzymes from chondrocytes may lead to some small inflammatory component. Generally, inflammation is only a secondary factor in OA.

The diagnosis of OA is usually made on clinical grounds, which includes pain and stiffness, loss of motion with crepitation in one or several joints, the appearance of bony proliferation at the joint, especially in the small joints of the

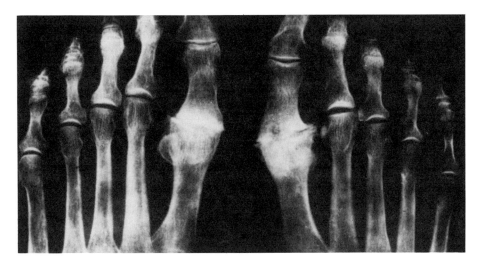

Fig. 4-1. Osteoarthritis: joint space narrowing of big toe with osteophytes at the first metatarsal phalanx is evident. Similar changes are apparent on the second and third toes.

distal interphalangeal joints (DIP) called Heberden's nodes, or the knees. The laboratory findings are nonspecific but radiographs should demonstrate joint space narrowing in an asymmetrical fashion and surface osteophytes. Later on, cysts, and eburnation of bone can follow (Fig. 4-1).

The ankle can be affected by primary or secondary OA. It begins as pain in the ankle and limited range of motion (ROM), usually dorsiflexion. Most often, it is a long-term sequela of trauma. OA of the subtalar joint usually begins with hindfoot pain and instability in walking on uneven ground. Occasionally, this may be associated with peroneal spasm. The first metatarsocuneiform joint and occasionally the second or third may be involved with degenerative changes, and a dorsal exostosis may develop which makes shoeing difficult. An associated biomechanical problem of abduction of the forefoot and flattening of the longitudinal arch may occur with a painful medical callosity. OA of the first MTP is the most commonly affected site in the foot. The joint usually is painful over the dorsum, enlarges, and loses ROM. Shoeing is often a problem, especially for women who chose to continue wearing shoes with high heels. Occasionally, first MTP OA may be caused by osteochondritis or trauma. DIP or PIP joint involvement of all the toes can be seen. The great toe is often involved. As the process progresses, mallet or hammer toe deformities may develop. The former is associated with flexion deformity of the PIP and the latter with a flexion deformity of the DIP. Pain is usually caused by a narrow shoe with a shallow toe-box pressing on the dorsal aspect of the toe in the hammer toe and the tip of the toes in the mallet toe. Treatment options include pharmacological interventions for control of pain; most frequently these are nonsteroid and antiinflammatory medicines. The efficacy of this treatment in terms of limiting progression of the process has been questioned.[4] Indeed, some suggest that it

TABLE 4-2. Criteria for RA

1. Morning stiffness.
2. Pain on motion or tenderness in at least one joint.
3. Swelling of one joint, representing soft tissue or fluid.
4. Swelling of at least one other joint (soft tissue or fluid) with an interval free of symptoms no longer than 3 months.
5. Symmetrical joint swelling (simultaneous involvement of the same joint, right or left.
6. Subcutaneous nodules over bony prominences, extensor surfaces, or near joints.
7. Typical roentgenographic changes that must include demineralization in periarticular bone as an index of inflammation; degenerative changes do not exclude diagnosis of RA.
8. Positive test for rheumatoid factor.
9. Synovial fluid; a poor mucin clot formation on adding synovial fluid to dilute acetic acid.
10. Synovial histopathology consistent with RA: a, marked villous hypertrophy; b, proliferation of synovial cells; c, lymphocyte/plasma cell infiltration in subsynovium; and d, fibrin deposition within or on microvilli.
11. Characteristic histopathology of rheumatoid nodules biopsied from any site.

Classic rheumatoid arthritis (RA) 7 criteria needed; definite RA, 5 criteria needed; probable RA, 3 criteria needed.

may hasten the process. Application of local treatment such as heat, cold, transcutaneous electrical nerve stimulation (TENS), ultrasound, and articular injection are often prescribed. Such measures have proven efficacy in pain control,[5-8] but few data have been presented to establish their efficacy in controlling disease process, particularly in OA.

RHEUMATOID ARTHRITIS

Rheumatoid arthritis is much less common than OA, and probably accounts for less disability on a population basis because of this. It causes more disability for individuals than OA, however, because of its systemic, polyarticular nature. The diagnosis is made clinically, using a set of criteria developed by Ropes et al for the American Rheumatism Association.[9] Table 4-2 describes the criteria and lists the number needed to establish differing levels of certainty. The prevalence of RA is 0.5 percent for women and 0.1 percent for men. It usually has an insidious onset with fatigue, malaise, morning stiffness, with diffuse musculoskeletal pain as the initial symptom. RA is usually symmetrical and often begins in the small joints of the hands and feet. Laboratory abnormalities include a moderate anemia that does not respond to iron replacement, as elevated sedimentation rate, and a positive rheumatoid factor (an IgM anti-IgG antibody). The synovial fluid can be of value because a cellular component (5–20,000) with RA cells often exists. Radiographs show a symmetrical pattern of abnormality, with juxtarticular osteoporosis and marginal erosions and very little bony repair. Pharmacologic treatment is often complex, and control of disease activity is not always satisfactory. Figure 4-2 is a general outline for medicinal treatment.

Vainio[1] has demonstrated that at some time during the adult lifetime of patients with RA, 85 percent will have foot problems. Foot pain is the common initial symptom, with metatarsalgia or first MTP pain. Occasionally, the adult with RA will note a widening of the forefoot and an inability to fit into the regular shoe size. The first changes occur in the forefoot, with redness and swelling of the MTPs and often a cocking up of the toes (Fig. 4-3). These physical findings correspond to the radiographic findings of juxtarticular osteoporosis, marginal bony erosion, and synovial proliferation. As the disease progresses, the MTHs often sublux, causing fixed cock-toe deformity and development of plantar callosity under the MTPs (Fig. 4-4). Often a hallux valgus deformity with associated bunions develops and the forefoot splays. Concomitantly, the hindfoot becomes more prone, either as a result of stretching or rupture of the posterior tibialis and/or ligamentous laxity in the midfoot comprising the longitudinal arch. The dynamic relationship between pronation at the hindfoot and development of hallux valgus has been well described.[10] Tendinitis of the Achilles, anterior tibialis, or toe flexors/extensors is not common in RA, but peroneal spasm frequently occurs and may be a significant pronatory force in the rheumatoid foot. Dynamically, one sees an apropulsive gait in which stride length is shortened, the amount of time spent standing on a single limb is decreased, foot contact is made with the entire foot rather than the heel, and roll off is markedly reduced.[11] Because many patients with RA are treated with steroidal preparations, skin fragility often occurs. Tissue breakdown over the crest of the toes at the apex of the hallux and over the malleoli can cause significant problems with shoeing and ambulation. Early in the course of the disease, the foot is quite flexible, but as the disease progresses and the proliferation phase decreases, fibrosis occurs and the foot loses its flexibility. Changes in the foot with RA, apparent on radiographs, are quite characteristic, including juxtarticular osteoporosis, erosion of the bone at the MTP joints, and some soft tissue swelling around the joints (Fig. 4-5). With time, the joints sublux, the toes become cocked, and the medial arch collapses. The tibiotalar joint is involved in less than 10 percent of patients, and its involvement occurs late in the disease process. Radiographs show uniform joint space narrowing and soft tissue swelling. A valgus or varus deformity can be seen. Rarely, there is bony ankylosis.

Occasionally, RA is associated with neuropathy as a result of vasculitis. This can lead to pain in the foot, anesthesia, or motor weakness. Nerve entrapment of the posterior tibial nerve has been reported[12] in as much as 14 percent of patients and may require surgical release. Finally, the presence of subcutaneous, rheumatoid nodules at the Achilles tendon or on the plantar surface along the flexor tendons can cause pain and difficulty in shoeing.[13]

In summary, in RA the foot is frequently involved. The involvement is primarily in the articular bony structure of the forefront and hindfoot, usually sparing tendon, bursae, and the structure of the midfoot. In a subset of RA patients, sensory neuropathy in a stocking distribution, nerve entrapments, and sensory motor neuropathy may occur.

JUVENILE RHEUMATOID ARTHRITIS

Juvenile onset rheumatoid arthritis (JRA) is not rare. It is characterized by joint swelling persisting for more than 6 weeks without known cause. It affects joints, tendon sheaths, and bursae and may affect other organ systems and

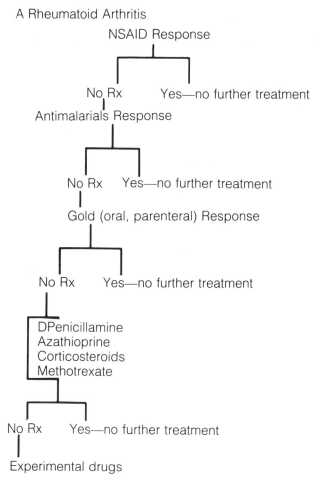

Fig. 4-2. Algorithims of pharmacologic management. (**A**) Rheumatoid arthritis, (**B**) gout (acute). (*Figure continues*).

growth abnormalities. There are three onset subtypes: systemic, polyarticular (involving many joints), and pauciarticular (involving a few joints). The systemic onset accounts for 20 percent of all JRA. It can begin at any age and affects males and females equally. Fever, rash, arthralgia, and myalgia are typical findings. Most patients later develop chronic polyarthritis. Approximately 40 percent of children with JRA have a polyarticular onset. Most of these patients are females aged more than 10 years. All joints in the body can be affected, and the arthritis is usually deforming. These children are often older at onset, develop the rheumatoid factor, and when the arthritis is positive, it most resembles the adult disabling and destructive form. The third subtype is that of the pauciarticular group, which is further divided into two groups: early childhood onset in girls under the age of 6 and later childhood onset in boys aged 10 years and older. Both groups tend to have mild disease, with chronic

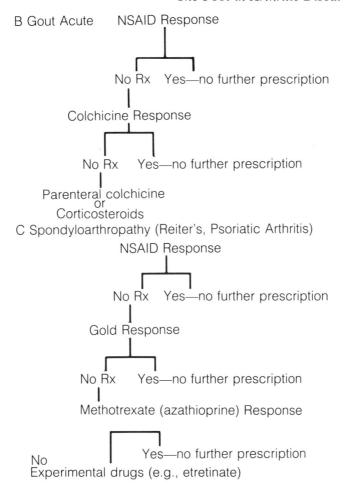

Fig. 4-2 (*Continued*). (**B**) gout (acute), (**C**) spondyloarthropathy (Reiters, psoriatic arthritis).

synovitis but usually without systemic symptoms and without major disability. One very important associated finding in girls who develop pauciarticular arthritis is the occurrence of iridocyclitis which can lead to blindness.

The diagnosis of JRA is usually made on clinical grounds, based on the criteria listed above. Often JRA is a diagnosis of exclusion, and the critical diagnoses that must be eliminated include other connective tissue diseases [systemic lupus erythematosus, (SLE), dermatomyositis, scheroderma], tumors, trauma, etc. The laboratory findings include a positive antinuclear antibody in a small number and a mild anemia. X-ray studies are often negative in the younger age group. Treatment differs from the adult management schema because of potential toxicities to the growing child. The basic pharmacological approach includes aspirin or nonsteroidal antiinflammatory drugs (NSAID), then gold or hydroxychloroquine and, last, steroids.

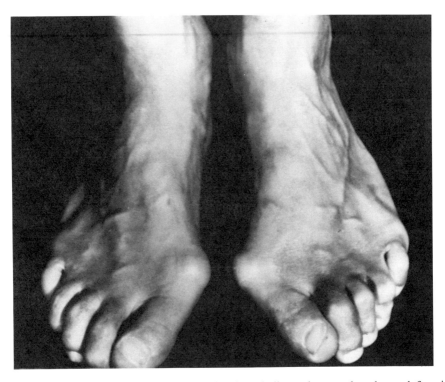

Fig. 4-3. Rheumatoid arthritis: widened forefoot, hallux valgus, and cock-toe deformities are apparent.

Any joint in the body can be affected in JRA, but 70 to 90 percent will make a good recovery from the arthritis without significant disability.[14] The process involves joints, tendons, and bursae, hence causing additional soft tissue inflammation early in the disease, often associated with contractures and fixed deformities over a short time. Growth retardation can occur if the disease is widespread or the patient is on corticosteroids, but this rarely happens in pauciarticular JRA. Premature closure of the epiphysis in the young arthritic may occur, and when it occurs in the foot, is usually in the metatarsals. When the foot is involved, as it frequently is, the MTP, interphalangeal (IP), tarsometatarsal, and tarsal joints are affected. Flexion contractures of the toes, with cock-toe deformity, subluxation of the metatarsal heads, and hallux valgus deformities result. Peculiar to JRA is tarsal joint involvement with fusion and a varus or valgus hindfoot deformity. Because this is particularly difficult to treat, prevention using night splints should be considered as an early intervention. True ankle joint abnormalities may occur following prolonged synovitis, and equinovarus contractures can occur if attention is not directed to foot positioning during those periods of inflammation. Other inflammatory arthropathies affect the foot. Specifically, those involving the spine are called spondyloarthropathies; psoriatic arthritis (PsA) and Reiter's syndrome belong to

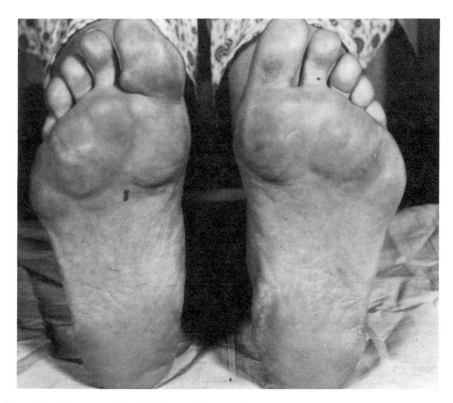

Fig. 4-4. Rheumatoid arthritis: swelling under metatarsal phalanges and rheumatoid nodule along the inner aspect of the big toe are apparent.

this group. They both have a high degree of back and sacroiliac joint involvement and usually are associated with arthritis of the foot. Another spondyloarthropathy, ankylosing spondylitis, similar in some respects to PsA and Reiter's, rarely affects the foot.

PSORIATIC ARTHRITIS

PsA is an asymmetrical, inflammatory polyarthritis. The diagnosis is made based on the existence of an inflammatory arthritis in a patient with psoriasis who lacks the rheumatoid factor. Approximately 80 percent of patients with PsA have pitting of the nails or a heaped-up appearance of the nail called onycholysis. Often the skin and nail changes precede the development of arthritis (Fig. 4-6). The laboratory is only minimally helpful in establishing the diagnosis and in differentiating PsA from RA. Soft tissue swelling occurs around the joint, and frequently an extension of the edema past the joint line is apparent. Clinically, this creates a sausage appearance of the digit (Fig. 4-7). In the small joints of fingers and toes, bone destruction may be quite extensive and

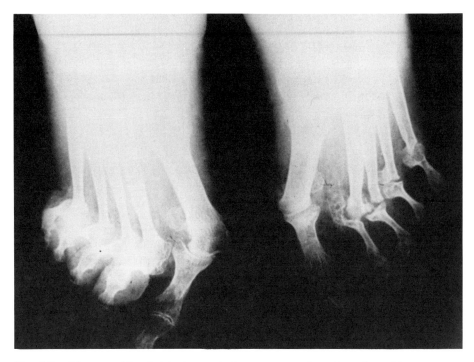

Fig. 4-5. Rheumatoid arthritis: juxtarticular osteoporosis and erosion of bone are apparent. There appears to be no bony reparative process.

create an appearance of joint space widening. Erosion is common; it may begin at bony margins, but then advances to the central portion of the bone, creating a pencil-like appearance. Bone on the other side of the joint may become saucerized, creating the classical pencil-in-cup deformity. Bone mineral is usually normal in PsA, and proliferation of bone may occur either as periostitis or at tendinous and ligamentous insertions, a finding that does not occur in RA. These typical radiograph findings are seen in the foot.

When PsA involves the foot,[15] which happens in virtually all patients, characteristic changes include sausaging of the toes, often only a few on each foot, which often progresses to a fixed flexion contracture of the DIP and PIP. In the rheumatoidlike PsA, metatarsophalangeal joint involvement occurs with subsequent MTP subluxation, cock-toe deformity, and MTP callosities. Because tendinitis and bursitis are common clinical features of the spondyloarthropathies, Achilles tendinitis, retrocalcaneal bursitis, and plantar fasciitis are frequently seen and are often initial symptoms. At times, the tarsal joints fuse. In general, the arthritis is quite severe, often rapidly progressive, and is associated with much swelling and redness and a great deal of pain. Shoeing is often a problem because of the sausaging of toes and the need for a deep toebox. Heal pain can be extremely difficult to control; hence, local injections of corticosteroids may be needed.

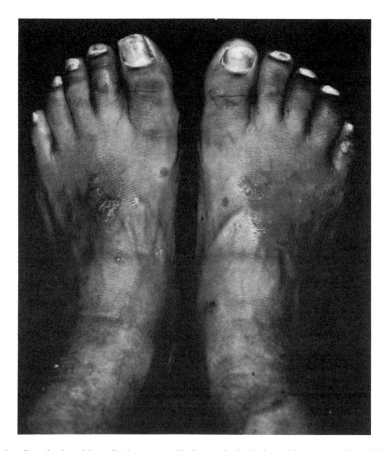

Fig. 4-6. Psoriasis with nail changes called onycholysis is evident on nails of big toes.

Pharmacological management of PsA is often necessary for those with more than a few joints involved and includes aspirin, NSAIDs, gold, and methotrexate.

REITER'S SYNDROME

Reiter's syndrome, one of the inflammatory spondyloarthropathies, classically consists of conjunctivitis, nonspecific urethritis, and polyarthritis. A skin rash, keratoderma blennorrhagicum, is also associated with Reiter's (Fig. 4-8). The appearance of Reiter's and PsA is similar; the laboratory and radiographic findings do not help distinguish the two arthritides. The clinical findings in the foot include pain and swelling in the midtarsal and MTP joints. The entire toe is often involved with redness, swelling, and the typical sausage appearance. The metatarsals may sublux quickly, leaving cock-toes whose IP joints fuse. Achilles tendinitis, with painful tender swelling at the insertion of the heel cord, is

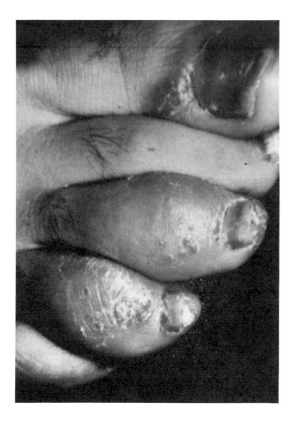

Fig. 4-7. Psoriatic arthritis: sausaging of third digit is evident.

characteristic. Calcaneal spurs, fasciitis, and periostitis of the calcaneus also commonly occur (Fig. 4-9). As in PsA, tendinitis often limits motion and function. Tendinitis of the peronei, posterior tibialis, and flexors and extensors of the toes, as well as of the Achilles tendon, has been reported. Treatment of foot problems is often conservative and local injections are used with good success.

INFLAMMATORY ARTHRITIS

True Gout

Inflammatory arthritis can also be caused by a variety of crystals: uric acid, calcium pyrophosphate, or hydroxyapatite. True gout is caused by monosodium urate crystals in the joint. These crystals are readily identified by their strong-negative birefringence when seen under the polarizing microscope and their irregular, needle-like shape. The crystals in the joints of patients with pseudo-gout have weak positive birefringence and are thomboid-shaped. Hydroxyapatite crystals can be seen only in aggregates and using the electron microscope.

Clinically, true gout is an acute, intermittent, mono- or oligoarticular arthritis. The pain is often so severe that the patient cannot tolerate the weight of

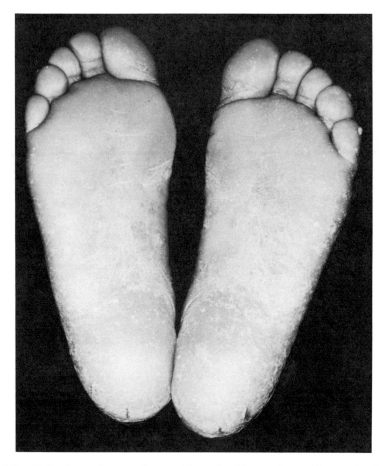

Fig. 4-8. Reiter's syndrome: plantar skin rash of keratoderma blennorrhagicum.

a sheet on the affected joint. The erythema is very intense, and the skin may subsequently peel. The first MTP is the site of the initial attack in more than 75 percent of cases. This particular arthritis is called "podagra." Subsequent attacks are frequently polyarticular. The next most common anatomic locations for arthritis to develop are instep, ankle, and heels. Gout occurs most frequently in middle-aged males. The laboratory findings are helpful in confirming the diagnosis when the serum uric acid is in excess of 8.0 mg/dl; but the diagnosis is dependent on identifying sodium urate crystals in the joint fluid. Radiographs reveal soft tissue swelling around the involved joint. With chronicity, tophi may become calcified or show up as lobulated soft tissue densities and adjacent extraarticular erosion involving the bony cortex (Fig. 4-10).

Treatment of the acute attack consists of colchicine or NSAIDs. Treatment of the chronic hyperuricemic state may require use of allopurinol to inhibit xanthina oxidase and block uric acid synthesis. Treatment often results in mobilization of urate deposits and restoration of normal bony structure.

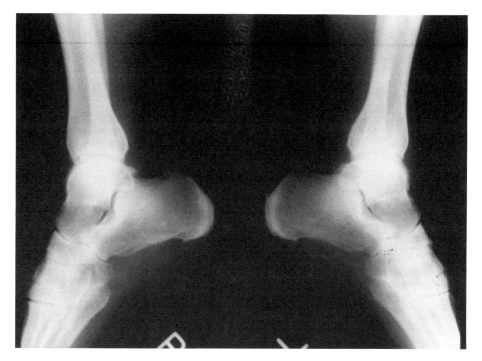

Fig. 4-9.   Reiter's syndrome: heel spur and calcification of Achilles tendon insertion.

Pseudogout

Pseudogout is really a cluster of clinical entities associated with calcium pyrophosphate crystals and takes three forms: sporadic form, a hereditary form, and a form associated with metabolic diseases such as diabetes, hyperparathyroidism, etc. Pseudogout is also associated with OA, RA, and gout. The diagnosis is made on the basis of joint fluid analysis, in which the calcium pyrophosphate crystal is identified, and through characteristic changes evident on radiographs. These include deposits of crystals, which are radioopaque, in hyaline cartilage, synovium, and tendon. Often degenerative joint changes occur, with joint space narrowing, bony sclerosis, and subchondral cysts as the disease progresses. These depositions can occur in any joint of the foot, but the first MTP, with development of hallux valgus is common in the hereditary form, whereas the ankle is more likely to be involved in the other types.

Attacks of pseudogout are usually managed with NSAIDs, with satisfactory control. Hydroxyapatite crystal disease has not been documented to occur in the foot.

The crystal-induced arthritides must be differentiated from joint infections. Almost any organism has the potential for settling in a joint. The presence of other systemic illnesses, such as diabetes, malignancies, alcoholism, RA, and various treatments such as immunosuppressive therapy or cortico-

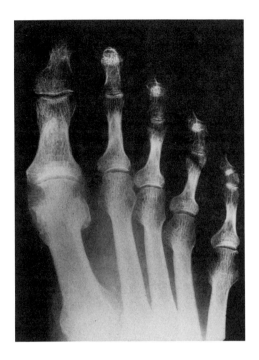

Fig. 4-10. Soft tissue deposition of gout crystals and erosion of bone of first metatarsal phalanx.

steroids may predispose toward development of a joint infection. A single hot, swollen, tender joint that has limited ROM should be suspected as a possibly infected joint. The lower extremity is more likely to be involved than is the upper, and larger joints are more likely to be infected than are smaller joints, but any joint can be infected in the right host. The ankle is the most commonly infected site in the foot. The synovial fluid usually reveals the diagnosis when the WBC count is high, with a large number of neutrophils and an organism cultured. The radiograph may show an articular effusion, periosteal reaction, and marginal bony erosion.

Such conditions are properly treated early with intravenous (IV) antibiotics, nonweightbearing and occasionally, joint drainage.

Neuropathic Arthropathy

Neuropathic arthropathy, or Charcot joint disease, is not an inflammatory arthritis. It results from loss of pain and proprioceptive responses and allows the joints to exceed normal ROM. Trauma, sometimes merely resulting from weightbearing, causes chronic breakdown of the bones and joints of the midfoot. The patient has a warm, swollen, nonpainful midfoot, possibly with associated soft tissue ulceration. The radiograph shows joint effusion, early in the course, followed by subluxation and then destruction of the articular surface and eburnation of the bony structures. Periosteal new bone may proliferate in

TABLE 4-3. Distribution of Joint Involvement in the Foot

	IP	MTP	Midtarsal	Hindfoot	Ankle	Achilles Tendon
Type of arthritis						
Adult RA	+	+++	+	++	+	+
Juvenile RA	+	++	++	+	++	+
OA	++	++	+[a]	+[a]	+[a]	+
PsA	+++	+++	+	++	+	+
Reiter's	++	++	+	++	+	+++
AS	+	+	+	+	+	++
Gout	+	+++[b]	+	++	+	+
CPPD	+	+	+	+	++	+

IP, interphalangeal; MTP, metatarsalphalangeal; RA, rheumatoid arthritis; OA, osteoarthritis; CPPD,
[a] Usually 2° to trauma.
[b] Especially first MTP.

an attempt to repair the defect. It is most often an associated finding of tabes dorsalis and diabetes mellitus. In the former, the ankle is most often the site affected; in the latter, the tarsal and the tarsometatarsal articulations are affected most often.

The Prone Foot

The prone foot, especially when it is subjected to excessive stress, as in athletes or in obese patients, may exert an unusually high amount of stress on midtarsal joints, leading to traction osteophytes. These occur in the talonavicular, navicular-cuneiform, and cuneiform-metatarsal joints. Tendons overlying these bones frequently develop tendinitis. Chronic excessive pronation results in stretch to plantar ligaments, capsule, and fascia.[16] This chronic stretch is believed to play a role in the etiology of heel pain and development of plantar spurs. Although these conditions are not arthritis, the role of excessive pronation in causing bony reaction (osteophyte) and tendinitis is worth commenting on and should be addressed with appropriate corrective steps both as a possible preventive measure or as concomitant treatment in management of the arthritic foot.

SUMMARY

The foot is often involved in the arthritic process. A careful examination can occasionally help in differentiating among the various types of arthritides (e.g., gout vs psoriatic arthritis on the basis of crystals in the former and nail abnormalities in the latter.) The distribution of joint involvement, summarized in Table 4-3, as well as the presence or absence of signs of inflammation can also help diagnostically and in planning appropriate interventions (e.g., polyarticular vs monoarticular involvement as occurs in RA vs OA). Finally, the ability to recognize dynamic relationships in the foot (e.g., relationship of pronation to development of hallux valgus) is important in maintaining alignment and possibly preventing future joint destruction.

REFERENCES

1. Vainio, K: The rheumatoid foot: A clinical study with pathological and eorntgenological comments. Ann Clin Gynaecol Fenn 45 (suppl. 1)5:107; 1956
2. Wright V, Moll JMH: Seronegative Polyarthritis. North-Holland, Amsterdam, 1976
3. Lawrence JS, Brenner JM, Brer F: Osteoarthritis. Prevalence in the population and relationship between symptoms and x-ray changes. Ann Rheum Dig 25:1, 1966
4. Palmoski M, Brandt K: In vivo effect of aspirin on canine osteoarthritic cartilage. Arthritis Rheum 26:994, 1983
5. Friedman DM, Moore MA: The efficacy of intraarticular corticosteroid for osteoarthritis of the knee. Arthritis Rheum 21:556, 1978
6. Benson TB, Copp EP, The effects of therapeutic forms of heat and ice on the pain threshold of the normal shoulder. Rheumatol Rehabil 13:101, 1974
7. Magora F, Aladjemoff L, Tannenbaum J, et al: Treatment of pain by transcutaneous electrical stimulation. Scand J Anesthesia 22:589, 1978
8. Clark GR, Willis LA; Stenner L, Nichols PJR: Evaluation of physiotherapy in the treatment of OA of the knee. Rheum Rehabil 13:190, 1974
9. Ropes MW, Bennett EA, Cobb S, et al: 1958 Revision of diagnostic criteria for rheumatoid arthritis Bull Rheum Dis 9:175, 1958
10. Root M, Orien W, Weed J: Abnormal Function of the Foot. Clinical Biomechanics, Los Angeles, 1978
11. Marshall RN, Myers DB, Palmer DG. Disturbance of gait due to rheumatoid disease. J Rheumatol 7:617, 1980
12. McGuigan L, Burke D, Fleming A: Tarsal tunnel syndrome and peripheral neuropathy in rheumatoid disease. Ann Rheum Dis 42:128, 1983
13. Bywaters EGL: Heel lesions of rheumatoid arthritis. Ann Rheum Dis 13:42, 1954
14. Hanson V, Kornreich H, Bernstein B, et al. Prognosis of juvenile rheumatoid arthritis. Arthritis Rheum 20:279, 1977
15. Sbarbaro JL, Katz WA: The feet and ankles in the diagnosis of rheumatic disease. In Katz WA, (ed): Rheumatic Diseases: Diagnosis and Management. Lippincott Philadelphia, 1977, 189
16. Furey, JGF: Plantar Fasciitis. J Bone Joint Surg [Am] 57:672, 1975

SUGGESTED READINGS

1.   Kelly WN, Harris ED, Ruddy S, Sledge CB, (eds): Textbook of Rheumatology. WB Saunders, Philadelphia, 1985
2.   Mann R: Osteoarthritis of the Foot and Ankle. In Moskowitz, Howell, Goldberg, Mankin, eds. Osteoarthritis, Diagnosis and Management, WB Saunders, Philadelphia, 1984
3.   Rana N: Rheumatoid Arthritis, Other Collagen Diseases and Psoriasis of the Foot. WB Saunders, Philadelphia, 1982
4.   Rana N: Gout. p. 1014. In Jahss, MH ed., Disorders of the Foot. WB Saunders, Philadelphia, 1982

5 | The Foot in Hemiplegia

Susan D. Ryerson

The ability to walk safely and independently is an important functional goal for patients with hemiplegia. A normal gait pattern implies both proximal control of the pelvis and hip and proper foot function, both of which may be impaired with hemiplegia. Loss of proximal motor control may alter the position and function of the foot biomechanically during swing phase of gait and during the initial contact of the foot with the ground. Altered biomechanics in the foot during stance phase may affect the muscular activity in the entire lower extremity. Thus, restoring or preserving proper foot mechanics is an important part of regaining the motor control necessary for ambulation.

In this chapter, abnormal lower extremity movement patterns and abnormal mechanical patterns in the foot in hemiplegia are discussed. The comparison between these abnormal components and the normal components of foot function are used to suggest principles for treatment and orthotic management of the foot in hemiplegia.

PATHOGENESIS OF DISEASE PROCESS

Hemiplegia, a paralysis of one side of the body, is the classic sign of cerebrovascular disease. Hemiplegia occurs with stroke or cerebrovascular accident, an impairment of the cerebral circulation from a thrombus, embolus, or hemorrhage. Although hemiplegia may be the most obvious sign of a stroke, other deficits are equally disabling, including sensory loss, impairment of speech, visual defects, cognitive loss, and perceptual dysfunction. These neurological deficits enable the physician to determine the size and location of the pathological process. Strokes can manifest themselves suddenly—in seconds, minutes, or an hour—or can "progress" slowly over days. A transient ischemic attack (TIA) is a stroke that occurs as a brief episode of neurological deficit that clears completely.

Of the three pathological processes that cause a cerebrovascular accident—thrombosis, embolus, and hemorrhage—atherosclerotic thrombosis is the most common cause. These atherosclerotic plagues form at the branchings and curves of the cerebral arteries. Because occlusion of an artery by a thrombus occurs over time, the process explains the difference between the stroke-in-evolution and the fully established stroke. A TIA is an indication of thrombotic disease. Adams states that cerebral vasospasm or transient systemic arterial hypotension may also be factors contributing to the onset of TIAs.[1]

An embolic infarction that causes a stroke can arise from the heart or from a carotid artery thrombosis. Cerebral embolism is a sign of cardiac disease. The branches of the middle cerebral artery are infarcted most often since the middle cerebral artery is a direct offshoot of the internal carotid artery. Embolic infarc-

Table 5-1. Clinical Symptoms of Stroke

Vessel	Possible Clinical Signs (Depending on region affected)
Middle cerebral artery	Contralateral paralysis and sensory loss
	Homonymous hemianopsia
	Aphasia (if in dominant hemisphere)
	Unilateral neglect, visual spatial disorientation—disturbed body image (nondominant hemisphere)
	Pure motor hemiplegia
	Dysarthria
Anterior cerebral artery	Contralateral hemiplegia with lower extremity sensory loss (arm affected to lesser degree than leg)
	Urinary incontinence, lack of spontaneity, gait apraxia
	Perseveration and amnesia
Posterior cerebral artery	Homonymous hemianopsia, cortical blindness
	Contralateral sensory loss—thalamic syndrome
	Weber's syndrome
	Contralateral ataxia, athetosis, or tremor
	Coma
Basilar artery	Cerebellar ataxia
	Nystagmus, vertigo, nausea, vomiting
	Contralateral loss of pain and temperature
	Hemiparesis of arm and leg
	Facial pain and numbness same side
	Ataxia
	Decreased gag
	Hiccups
Complete basilar artery syndrome	Coma
	Quadriplegia
	Cranial nerve abnormalities
	Bilateral cerebellar ataxia

(Adapted from Adams RD, Victor M: Principles of Neurology. McGraw-Hill, New York, 1981.)

tions occur more quickly than thrombotic obstructions, which result in the formation of less collateral blood supply and consequently more damage to the tissue distal to the infarct.

The third process, intracranial hemorrhage, that leads to a stroke can be divided into three types: hypertensive, ruptured saccular aneurysm, and atrio-ventricular (AV) malformation.

The precise mechanism of intracerebral hemorrhage is not known. With hemorrhage, the stroke occurs quickly, without warning, or evolves rapidly. The neurological signs following hemorrhage vary as a result of the bleeding into surrounding brain tissue and of the rise in intracranial pressure.

Saccular or berry aneurysms are small, thin-walled pouches that develop in the vascular walls of the major cerebral arteries, especially the anterior portion of the Circle of Willis.[1]

AV malformations are developmental abnormalities that result in a spaghetti-like mass of dilated arterio-venous fistulas in the brain tissue. The walls of these vessels are thin and abnormally arranged.

Clinical Findings

The symptoms resulting from a stroke depend on the site and size of the lesion and the amount of collateral circulation. Unilateral neurological deficits occur when the carotid vascular system is interrupted, and bilateral deficits occur when the basilar vascular system is compromised. Table 5-1 describes the clinical symptoms of stroke according to the vessels involved.

PERTINENT ANATOMICAL CONSIDERATIONS

Following a cerebrovascular accident, the client with a hemiplegia experiences a change in the postural tonal state and a loss of motor control. As the client learns to function in antigravity positions, the predictable patterns of motor return, the laws of biomechanics, and gravity alter the relationship of body segments. The foot, being the last link in the lower extremity kinematic chain, is influenced by the loss of motor control and change in alignment of the trunk, pelvis, hip, and knee. These new anatomical relationships must be considered when evaluating and treating the foot of the client with a hemiplegia.

Three lower extremity hemiplegic patterns have been described that influence the control and alignment of the ankle and foot. These patterns have been explained either by their biomechanical or kinesiological attributes or by their centrally programmed motor control characteristics.[2,3] Although the patterns have been separated into three groups, overlap or progression from one pattern to the next exists as recovery progresses.

Pattern I

In the acute stage of recovery or following a severe stroke, the client's motor control state is one of low postural tone and little motor activity. The influence of gravity and the laws of biomechanics greatly influence these clients' movement patterns. With severe loss of motor control, the spine will laterally flex towards the affected side as a result of the pull of gravity during stance. The upper trunk will be laterally flexed over the lower trunk and the rib cage will begin to rotate. In sitting, the pelvis becomes posteriorly tilted as a result of the loss of antigravity control. As the client attempts to assume a standing position, the pelvis will anteriorly tilt and list downwards on the affected side. As a result of this position, and the loss of motor control (Fig. 5-1) the hip and knee will flex (Fig. 5-1). This hip and knee flexion combined with an inability to bear weight on the affected side places the ankle in plantarflexion. Because the calcaneus becomes nonweight bearing, any weight that is placed on the leg will be borne by the forefoot (Fig. 5-2).

As functional training for activities such as transfers, standing, and walk-

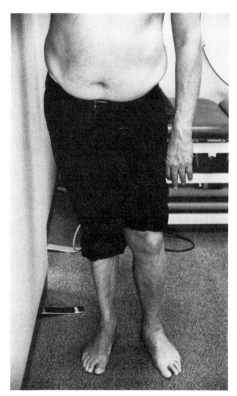 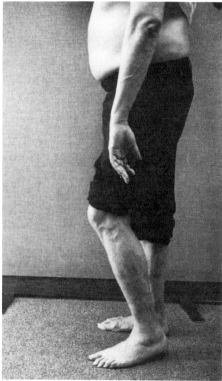

Fig. 5-1. Pattern I, left hemiplegia: pelvis lists downward on left.

Fig. 5-2. Pattern I, left hemiplegia: pelvis falling into anterior tilt; hip and knee flexion with a nonweightbearing calcaneus.

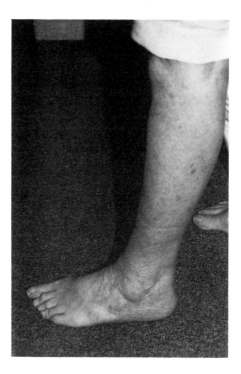

Fig. 5-3.   Knee moving into recurvatum, with calcaneus nonweightbearing.

ing is begun, these clients are often encouraged to put the heel down on the ground. If this is done without correction of the proximal trunk and hip problems, the knee will move into recurvatum and the ankle will continue to move in the direction of plantarflexion (Fig. 5-3).

If this movement pattern and abnormal alignment remain uncorrected in stance and swing, the client with hemiplegia will develop a soft tissue contracture of the gastrocsoleus muscle group and a loss of ankle dorsiflexion range (Fig. 5-4 A and B). Subtalar joint motions as well can become restricted in combination with ankle joint involvement.

If the client is encouraged to place weight on the affected lower extremity without a correction of subtalar joint alignment, the midfoot will pronate and the forefoot will move into relative abduction. The longitudinal and transverse arches of the foot will collapse and the toes will "claw".

To summarize, the common foot and ankle problems resulting from this pattern include (1) loss of ankle joint dorsiflexion, (2) a nonweight bearing calcaneus, (3) an everted calcaneus, and (4) an abducted forefoot.

Pattern II

As recovery occurs or with a less severe stroke, incomplete firing patterns with emerging spasticity become evident. Motor return causes an imbalance of control between trunk flexor and extensor muscle groups. Spinal extensor

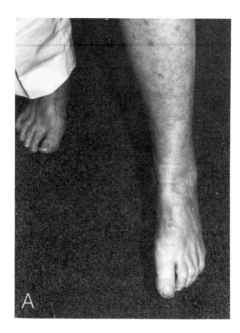

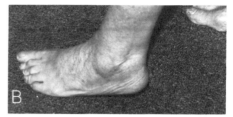

Fig. 5.4. (**A**) Pattern I, swing: foot is plantarflexed. (**B**) Pattern I, stance: Forefoot accepting weight; nonweightbearing calcaneus.

patterns are more available to the client than are spinal flexor patterns. Clients use these extensor patterns unilaterally as they attempt functional activities. This unilateral use of extensor patterns results in ipsilateral flexion and contralateral rotation in the cervical spine, rotation of the thoracic vertebrae to the affected side, and rib cage rotation backwards on the affected side (Figs. 5-5 A and B). In standing, strong activity of the low back extensors and the pelvic hikers cause the pelvis to be anteriorly tilted and elevated (listed upwards). The knee will extend unless the client has been taught to push the knee into flexion. If the knee moves into recurvatum, the ankle will plantarflex and the talus moves anteriorly relative to the calcaneus. If soft tissue tightness develops, ankle dorsiflexion range is lost. As the client tries to move over the foot, the midtarsal joint will dorsiflex and a strong force downward occurs across the forefoot. The forefoot will move into relative abduction.

These clients use this lower trunk extension and pelvic hiking to initiate swing phase of gait (Fig. 5-6). This pelvic hiking prevents any lower trunk rotational component from occurring. The hip and pelvis become a unit (with no disassociation present), the knee is extended stiffly, and the ankle is "pushed" into plantarflexion as the client attempts to swing the leg forward. As the client tries to clear the foot from the floor, the midfoot will begin to supinate and the forefoot may adduct as a result of unbalanced motor control.

At heel strike, the client's forefoot strikes the ground first (Fig. 5-7A). When body weight is placed on the foot, the calcaneus everts and the midfoot collapses and weight is transferred back toward the heel (Fig. 5-7 B and C). However, the calcaneus may not be in a position to bear significant weight. As weight shift during stance is attempted, the knee remains in recurvatum, hip

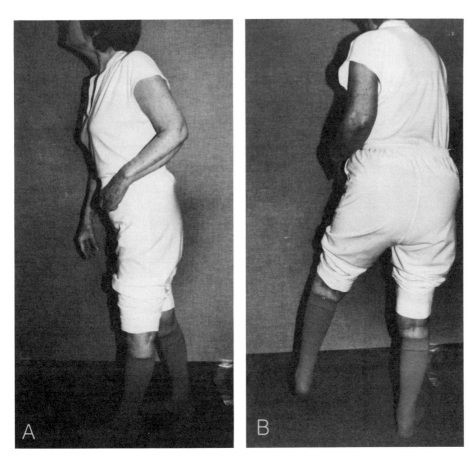

Fig. 5-5. (**A** and **B**) Pattern II, left hemiplegia: rib cage rotation backwards.

extension is blocked, and the pelvis is not able to initiate a forward diagonal movement pattern. Therefore, these clients compensate with either the upper trunk or the unaffected side to initiate weight shift over the stance limb. The pelvis stays elevated, anteriorly tilted and rotated backwards. The hip is in relative flexion and varying degrees of internal rotation. There is a strong, rigid push of the leg into the ground. The foot assumes the same position as described in standing.

The toes of such clients claw severely for one of two reasons:

1. The loss of the arches of the foot allows the heads of the metatarsals to depress and the phalanges hyperextend proximally and flex distally.[4]

2. When these clients attempt to move their trunk and pelvis forward during gait, compensations occur that shift the center of gravity outside the base of support. This causes the body to recruit an equilibrium reaction and as part of the equilbrium reaction, the toes claw.

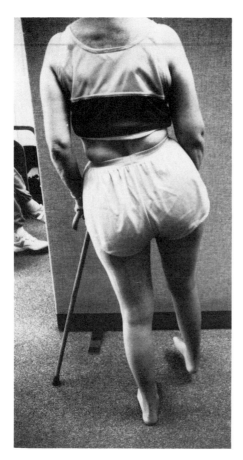

Fig. 5-6.   Pattern II, right hemiplegia: initiation of swing phase by hiking pelvis.

The common foot and ankle problems resulting from this pattern include (1) loss of ankle dorsiflexion, (2) an everted calcaneus with medial midfoot collapse, (Fig. 5-7B, C) and (3) toe clawing.

Pattern III

The third movement pattern is characterized by abnormal coactivation of muscles. This gives the appearance of ''mass flexion'' during movement of the lower extremity. The trunk control in clients with this lower extremity pattern contains elements of both flexor and extensor patterns, but the control of these patterns is not integrated enough to allow selective movement patterns; i.e., lateral flexion, upper or lower trunk rotation, or counter rotation. Such clients recruit flexor patterns during swing phase of gait and extensor patterns during stance. Recruitment of distal motion is used to reinforce the proximal motions, especially during nonweightbearing movements.

Clients who move with this third control pattern initiate the swing phase

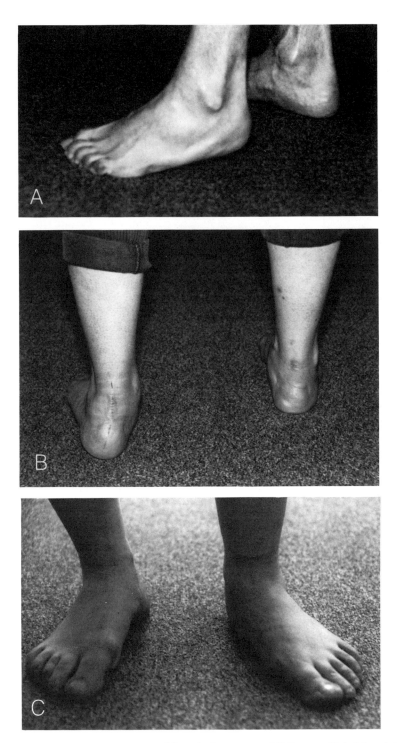

Fig. 5-7. (A) Forefoot strikes ground first during stance. (B) Pattern II, left hemiplegia: stance phase, calcaneal eversion; (C) pattern II, left hemiplegia: stance phase, midfoot pronation.

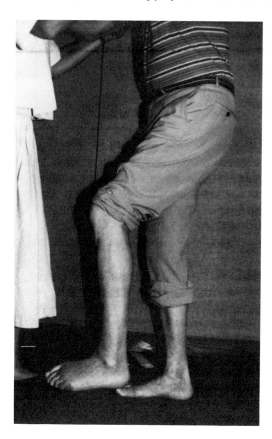

Fig. 5-8. Pattern III, left hemi-plegia: use of posterior pelvic tilt to initiate swing.

with a posterior pelvic tilt (Fig. 5-8). The hip moves into relative flexion, but the most noticeable hip movement is abduction. The foot strongly supinates: the calcaneus inverts with midfoot supination and forefoot adduction. If this distal component is strong enough, the foot will stay "locked" in supination and the body weight will be accepted onto the lateral border of the forefoot at the heel strike portion of stance (Fig. 5-9 A–C).

Over time, the midfoot may begin to shift dorsolaterally (Fig. 5-10).

Once weight is on the lateral border of the foot, two situations are possible:

1. If the foot is rigidly locked in supination, the client will move through stance on this narrow "razor-edged" foot. This occurs when strong spasticity is present. When the foot is on the ground, the supination component of the rearfoot results in a lateral rotation movement of the tibia on the foot. The pelvis will rotate backward on the affected side and the rib cage will compensate according to the amount of control present.[5]

2. If the foot is not rigidly locked in supination, the client will land on the lateral border of the forefoot. The weight will be forcefully transferred medially in an attempt to place the foot flat on the floor (Fig. 5-11 A–C). The midfoot will collapse medially, and the heel, while it may be in contact with the floor, never

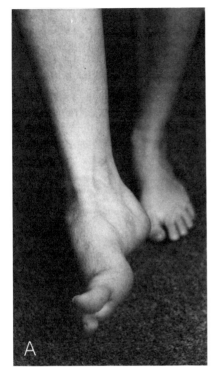

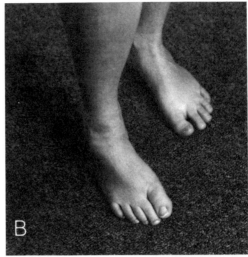

Fig. 5-9. Pattern III. (**A**) Right hemiplegia: foot supinates severely during swing. (**B** and **C**) Right hemiplegia: foot stays locked in supination during stance.

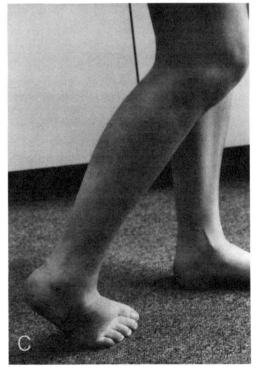

accepts body weight. This foot may become hypermobile due to the interplay between these two forces: strong supination during swing and strong pronation during stance. Clawing of the toes is present[6] (Fig. 5-12).

Common foot problems resulting from this pattern include the following:

1. Inverted calcaneus
2. Excessive lateral rotation of the tibia on the foot
3. Excessive forefoot adduction

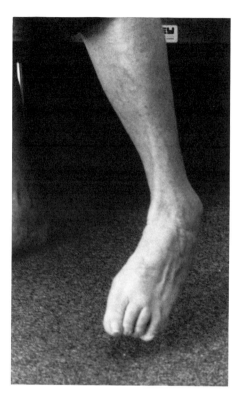

Fig. 5-10. Left hemiplegia: midfoot subluxes dorsolaterally.

SPECIFIC EXAMINATION PROCEDURES

An evaluation of the functional capabilities in the foot following a stroke can be divided into five distinct but interrelated parts: (1) dynamic gait evaluation; (2) assessment of the mobility of the subtalar joint, midfoot, and forefoot in sitting and standing; (3) assessment of the location and degree of posturing during walking; (4) amount of active control; and (5) assessment of the amount of manual correction required during standing and walking necessary to obtain neutral foot and ankle alignment.

Dynamic Gait Evaluation

A dynamic gait evaluation is performed to ascertain the relationships of the trunk, hip, knee, ankle, and foot. In hemiplegia, the key elements of the gait evaluation include: (2) the initiation (lift-off) of swing, (2) the position of the foot at initial contact, and (3) the initiation and direction of weight shift during

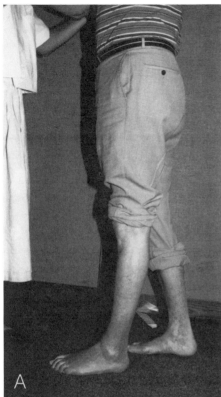

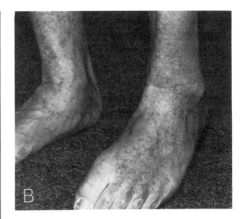

Fig. 5-11. (A) Pattern III, left hemiplegia: use of lumbar extension to stabilize trunk during stance; body weight is transferred back in an attempt to place foot on floor. (B and C) Metatarsals accept weight initially, and the body weight is then transferred medially and backwards in an attempt to place foot flat on floor.

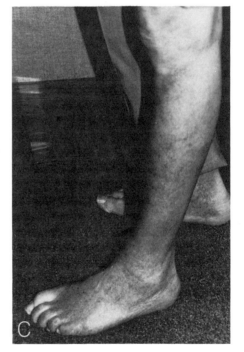

midstance. Differentiation between active control and posturing should be made by the evaluator during all phases of the gait cycle.

Mobility

Foot problems in the client with hemiplegia may become evident when the client attempts to stand or walk. In sitting, however, mobility problems appear mild or minimal. This situation exists when proximal control is poor and the foot postures or becomes immobile during movement as a result of the biomechanical influences of the poorly aligned kinematic chain structures (i.e., trunk,

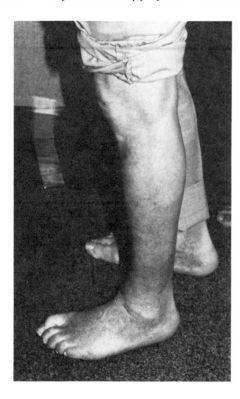

Fig. 5-12.   Pattern III, toe clawing.

pelvis, and hip). Therefore, the foot should be evaluated for problems of immobility, hypermobility, or posturing in sitting, as the client rises to stand and in standing.

Common problems of mobility in the foot of the hemiplegic client include:

1. *Ankle joint:* When measuring ankle joint range in sitting or in standing, it is important to remember that dorsiflexion can also occur at both the subtalar joint and the midtarsal joint.[5] If the calcaneus has shifted into plantarflexion from poor dorsiflexion control or from tight or spastic posterior calf muscles, the talus and distal tibia may not be aligned correctly on the calcaneus. Therefore, to evaluate available ankle joint motion, the calcaneus should be brought into correct alignment with the talus and tibia. Then, ankle joint range can be assessed.

2. *Subtalar joint:* A nonweight bearing evaluation of subtalar joint position and mobility must be followed by an evaluation of subtalar joint mobility and position during stance and swing. In sitting, clients who use pattern I or II may present with a pronated subtalar joint. Clients who use movement pattern III may exhibit excessive supination. The position of the subtalar joint during swing phase and stance phase of gait will be determined by the amount of motor control available and the degree of posturing present, as discussed in the previous section.

3. *Midtarsal joint:* During stance phase of gait, if ankle joint dorsiflexion is insufficient; the forefoot strikes first and becomes rigidly planted on the floor. As a consequence, pronation around the oblique axis of the midtarsal joint can provide dorsiflexion in the midfoot region. During swing phase of gait, the midtarsal joint supinates to varying degrees depending on the amount of motor control present and the alignment of the ankle joint, the subtalar joint and the forefoot. The midtarsal joint is a prime site for transverse and sagittal plane deformities because of the interplay between pronation and supination forces during the gait cycle.

4. *Forefoot:* In hemiplegia, a nonweightbearing evaluation of the relationship between the forefoot and rearfoot may be within normal limits. However, during the various phases of the gait cycle, the amount of apparent forefoot abduction or adduction may appear excessive. In stance, the forefoot abduction that is seen with subtalar joint pronation is not the result of the forefoot actively moving into abduction, but is the result of the forefoot being rigidly planted on the floor and the calcaneus and midfoot continuing to move on the planted forefoot.[3] If trunk, pelvis, and hip control is poor, the apparent abduction of the forefoot will be greater because the control of the rearfoot will be less. In swing, the amount of forefoot adduction will be greater as the subtalar joint postures in more supination and as the strength of unbalanced distal return increases.

Posturing

Distal posturing in the foot occurs in hemiplegia in two ways. First, as the foot attempts to make contact with the ground, the ankle can push strongly into plantar flexion. As the forefoot strikes the ground first, the posturing produces subtalar joint pronation resulting in calcaneal eversion with forefoot abduction.

Second, the foot can be pulled into a supination posture during nonweight bearing. Usually, ankle joint dorsiflexion is limited due to soft tissue tightness or spasticity. If the ankle joint remains in plantarflexion, the posturing pulls the calcaneus into inversion (the line of pull of both the anterior and posterior tibialis are medial to the subtalar joint axis), the midfoot dorsiflexes and supinates with relative adduction of the forefoot.

The strong extension/pronation posturing usually occurs during stance phase of gait and the supination posturing is present during swing phase, but each posturing pattern, if strong enough, can be present throughout both gait phases.

The location, direction and force of the posturing should be noted. If these postures are allowed to persist, a decrease in range of motion (ROM) or soft tissue contracture will result. During standing, if these postures can be controlled manually with little to moderate effort, normal alignment will be easily maintained in appropriate bracing with foot control. If maximal effort is required to hold the correct foot and ankle alignment, the bracing will need to hold the ankle and foot more securely until the posturing decreases and balanced motor control develops.

Active Control

Active movement patterns in the ankle and foot should be noted descriptively by joints and position (supine, sitting, standing, walking) since the effect of gravity and amount of trunk control will influence the motor control of the foot and ankle. The evaluation should note if the movement can be initiated, "held" when placed in varying degrees of the movement arc, and whether the movement can be completed through available joint range. If alignment of the foot is disturbed, active movement of individual foot muscles may be impaired. It is important to align the foot manually however, and then to ask the client to attempt the desired motion again. This allows the evaluator to determine if loss of control is preventing the movement or if the loss of alignment is preventing or hindering the movement from occurring.

Manual Correction

As noted in the preceding section, manual correction of posturing or malalignment, whether from imbalance of motor control or loss of ROM, is an important part of the assessment process. It gives the evaluator an idea of the amount of control that needs to be built into an orthotic device and provides an assessment of the interaction between loss of control and degree of posturing.

MANAGEMENT

Treatment: Motor Reeducation

Treatment of motor control deficits in the lower extremity in the client with a hemiplegia should focus on reestablishing normal movement patterns for functional activities and prevention of greater disability from secondary complications. During standing and walking the foot is required to move in response to the supporting surface. If foot control or alignment is not optimal, normal movement patterns in the joints above the foot will be difficult to achieve.

Establishment of trunk control provides the client with the ability to shift weight over the extremities. This weight shift then frees the extremities for functional activities and, in the case of the lower extremities, weight shift frees the leg and foot to "step." At the same time, reeducation of control patterns in the foot and ankle provides the base on which proximal control can be developed and refined. Reestablishment of proximal control in hemiplegia will also decrease posturing patterns in the foot.

Weightbearing

Establishment of the ability to accept weight is the most critical treatment objective for the foot in clients with hemiplegia. The foot must be able to accept weight, come in total contact with the ground, and remain "fixed" yet adapt-

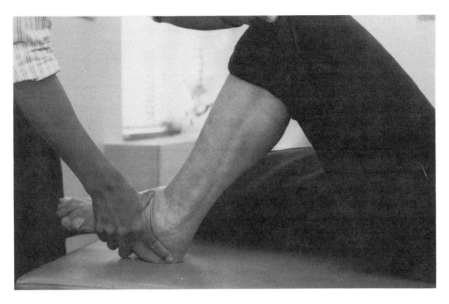

Fig. 5-13.   Client is taught to accept weight on heal during early treatment.

able as the body and limb move over the foot. The foot can be prepared to accept weight in the early stages of recovery through bed mobility activities (Fig. 5-13) and as the client learns to sit and transfer. While in the sitting position, the hemiplegic client should be encouraged to place both feet firmly on the floor. As weight shift in sitting is practiced, anterior and posterior trunk movement will shift weight from the heel to the ball of the foot, and lateral trunk movements will shift weight from the lateral side to the medial side of the foot. An important activity for the initiation of normal standing is the ability to accept weight on the heel. As the body moves forward and up from a chair, ankle joint dorsiflexion allows the proximal tibia to move forward over the foot (Fig. 5-14). As the body rises to stand, and the heel accepts body weight, an equilibrium reaction may help encourage active ankle dorsiflexion and toe extension. During transfer activities, the foot must be able to respond to lateral and rotational movement of the lower extremity.

In standing with feet parallel and in step-stance positions, the client with hemiplegia must learn to move the body over the foot. While the foot must be able to respond to lateral and rotational lower extremity movement patterns, the ability of the ankle and foot to allow and to control anterior and posterior body movements is critical for ambulation (Fig. 5-15 A and B). Weight shift in stance occurs with a forward diagonal movement over the foot. When appropriate foot and ankle control or mobility does not exist, the tibia cannot move forward over the foot. In this situation, if standing is attempted, the knee moves into recurvatum and the pelvis rotates backward in the transverse plane.

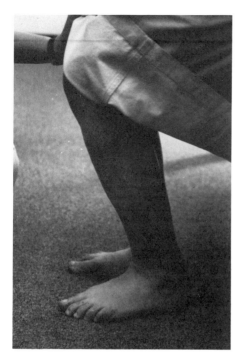

Fig. 5-14.   Ankle joint dorsiflexion is necessary as the body prepares to rise to stand.

Nonweightbearing Control

Along with reeducation of the foot in a weightbearing position, the foot needs to learn how to move in space. To accomplish swing phase of gait, the hemiplegic client must learn to control the foot and ankle enough to allow the foot to clear the ground (Fig. 5-16). Because in many cases the calcaneus is nonweightbearing and therefore is in some degree of plantarflexion, reestablishment of calcaneal alignment and control must precede correction of the midfoot and forefoot posturing.

ORTHOTIC MANAGEMENT

Orthotic management should be an integral part of treatment for the client with hemiplegia. Bracing can be used to improve the quality of motor control as well as for safety. The use of orthotic devices should not be considered an end-stage activity, but should be dynamically modified as recovery occurs. A well-designed orthosis allows correct alignment of the foot and ankle and will reinforce more normal alignment and control of the knee, hip, pelvis, and trunk. An ankle-foot orthosis (AFO) will contribute to the improvement of proximal motor control by providing a more normal sensory-motor base for the entire body. In hemiplegia, ankle foot orthoses can provide maximal control, as with a solid ankle type brace, or they can control the foot but allow ankle motion, as with an articulated brace.

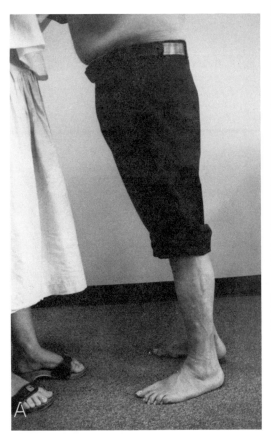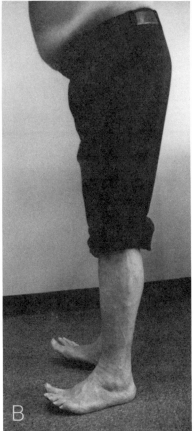

Fig. 5-15.   (**A**) Anterior weight shift in standing over a weightbearing foot; (**B**) Posterior weight shift in standing over a weightbearing foot.

Reasons for Bracing

Indications for bracing the ankle and foot in clients with a hemiplegia center around problems in control in stance, problems in swing, or a combination of loss of control in stance and swing.

The most common stance control problem is excessive pronation. The foot can be either collapsed into pronation due to the forces of body weight superimposed on a severe loss of motor control or it can be pushed into pronation by abnormal posturing. The goals for preventing excessive pronation in stance through the use of orthotic devices include:

1.   Preventing the ankle joint from inappropriately plantarflexing while maintaining the subtalar joint in neutral with special consideration given to the increased amount of force present in standing.

2.   Providing for sufficient ankle joint motion. A plastic custom-molded

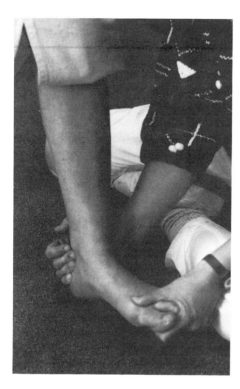

Fig. 5-16. Left hemiplegia: training the foot to move in space.

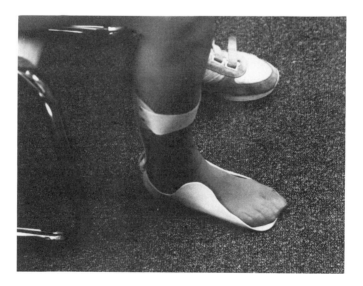

Fig. 5-17. Ankle-foot orthosis with high lateral border to control midfoot dorsolateral migration.

solid ankle AFO can be trimmed back to allow increased ankle joint motion as soon as the client develops appropriate motor control.

3. Maintaining a neutral rearfoot alignment with a long lateral border to prevent the forefoot from abducting. This correction of the forefoot on the rearfoot will influence the midfoot and help prevent excessive pronation.

4. Maintaining an appropriate calcaneal inclination by supporting the sustentaculum tali. This will prevent the loss of the longitudinal arch and decrease the amount of toe clawing.[7]

During swing phase, distal posturing produces varying degrees of calcaneal inversion, midtarsal joint supination, and forefoot adduction. This pattern is present in a mild form in clients who use movements from pattern II and is present in a moderate to severe form in clients who use movements from pattern III. If the supination pattern during swing is severe, the foot may become locked in this supinated position and remain there during stance. The goals for orthotic control here include:

1. Preventing the calcaneus from inverting and maintaining subtalar joint neutral, with special consideration given to the amount of force produced during the swing phase.

2. Providing appropriate ankle joint control. With these clients, a solid ankle is used to help prevent the strong posturing and is used until a portion of the distal posturing decreases.

3. Controlling midfoot supination with a high lateral border (Fig. 5-17).

4. Maintaining neutral rearfoot alignment with a long medial border to prevent the forefoot from adducting. This correction of the forefoot on the rearfoot will influence the midtarsal joint and help prevent the excessive supination.

If the client demonstrates excessive pronation in stance and excessive supination in swing, combinations of these features are used.

FOOT CONTROL VS ANKLE-FOOT CONTROL

The decision of whether or when to brace a client with a hemiplegia is a difficult one. The ankle-foot complex needs to be braced in the following cases:

1. Clients whose ankle and foot falls into plantarflexion during swing phase.

2. Clients who display a severe loss of trunk and pelvic control but display some motor control in the lower extremity.

3. Clients with poor subtalar joint alignment and severe posturing in the midtarsal joint.

4. When reestablishment of pelvic and hip control is a goal of treatment but the heel does not strike the ground during the initial contact phase of stance.

A foot orthosis is indicated when:

1. Hip and knee control are present, but the weight of the body pushes the foot into excessive pronation in stance.
2. Return is occurring in the acute recovery phase. Minimal bracing will insure heel contact and prevent the weight of the body and the incomplete motor control from setting up abnormal patterns in the foot mechanically.

Influences of Normal Ankle-Foot Alignment on Goals of Therapy

When the client with hemiplegia whose foot and ankle have been in poor alignment is braced appropriately, treatment goals will be changed. Initially, with the foot and ankle held in good alignment, the client will be standing on what is perceived to be a "new" base of support. The client will have to learn to control the trunk, pelvis, hip, and knee in a different way. With this new balance adjustment, it may take a few days before the body feels "stable" again. Treatment time will have to be directed at teaching the body to move over this newly aligned base of support.

An increase in the sensory motor experience will be noted by the client as a result of strong heel contact and an aligned foot during midstance. Clients experience this new sensation as a feeling of pressure in the heel and in the hip. They often say that they feel taller on the hemiplegic side as a result of the heel strike at stance. Treatment goals should be appropriately modified to take advantage of this new learning experience.

Because correction of the alignment of the foot affects control and alignment of the entire body, a decrease in the amount of upper extremity posturing will be noted.

Although bracing the foot and ankle will decrease posturing and help reestablish more proximal motor control, clients should be trained to reeducate the foot and ankle outside the orthotic device.

As is true with any disability, the results of treatment depend on the ability of the therapist to evaluate and treat appropriately the motor dysfunction and the biomechanical imbalances in the entire kinetic chain.

REFERENCES

1. Adams RD, Victor M: Principles of Neurology. McGraw-Hill, New York, 1981
2. Knutssen E, Richards C: Different types of disturbed motor control in gait of hemiparetic patients. Brain 102:405, 1979

3. Perry J: Clinical gait analyzer. Bull Prosthet Res Fall: 188, 1974
4. Kapandji IA: The Physiology of the Joints: Lower Limb. Churchill Livingstone, Edinburgh, 1970
5. Root ML: Orien WP, Weed JH: Clinical Biomechanics: Vol. 2. Normal and Abnormal Function of the Foot. Clinical Biomechanics, Los Angeles, 1977
6. Gould JA, Davies GJ: Orthopedic and Sports Physical Therapy. CV Mosby, St. Louis, 1985
7. Jordan RP, Resseque BA, Cusack J: Dynamic Components of Foot Function. Langer Biomechanics Group, New York, 1984

6 | The Insensitive Foot

James A. Birke
David S. Sims

Plantar ulcers are associated with many different diseases, including diabetes mellitus and Hansen's disease. A common misconception is that plantar ulcers are caused by specific diseases. This misconception has resulted in the belief that ulcers cannot be prevented. A comparison of those diseases associated with plantar ulcers has shown loss of plantar sensation to be a common factor.[1] The lack of a pain warning system and stress on the plantar surface of the foot predispose the foot to injury. If these factors are recognized, ulcers are viewed as preventable and treatable injuries.

Many physical therapists are presently involved in treatment of foot ulcerations and prosthetic management of secondary amputations. The purpose of this chapter is to provide the therapist with a broader knowledge of methods used in prevention and management of plantar ulceration. We hope that this material will provide a concise but comprehensive approach to management problems and enable the physical therapist to assume a greater role in the coordination of care for the patient with insensitive feet.

MECHANISMS OF INJURY

Plantar ulcerations in the insensitive foot are caused by one of three possible mechanisms of injury: ischemia, direct trauma, or repetitive stress.[2] Ischemia occurs when blood flow to the tissues of the foot is blocked. Low levels of pressure (1 to 5 psi) will cause ischemia, but tissue damage does not occur until this stress has been sustained for several hours. Ischemic injury in the insensitive foot is most often caused by tight shoes or dressings. The second mechanism of injury is direct trauma. High stress of about 1,300 psi is required to break normal soft tissue. Plantar ulcers from direct trauma occur only if a patient steps barefoot on a sharp object or a nail penetrates the shoe. The most common cause of injury to the insensitive foot is repetitive stress. Moderate pressures (about 20 psi) repeated thousands of times a day have been shown to result in ulceration of the rat footpad. The normal foot is subjected to similar pressures during walking. A person with normal sensation who develops abnormal stress on the foot immediately changes the way of walking in an attempt to shift the stress to other areas. If this is not adequate to alleviate the pressure, increased pain develops causing the person to remove the source of irritation or stop walking. The person with an insensitive foot behaves much differently and in the absence of pain will continue to walk on an inflamed area of the foot, resulting in further injury and ulceration. Inflammatory autolysis resulting from release of lysosomal enzymes may be an additional cause of tissue necrosis.

PREVENTION OF PLANTAR ULCERATION

Plantar ulcers may be prevented by use of regular foot screening examinations, protective footwear, patient education, and surgical correction of selected deformities. The primary purpose of these tools is to detect areas of high tissue stress early and redistribute the plantar pressures.

Foot Screening

A foot screening examination is by definition a concise evaluation for the purpose of identifying critical factors that may predispose an individual to injury. These critical factors are then used to categorize the patient according to the level of risk of plantar ulceration. Treatment planning is based on the derived patient risk category (Fig. 6-1).

Patient Interview

The screening examination is begun by interviewing the patient to obtain a brief history. Two special questions should be asked of all patients: (1) Has there been any change in your strength or sensation since your last visit or within the past six months? (2) Have you ever had an ulcer on the bottom of your foot? A recent change in strength or sensation may indicate an impending neurologic crisis. Careful medical management is required during periods of change to prevent major disability secondary to peripheral nerve damage.[3] Patients with a positive history of plantar ulceration are very likely to ulcerate again if protective measures are not taken. This susceptibility is owing to the fact that extremely high stress is concentrated in the healed scar, which is less compliant than the surrounding tissues.[4]

Strength Testing

Evaluation of muscle strength, with the exception of plantarflexion, may be performed with the client in the sitting position. Selected muscles are tested to determine the extent and distribution of possible weakness. The most common patterns of weakness are involvement of a major terminal nerve or neuropathy limited to distal motor branches. Occasionally a coexisting radiculopathy may be present.

The common peroneal nerve is the most frequently damaged lower extremity motor nerve in both Hansen's disease and diabetes mellitus.[5,6] Damage usually occurs in the nerve segment at the fibular head. This site is extremely vulnerable to trauma due to the superficial location of the nerve. In addition, Hansen's bacilli thrive in the cooler, more superficial portions of the nerve, thus producing greater localized damage.[7,8]

Peroneal innervated muscles that are routinely tested include the anterior tibialis, peroneus longus, and extensor hallucis longus. Determination of peroneus longus and anterior tibialis muscle strength will allow the examiner to check the integrity of the superficial and deep motor branches of the peroneal nerve, respectively. The extensor hallucis longus provides an index of distal motor function. Atrophy of the extensor digitorum brevis muscle is another important sign of distal motor involvement.

The tibial nerve is the largest terminal branch of the sciatic nerve. Major functional deficits in this nerve are rare due to the deep position of the tibial nerve throughout most of the leg; its deepness provides protection from trauma.

Tibial innervated muscles that are routinely tested include the gastrocnemius-soleus group, the posterior tibialis, and the flexor hallucis longus. Evaluation of gastrocnemius-soleus strength provides an index of proximal motor function. Determination of the strength in the tibialis posterior is important since this muscle is frequently transferred to the anterior ankle to substitute for lost dorsiflexion. Good (grade 4) muscle strength must exist preoperatively since the functional strength will usually be one muscle grade less after the operation owing to alteration of the muscle length tension relationship.[9] The flexor hallucis longus strength and estimation of plantar intrinsic muscle bulk provide an index of distal tibial motor function.

Manual muscle testing techniques may be used to assess muscle strength. These procedures are outlined in detail in standard textbooks.[10] The most common method of grading strength is to assign a number from 0 to 5 as recommended by the Medical Research Council.[11] Alternatively, handheld dynamometry may be performed to provide more quantitative data.

Skin Inspection

Inspection of the skin should be performed with the patient lying supine. Disturbances of temperature, color, volume, and texture, and the presence of

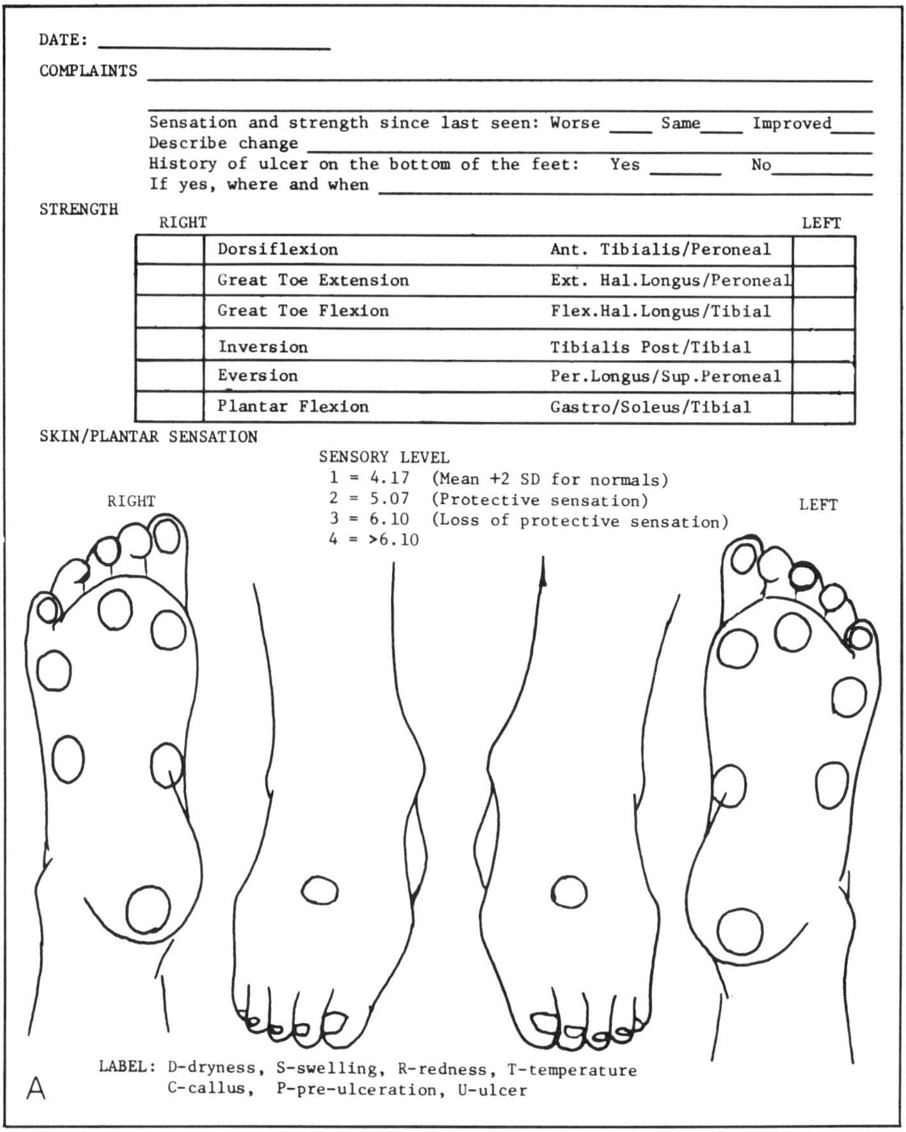

DATE: _____

COMPLAINTS _____

Sensation and strength since last seen: Worse ____ Same____ Improved____
Describe change _____
History of ulcer on the bottom of the feet: Yes _____   No_____
If yes, where and when _____

STRENGTH

RIGHT			LEFT
	Dorsiflexion	Ant. Tibialis/Peroneal	
	Great Toe Extension	Ext. Hal.Longus/Peroneal	
	Great Toe Flexion	Flex.Hal.Longus/Tibial	
	Inversion	Tibialis Post/Tibial	
	Eversion	Per.Longus/Sup.Peroneal	
	Plantar Flexion	Gastro/Soleus/Tibial	

SKIN/PLANTAR SENSATION

SENSORY LEVEL
1 = 4.17 (Mean +2 SD for normals)
2 = 5.07 (Protective sensation)
3 = 6.10 (Loss of protective sensation)
4 = >6.10

RIGHT   LEFT

LABEL: D-dryness, S-swelling, R-redness, T-temperature
C-callus, P-pre-ulceration, U-ulcer

A

Fig. 6-1. Foot screening form.

any open woulds should be carefully recorded. Early identification and treatment of problems will limit the extent of injuries.

The entire surface of the foot and ankle should be scanned using the hand to locate any areas of temperature disturbance. Most individuals can more easily detect minor temperature differences using the skin of the first dorsal web space. Always compare one side of the body to the other since large diurnal changes occur in absolute distal limb temperature. The difference in temperature should normally be within 1°C.[12] This level of accuracy may be

DEFORMITIES:

	RIGHT	LEFT		COMMENTS
	——	——	Hammer/claw toes	_____
	——	——	Bony prominence	_____
	——	——	Limited great toe	_____
	——	——	Equinus	_____
	——	——	Foot drop	_____
	——	——	Partial foot resection	_____
	——	——	Complete foot amputation	_____

(Check if deformities are present)

	RIGHT	LEFT		COMMENTS
	——	——	Ankle brachial vascular index	_____

FOOTWEAR:

   Type: Standard _____ Special _____ Describe _____

   Fit: Adequate _____ Inadequate _____ Describe _____

ASSESSMENT: RISK CATEGORY (Check appropriate category)

   _____ 0 (No protective sensory loss)

   _____ 1 (Protective sensory loss)

   _____ 2 (Sensory loss and history of ulceration)

   _____ 3 (Sensory loss, history of ulceration and deformity)

   _____ 4 (Charcot foot)

PLAN:

   _____ Patient education (inspection, skin care, footwear)

   _____ Special footwear _____

   _____ Referral (medical, surgical, orthotic)

   _____ X-ray

   _____ Other _____

                              _____
                                      (Signature)

B

Fig. 6-1. (*Continued*).

achieved with the unaided hand. Any areas of perceived difference should be documented by performing spot temperature recordings. A handheld infrared thermometer or thermocouple is ideally suited for this purpose (Fig. 6-2). Local increase in temperature, possibly accompanied by redness, denotes inflammation. Tissue inflammation may be caused by high stress or deep infection. An abnormal decrease in temperature, if an obvious injury exists, is strongly suggestive of arterial insufficiency.

   Limb volume should normally be symmetrical, with clear definition of

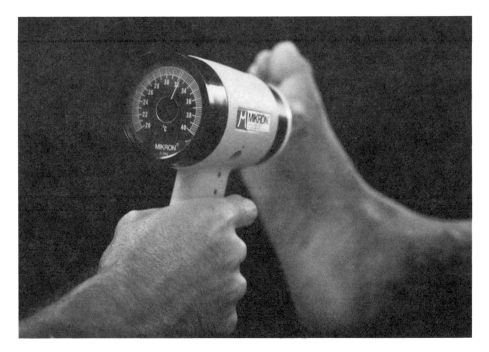

Fig. 6-2.   Infrared thermometer (Mikron Instruments, Midland Park, NJ).

anatomical contours. Differences in limb volume may be secondary to muscle atrophy or swelling. Muscle atrophy will usually be accompanied by weakness. Two common patterns of swelling exist. The first is generalized pitting edema of the foot and leg. This pattern of swelling may be caused by many different diseases and predisposes the individual to stasis ulcerations of the leg. Pitting edema is easily controlled by use of elastic support stockings. A second pattern is swelling isolated to the foot and ankle. This pattern is suggestive of injury, and a neuropathic (Charcot) fracture must be considered as the etiology. Predisposing factors to the development of Charcot fractures include recent prolonged bedrest, immobilization, or infection in the presence of a sensory neuropathy.[13] Radiographs should be obtained to determine the integrity of the foot skeleton (Fig. 6-3A). Neuropathic fractures should be treated immediately to prevent rapid total destruction of the bones of the foot and ankle.

Skin hydration is regulated by secretions from the sweat glands located in the dermis. These structures are innervated by the sympathetic nervous system.[14] Most of the sympathetics to the foot are contained within the tibial nerve. Damage to the sympathetic axons will result in decreased ability of the skin to sweat (Fig. 6-4). This will produce dry, noncompliant skin that is more susceptible to injury.[15]

The plantar surface of the foot should be inspected for any signs of high stress. Two common patterns of stress exist. The first pattern is associated with frictional skin lesions. This type of stress (primarily shear) usually results in a

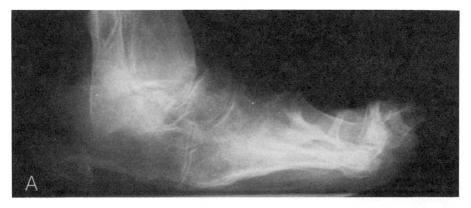

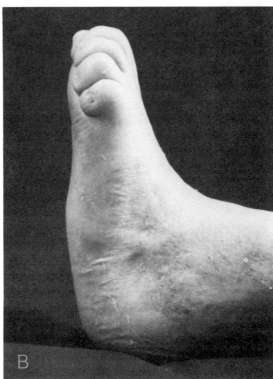

Fig. 6-3. Charcot foot. Radiographic evidence of midfoot collapse (**A**) resulting in rocker bottom foot deformity (**B**)

superficial blister with little or no advance warning of a problem. Fortunately, this type of wound is easily managed. The second pattern of skin lesions is associated with repetitive stress (normal and shear). A callus lesion is an early sign of an impending problem. Thickening of the keratinized layer of the skin is a compensatory mechanism in response to local stress. This response is initially helpful in preventing ulceration; as the callus lesion thickens, however, it becomes an additional source of high stress. Continued walking will produce a local inflammatory response. The increase in skin temperature is a second

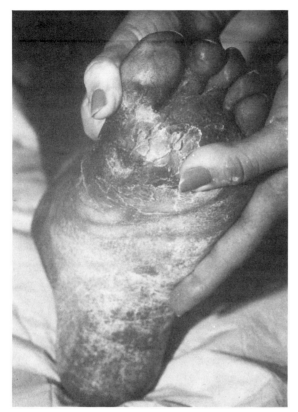

Fig. 6-4. Dry noncompliant skin.

warning sign. This is followed by a preulcerative lesion. Preulceration is characterized by a subcutaneous hematoma. Failure to recognize this final warning sign will lead to a full-thickness ulcer.[16,17] The most frequent sites of plantar ulceration are the great toe, the first metatarsal head (MTH), and the fifth MTH.[18,19] During the examination, the index of suspicion should be greatest for these areas. Dense callus lesions should be trimmed sufficiently to allow inspection of the underlying tissues.

Sensation Testing

Evaluation of plantar sensation should be performed following skin inspection. The normal foot is protected from major injury by an intact pain warning system. Diminished or absent plantar sensation places the foot at high risk of injury. Also, the extent of the damage is frequently underestimated by the patient and the clinician due to the minimal pain. Quantitative assessment of sensation allows the clinician to determine a functional level of sensation below which the patient must be taught protective measures to prevent problems.

Semmes-Weinstein monofilaments are used to assess the plantar sensation. Test probes consist of a nylon monofilament mounted in a square plastic handle. The manufacturer supplies 20 different monofilaments from 1.65 to 6.65. Monofilament numbers originally indicated the common logarithm of ten times the monofilament buckling force in milligrams. In reality, the numbers are only approximate and therefore should be considered as nominal values. Filaments 4.17, 5.07, and 6.10 provide a measurement scale for the foot that is reliable at the 95 percent confidence level.[20] Interpretation of test results is based on a recent study of normal subjects and patients with a history of plantar ulceration. The mean plantar sensory threshold plus 2 SD in normal subjects was the 4.17 monofilament. Testing was performed on 72 Hansen's disease patients and 21 diabetic patients with a history of ulceration. All individuals tested were accustomed to wearing shoes most of the time. None of the pa-tients could feel the 5.07 monofilament in the area of skin surrounding the previous ulcer. This filament was selected as the functional definition of protec-tive sensation.[21] The next available monofilament on the scale, 6.10, was de-fined as loss of protective sensation. Inability to feel the 6.10 filament is consid-ered loss of local pressure sensation.

Testing is begun by touching an area of the body with known good sensa-tion. This area becomes the reference point by which all subsequent stimuli will be judged. Nine different sites are tested on the plantar surface of each foot. These sites correspond to the most frequently injured areas of the foot. Fila-ments should be applied, from smallest to largest, perpendicular to the skin with sufficient force to cause a "C-shaped" buckling without the tip slipping laterally (Fig. 6-5). The rate of application and removal of the probe should be approximately constant at one second. Patients should be instructed not to attempt to localize the area touched on the foot but merely to respond "yes" whenever a stimulus is felt.[22] The testing order between sites and the time interval between successive stimuli should be randomized to prevent patient guessing. If the patient's responses are erratic, the reference point should be touched again to reinforce the correct response. The smallest filament at which the patient responds correctly is defined as the site threshold. A number from 1 to 4 is assigned to filaments 4.17, 5.07, 6.10, and > 6.10, respectively. If any site has a threshold greater than 2 (5.07), the entire foot is considered to have lost protective sensation. A composite score consisting of the sum of the ranked thresholds for all nine plantar test sites may also be used to provide an overall index of foot sensation.

Deformity Identification

Mechanical imbalance, joint stiffness, or bony prominences are all consid-ered deformities. These abnormalities rarely cause skin ulcerations if normal sensation exists. Deformity in the insensitive foot greatly increases risk of injury.

Mallet, hammer, and claw toes comprise a group of related digital deformi-ties.[23] A mallet deformity consists of a flexion contracture of only the distal

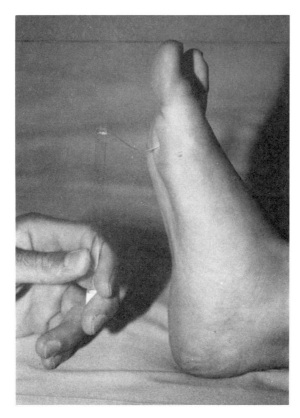

Fig. 6-5. Technique of applying Semmes-Weinstein monofilament to the skin deformity.

interphalangeal (IP) joint of the toe. This abnormality rarely causes any disability. Combined flexion contractures of the proximal and distal IP joints will produce a hammer toe deformity, resulting in weightbearing on the tip of the toe. The tissue of the toe pulp is not capable of tolerating stress of this magnitude and will eventually ulcerate. Attempts to prevent ulceration through the use of footwear are usually unsuccessful. Surgical evaluation of the deformity is recommended as soon as a callus lesion is evident. Claw toes are characterized by an extension contracture of the metatarsalphalangeal (MTP) joint and flexion contractures of the IP joints. The primary problem associated with this deformity is dorsal IP joint skin lesions due to shoe pressure. A secondary problem is prominence of the MTH due to plantarflexion of the metatarsal and dislocation of the plantar fat pad.[24] These problems can usually be managed successfully with appropriate footwear.

Hallux abducto valgus and hallux limitus are common abnormalities involving the first MTP joint. Hallux valgus may be caused by abnormal foot pronation or a congenitally large first-second intermetatarsal angle. The primary deformity is lateral drifting of the great toe. Secondary deformities include a dorsal medial bunion and overlapping toes. Management should be

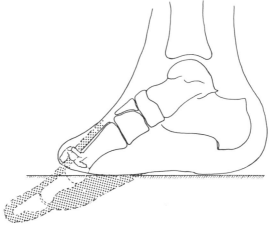

Fig. 6-6. Tracings of superimposed radiographs showing hidden equinus in a shortened foot as compared with a contralateral normal foot.

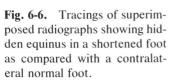

directed toward accomodating the existing deformity and eliminating any factors contributing to the progression of the deformity. A limited hallux creates high stress over the plantar tip of the distal phalanx. This deformity is probably the major cause of great toe ulcerations in the insensitive foot. Compensation for the stiff first MTP joint may occur in the IP joint through stretching of the capsule and ligamentous structures, resulting in ulceration over the condyles of the IP joint instead of the tip of the great toe. The preferable treatment would be to provide a rigid shoe to eliminate the need for extension at the first MTP joint.

Uncompensated varus deformities of the forefoot or rearfoot are the primary cause of fifth metatarsal head ulcers. These deformities may be due to a primary osseus lesion or are acquired following muscle paralysis. A varus attitude of the foot creates extremely high stress over the lateral forefoot. The use of a medially posted foot orthotic device, high quarter shoes, and a lateral sole flare may decrease the forefoot stress to a tolerable range. In extreme cases, a surgical evaluation may be required.

Equinus is the most frequently encountered abnormality of the talocrural joint. This passive restriction to dorsiflexion is usually secondary to a dropfoot deformity from peroneal nerve damage. The unopposed tension of the posterior leg compartment muscles will cause a progressive loss of range of motion (ROM). A combined lesion of the superficial and deep peroneal motor nerve will result in a coexisting subtalar varus deformity. Ankle dorsiflexion should be evaluated with the subtalar joint in a neutral position to obtain a true measurement of the motion available at the talocrural joint. A stress lateral radiograph may be needed to evaluate the amount of equinus present in a shortened foot (Fig. 6-6). If anterior leg compartment muscle weakness exists, an ankle foot orthosis should be used to maintain proper ankle joint alignment in the sagittal plane. External attachment of the orthosis to the shoe is preferred to prevent irritation of insensitive skin. Permanent correction of the dropfoot deformity by tendon transfer should be considered after sufficient time has elapsed for possible nerve recovery. An Achilles tendon lengthening is usually performed simultaneously to provide a better balance of tension. Extrinsic toe flexors should also be elongated if full toe extension is not possible with the ankle in approximately 10° of dorsiflexion. Delayed treatment of a dropfoot deformity may require bony subtalar surgical procedures to achieve a plantigrade position of the foot. This will usually result in some loss of foot length and a lower extremity length discrepancy.

Resections of the great toe and first ray will create a functional varus deformity of the forefoot. Abnormal subtalar pronation will then result to compensate for the forefoot position. Skin lesions over the second MTH frequently occur as the stress is transferred proximally and laterally (Fig. 6-7). Restoration of medial foot stability through use of orthotic devices will minimize occurrence of transfer lesions.

A shortened foot is usually caused by repeated osteomyelitis of the metatarsal bones. Loss of foot length greatly increases the plantar stress owing to a shortening of the toe lever and a loss of surface area. A short toe lever will decrease the passive dorsiflexion moment at the ankle during late stance. Lack of stretch on the posterior leg compartment structures eventually leads to the development of an equinus deformity. Loss of plantar surface area also causes tissue destruction by increasing local pressure. Foot amputation is occasionally necessary in order to improve function. The decision to amputate should be made prior to involvement of the plantar calcaneal fat pad. This will provide the option of performing a Symes amputation, which is considerably more functional than a standard below-knee amputation.

The endstage of a neuropathic fracture (Charcot fracture) is a rocker-bottom foot deformity (see Fig. 6-3B). Collapse of the tarsal bones is responsible for the characteristic rocker appearance. This type of foot is difficult to manage even with custom footwear. Chronic joint instability or recurrent ulcerations may require surgical revision or amputation.

Footwear Inspection

Footwear is the primary line of defense between the foot and the environment. For footwear to be effective it must be of the proper style, must fit well, and must be in good repair.

An enormous variety in shoe styles is available today. Many of these styles are inappropriate for even the normal foot. The most important style criterion is that the shoe should fit the shape of the foot. This will usually result in the selection of a shoe that has a rounded or squared toe box. The uppers should be made of calf leather or nylon. These materials will mold to the foot during use to accommodate minor shape incongruencies. Lace or strap closures are preferred over a loafer style. They will provide adjustment to accommodate changes in the volume of the foot or stretching of the shoe. Finally, a wedge-type sole will provide a more stable platform for walking than a conventional

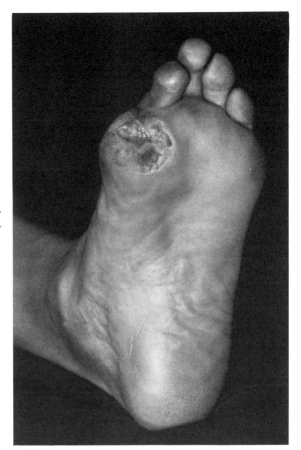

Fig. 6-7. Stress transfer lesions secondary to digital amputation.

heel and sole design due to the fact that the entire bottom surface of the shoe is in contact with the ground. Increased stability will result in decreased stress on the tissues of the foot.[25]

The criteria for selecting sandals is similar to that used for shoes. All sandals should have a forefoot and heel strap. This strap arrangement will minimize sliding of the foot within the sandal.

Proper style footwear is of limited usefulness if the fit is poor. The most common fitting error is selection of a shoe which is too narrow. This may occur in the patient with an insensitive foot due to the increase in the sensory threshold. If the patient cannot feel the shoe, he or she assumes that the footwear is too loose (P. W. Brand and W. C. Coleman, personal communication). A shoe of the proper width should wrinkle slightly when the vamp is pinched between the thumb and index finger. There should be no more than $\frac{1}{4}$ inch between the lateral border of the shoe and foot. Shoe length should be checked to insure that there is at least $\frac{1}{2}$ inch beyond the longest toe. Also, the shoe break (bend) should match the position of the MTP joints as closely as possible. A long shoe will produce skin irritation on the dorsum of the toes due to a mismatched shoe break. The toe box should provide at least ¼-inch clearance between the toes and the top of the shoe. Additional clearance may be needed if claw toe deformities are present.

Soft polyethylene materials used in the fabrication of sandals and shoe insoles present special fitting problems. Although these devices may be of the proper length at the time of fabrication, wear compression of the material will cause the footwear to become functionally too short. This problem should be corrected immediately be removing the material distal to the toes to allow freedom of toe movement or by replacing the device. In general, polyethylene sandals or insoles will need to be repaired or replaced approximately every 6 months. Worn outersoles should be repaired promptly to maintain proper foot balance. Torn linings or badly distorted heel counters require shoe replacement.

Noninvasive Vascular Testing

A vascular screening examination should be performed routinely on patients with diabetes mellitus if a foot wound exists to rule out the possibility of arterial disease. In addition, dysvascular problems should be suspected in the nondiabetic patient if a wound is located in a nonweightbearing area of the foot or if wound healing is delayed despite appropriate treatment. The purpose of the examination is to predict the probability of wound healing, not to localize the anatomical site of the suspected arterial lesion.

Segmental systolic blood pressures are obtained at the brachium and ankle with the patient supine, using a standard adult pneumatic cuff (12.1 × 22.2 cm) and an ultrasound Doppler unit (Fig. 6-8). Doppler monitoring is usually performed at the radial and dorsalis pedis artery, but other sites may be used to obtain the best quality signal. Foot wound healing is likely if the ankle systolic pressure is greater than or equal to 55 mm Hg (greater than or equal to 80 mm Hg in the diabetic patient) or the ankle-brachial pressure ratio (ankle-brachial index) greater than or equal to 0.45.[26,27] These criteria are considered valid since most dysvascular amputations are performed because of large vessel involvement regardless of disease category.[28]

Occasionally, an ankle systolic pressure may not be obtainable or may be greatly elevated owing to the inability to occlude a noncompliant artery. In such cases, segmental pneumatic plethysmography may be used to provide an estimate of the regional circulation.

Foot Risk Categories

On completion of the screening examination, the patient is categorized according to the level of risk of foot injury. Five categories have been developed by the authors based on several simple criteria (Table 6-1). The primary

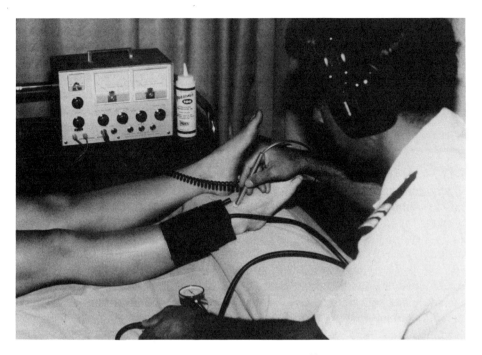

Fig. 6-8. Measurement of ankle systolic pressure.

criterion is loss of protective sensation, which is defined as the inability to feel the 5.07 monofilament at any test site. Additional criteria include a positive history of plantar ulceration or the presence of a deformity.

The previously ulcerated foot will remain more vulnerable to skin damage for life owing to the high stress concentrated in the healed scar. This susceptibility to reulceration precludes assignment of the patient to a lesser risk category after wound healing. Deformity in the presence of protective sensation rarely results in skin ulceration. Loss of protective sensation, history of ulceration, and deformity would result in a risk category of three. Surgical correction of the deformity would reduce the level of risk to category two. The Charcot foot deformity presents the highest risk of ulceration. This group of patients requires careful management to prevent recurrent problems.

Patient Education

Prevention of foot injuries is a shared responsibility between the clinician and the patient. The therapist needs to provide specific guidelines to the patient regarding foot self-inspection, skin care, and selection of proper footwear. Daily preventive care by the patient will prevent catastrophic injuries through early identification of problems.

Effective patient education depends on message content, presentation me-

Table 6.1. Foot Risk Categories

Category	Protective Sensation[a]	HX Ulcer	Deformity
0	Yes	No	Yes/no
1	No	No	Yes/no
2	No	Yes	No
3	No	Yes	Yes
4	No	Yes/no	Charcot

[a] Monofilament $\leq$ 5.07.

dium, and time of delivery. Clear, simple language should be used for all educational materials. Consistency in the message is mandatory to eliminate patient confusion. If a patient receives conflicting information from different sources, the credibility of the educational program is greatly jeopardized, and this will ultimately result in patient noncompliance. Numerous methods are available for presenting educational materials. Videotape is an ideal medium because the program can be presented to the patient without the therapists' attendance. This insures that the educational program is readily available even during peak clinic hours. Also, the same message is delivered during every viewing. Patient acceptance of information is often determined by the timing of the educational program. The most effective time to promote patient behavioral changes is immediately after a treatment success, such as healing of a chronic plantar wound. During this time, the patient is more likely to comply with instructions because the clinician is perceived as credible.

Self-Inspection

The lack of a pain warning system in the insensitive foot may lead to injuries. Daily self-inspection is an alternative method of protecting the feet in the absence of normal sensation. The socks and feet should be examined in the evening prior to going to bed. Stains on the socks may indicate the presence of an open wound. All surfaces of the feet should be thoroughly inspected for signs of high stress such as callus, redness, blisters, or open wounds. Toes should be checked for thickened, ingrown, or long nails. The area between the toes should also be carefully examined for signs of maceration, a common problem. For a patient with poor vision or limited flexibility, a magnifying mirror may be useful.

Following visual inspection, the skin temperature of the foot should be checked using a sensitive part of the hand or forearm. The temperature should be compared with the contralateral side. Increased local temperature may indicate a pressure problem. If temperature is elevated the next morning, the patient should seek medical advice.

Next, the feet should be checked for areas of deep tenderness by palpating the areas shown in Figure 6-9. Local tenderness may indicate that an area has been injured by high pressure; such a region would be extremely vulnerable to

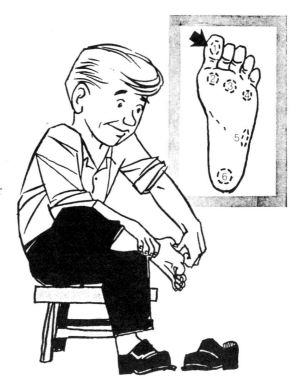

Fig. 6-9. Palpation sites for deep tenderness.

further damage. A combination of increased temperature, redness, swelling, and tenderness may indicate a deep infection or neuropathic fracture requiring immediate treatment.

Patients should inspect socks and shoes prior to donning them. Socks should be in good repair and free of wrinkles. The inside of the shoes should be checked for protruding nails, ridges, torn linings, or foreign objects. Insoles should be examined for signs of excessive wear or improper positioning within the shoe. Finally, the outside of the shoe should be checked for signs of excessive or uneven wear.[29]

Skin Care

Damage to the sympathetic axons in neuropathic diseases will result in inability to sweat, causing dry, cracked skin and greatly increasing probability of an open wound. Replacement of lost moisture will help to prevent skin injuries. The ideal method is to soak the feet for 10 minutes in lukewarm water every day.[30] The skin should not be dried after soaking but instead excess water should be shaken off and mineral oil or vaseline should be immediately applied. The oil should be massaged into all surfaces of the feet except between the toes where excessive moisture is a common problem. A more practical approach to moisturizing dry skin is to apply oil to the skin using a squeeze bottle after bathing or showering. As in the soaking method, the oil must be applied before drying so that the water is trapped against the skin.

Proper nail care is also an important part of preventive skin treatment. Toenails are a specialized form of skin and must be cared for on a regular basis to prevent ingrowing. The nails should be trimmed straight across approximately once a month. Rough edges should be smoothed with an emery board. If the nails are extremely thick or deformed, a medical professional should assist in the care.

Callus reduction is another important technique in the management of the insensitive foot. Callus is a normal response to increased stress on the skin. Regular callus care is required to prevent additional pressures on the foot from excess thickness. The safest method to reduce callus thickness is to use a skin file or sandpaper. Cutting with knives or razors should be avoided to prevent injury. File or sand the callus using slow strokes in one direction only. A properly filed callus will feel soft to the touch. If the callus lesions are extremely thick, several days may be required to reduce the callus sufficiently without causing injury to the surrounding skin.

Despite their best efforts, patients may occasionally injure their foot. If a wound does occur, the area must be kept clean and the foot rested. Hand washing before and after wound care will prevent infection. Small wounds should be cleaned with soap and water and then gently dried with a clean towel. Peroxide may be applied directly to the wound opening to clean the area further. A topical antiseptic such as betadine should be applied, followed by a light gauze dressing. A bulky dressing inside a shoe will cause pressure and further injure the wound site. The wound should be rested by minimizing movement and eliminating weightbearing, especially if the wound is on the plantar surface. Crutches or a walkerette may be used to eliminate weight on the bottom of the foot. A plaster walking cast is an alternative method of reducing plantar foot pressures. Large wounds or wounds that do not show signs of healing within a few days should be immediately reported to a medical professional.[31]

Footwear Selection

A person with normal pain sensation can wear most shoe styles with little risk of injury. If the ability to feel pain is lost, poorly designed or improperly fitting shoes may cause serious foot injuries. Patients should be encouraged to select shoes that conform to the shape of the foot. Wedge crepe-soled oxfords or running shoes are highly recommended.

A shoe must be properly fitted to provide adequate protection to the foot. Patients should be instructed to check for proper width, length, and depth of shoes prior to purchase. Oversized shoes can also cause foot injuries by friction due to sliding.

Some footwear styles should not be worn by individuals with insensitive feet. Thongs can cause blistering between the toes. Narrow-toed shoes will cause excessive pressure on the sides of the foot. Plastic uppers will also cause foot pressure because the material will not stretch. High-heeled shoes will greatly increase the stress on the ball of the foot.

A special insole is often needed to protect the insensitive foot. A shoe with extra depth will allow room for an insole when the client is fitted with the normal shoe size and is the preferred type of shoe. Good quality running shoes are an alternative choice. In some cases, an irregularly shaped foot may require a custom shoe. A person who has had a foot ulcer in the past may also require a special sole called a rigid rocker. The rocker sole is designed to decrease the pressure under the ball of the foot during walking.

Activities of daily living (ADL) must be adjusted to meet the special needs of the insensitive foot. To protect the feet, the patient must never go barefoot. Walking in socks or on carpeting does not offer adequate protection. A pair of soft molded sandals should be kept near the bed for night use. When showering, a pair of water-resistant sandals should be worn to protect the feet, particularly if the patient has had a previous plantar ulcer. Individuals should own at least two pairs of well-fitting sandals or shoes. Pairs should be worn on alternate days to provide different weightbearing patterns and prolong the life of the footwear. Patients should never walk long distances (relative to the normal activity level) without a rest. This will minimize the possibility of foot injury, and should avoid running or jogging because these activities greatly increases stress on the feet.

New shoes should always be broken in slowly. In general, shoes should not be worn more than 2 hours a day for the first week. Afterwards, the patient should change into an older pair of shoes or sandals. Careful foot inspection is required during the break-in period. If a problem occurs, the patient should not wear the shoes until checked by the therapist. New shoes may require adjustments to ensure a proper fit. These adjustments can usually be made by a shoe repair shop. Footwear will need to be repaired or replaced periodically. Worn soles and heels can be repaired. Insoles must be replaced every 6 months to remain effective. Torn linings or badly distorted uppers require shoe replacement.[32]

MANAGEMENT OF PLANTAR ULCERATION

Ulcer Treatment Scheme

Successful management of plantar ulcerations requires a clear, organized team approach focusing on the causes of tissue breakdown. Plantar ulcerations have been shown to occur at the areas of high pressure on the bottom of the foot.[18,19,33] The primary mechanism of injury in the insensitive foot has been identified as repetitive stress.[1,4] A successful treatment approach must be aimed at reduction of foot pressure to promote healing and prevent reulceration. A model for treating plantar ulcers is shown in Figure 6-10. This model describes a four-level treatment process. The levels include wound care, meth-

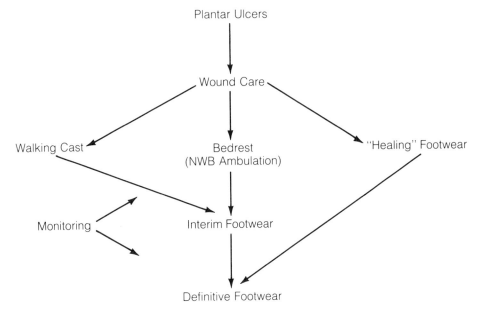

Fig. 6-10.   Treatment scheme for plantar ulcers.

ods of pressure reduction, interim footwear, and definitive footwear. Monitoring stress on the foot is also an important complement of the treatment process.

Wound Care

The first level of plantar ulcer management is wound care. Whirlpool and application of topical agents has been the traditional approach in treating plantar ulcers. This approach alone probably plays only a small role in healing a plantar ulcer. Wound care procedures should include evaluating, cleaning, and dressing the ulcer. Topical agents are an important adjunct to treatment but should not be the primary focus of care. The patient must understand that there is no ulcer medication worth walking to get.

On initial examination, the wound should be probed with a sterile instrument to determine whether there is penetration to bone or joint. Ulcerations involving these tissues will be more difficult to heal, and a surgical consultation may be needed.[2,34] Necrotic bone in the ulcer will retard healing and often is expelled by the body spontaneously; however, it may require surgical excision. A reliable sign indicating that the wound penetrates to joint is identification of a clear, bubbly fluid at the time of probing. We believe that joint fluid impedes healing owing to the presence of lytic enzymes. If purulent drainage is present, a culture should be taken. This will aid the physician in selecting appropriate antibiotic therapy.

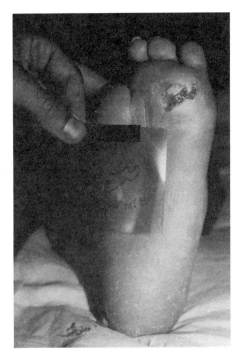

Fig. 6-11. Use of exposed radiograph for serial measurements of plantar ulcers.

Ulcer size is easily recorded by tracing the wound circumference on a piece of sterilized exposed x-ray film (Fig. 6-11). The tracing provides an accurate record of the progress of wound healing and is an excellent tool for reinforcing compliant behavior because the patient can see positive treatment gains.

Cleaning is the next step in wound care. Necrotic tissue should be debrided from the ulcer base. The presence of devitalized tissue promotes the growth of bacteria. Callus typically forms along the border of the ulcer site, impeding the growth of epithelium and delaying wound healing.[35-37]This hypertrophic border should be trimmed to good epithelium with a sharp blade. Swabbing with peroxide is an excellent method of mechanically cleaning the ulcer. Routine whirlpool soaks are not recommended because they may contribute to dependent edema.

Last, a topical antiseptic such as betadine is applied to the ulcer on a thin sterile dressing. We commonly use a 2 × 2 gauze and secure it with a small wrap of Kling or tubular gauze. Bulky dressings will increase pressure on the foot if the patient walks in shoes.

Methods of Reducing Pressure

Wound care alone is often not sufficient for healing the plantar ulcer. The reason is that wound care does not direct treatment at the cause of plantar foot ulcer, pressure on the bottom of the foot. Alternative ways to reduce foot pressure need to be developed to meet the needs of individual patients.

Bedrest

The management scheme provides three alternative ways of minimizing or eliminating pressure on the bottom of the foot. The best, but often the least practical, way to eliminate pressure on the ulcerative foot is bedrest.[4] Absolute bedrest can completely eliminate pressure on the plantar surface of the foot, but is dependent on full patient compliance for success. If the patient simply walks a few steps on the unprotected foot to go to the bathroom, all benefits of the day's recumbency may be lost. Crutches or a wheelchair must be used to maintain a nonweightbearing status when the patient is out of bed.

Walking Casts

Walking casts have been successfully used in the management of plantar foot ulcerations since the 1930s. Brand introduced the total contact cast design in the United States in the 1960s.[38-41] This design is currently used by many medical centers in this country. The cast must be carefully applied to the foot and leg to ensure a snug fit. If a total contact fit is achieved, walking pressures will be distributed to all parts of the foot and leg. The cast must be changed immediately if loosening or damage occurs to prevent secondary skin lesions on the foot and leg. Total contact casts are recommended only for healing of plantar ulcerations owing to foot insensitivity and have not been recommended for leg ulcers (stasis ulcers) or vascular lesions. Relative contraindications in casting an ulcerative foot include cellulitis, edema, and fragile hypotrophic skin. Antibiotics and bedrest should be used to treat patients with active cellulitis. The cast may be applied after the infection is localized. A 24-hour period of bedrest and elevation has been recommended before casting when edema is present. The use of a Jobst compression pump (Jobst Institute, Toledo, OH) for approximately 2 hours is another method of reducing swelling prior to casting. Residual edema will quickly decrease inside the cast due to enhancement of the muscle pump mechanism within the rigid plaster wall.[42,43]

Plantar walking casts are effective in reducing pressure on the bottom of the foot.[44-46] In a study of six normal subjects, walking pressures were reduced 75 to 85 percent, respectively, under the first and third metatarsal head (MTH) areas of the foot (Fig. 6-12). Reductions in pressure were noticeably less over the fifth MTH and heel. It is our experience that fifth MTH and heel ulcers do not heal as quickly as those in other areas, and this study provides an explanation for this observation.

The total contact cast technique uses minimal felt padding over the dorsum of the foot and leg and the malleoli and foam padding over the toes (Fig. 6-13).

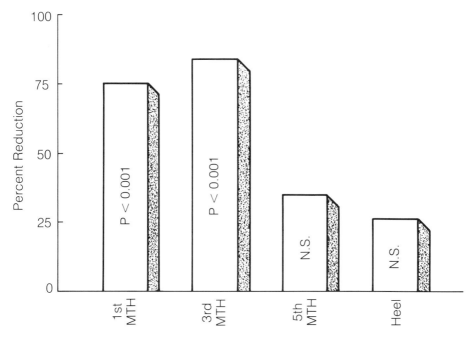

Fig. 6-12. Reduction of pressure walking in casts compared to shoes for each of four transducer sites. (Redrawn from Birke J, Sims D, Buford W: Walking casts: Effect on plantar foot pressures. J Rehabil Res Dev 22:18, 1985.)

Additional padding may be placed over bony prominences and the posterior heel. Care is taken to apply the plaster loosely around the irregular surfaces of the foot and leg so that total contact molding can be achieved. The inner layers of plaster are continuously rubbed until set. Additional layers of plaster are then applied for reinforcement. The toe area is covered so that foreign objects will not enter the cast and damage the foot. In addition, a ¼-inch board and rubber walking heel are applied to the bottom of the cast. A plywood board helps to dissipate the forces evenly throughout the cast during walking. The initial cast is changed after 1 week or sooner if loosening occurs. Remember that loose casts result in secondary skin breakdown. Subsequent casts are applied for 2-week intervals until healing occurs. Most ulcers will heal after 6 to 8 weeks.

Healing Footwear

Healing footwear include shoes, sandals, or other devices modified to relieve the pressure in the area of the ulcer.[47] Three types of healing footwear have been used successfully for Hansen's disease and diabetic patients. The first is the cutout sandal. The sandal footbed is completely cut out, leaving only the outer sole intact (Fig. 6-14). The relief must be of adequate depth to elimi-

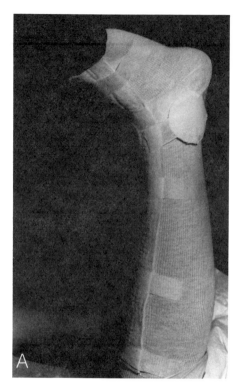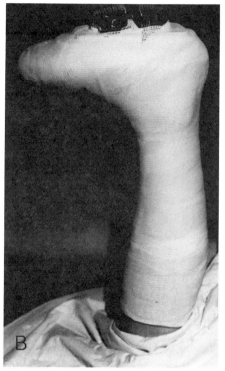

Fig. 6-13. (**A**) Padding technique for a total contact cast. (**B**) Finished total contact cast.

nate totally any weightbearing contact of the ulcer during walking. Moreover, the edges of the relief must be rounded to minimize shear stress on the border of the wound. Careful monitoring by the patient or a health professional is needed to ensure that the sandal footbed material does not compress, resulting in reoccurrence of ulcer pressure.

Another type of healing footwear is felted foam (Stein Foot Specialty, Union, NJ).[48] This technique works best on superficial ulcerations. The material consists of a thin layer of felt bonded to a layer of $\frac{1}{4}$-inch latex foam rubber. One or two layers of material is trimmed to fit the shape of the involved area of the foot. A cutout is made in the foam slightly larger than the ulcer and extended distally approximately $\frac{3}{4}$ inch (Fig. 6-15). The felt side is then attached directly to the surface of the foot using rubber cement. A piece of thin sterile gauze with a topical antiseptic may be placed on the ulcer within the foam relief area. Kling or Fabco bandage (Fab, Springfield, MA) is used to secure the felted foam pad to the foot. The pad may remain in place for as long as 1 week, at which time the foam is usually compressed. Original thickness may be restored by applying an additional layer of felted foam material or a new pad. We have not observed any allergic reactions resulting from the use of rubber ce-

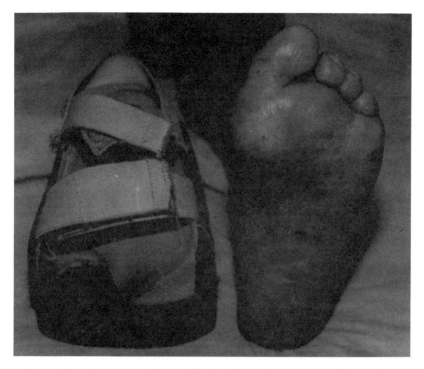

Fig. 6-14.   Cutout sandal used for healing a first metatarsal head ulcer.

ment in contact with the skin. A plastazote sandal or cast boot must be used for walking because of the bulky nature of the felted foam.

The last type of healing footwear is the walking splint (Fig. 6-16). A sci-foam relief pad (Contemporary Products, Corona, CA) is placed over the ulcer area. Plaster splints are molded carefully over the foot and posterior aspect of the leg, as if one were making a posterior resting splint. Scotchcast (3M, Orthopedic Products, Atlanta, GA) is used to reinforce the plaster and attach a walking heel. After the plaster dries, betapile and velcro straps are attached. The walking splint immobilizes the foot like a cast but allows removal for daily wound care and sleeping. This device has been effective in healing plantar ulcers in cases with marked deformity, particularly the shortened foot.

Crutches

The use of crutches, partial weightbearing, is an adjunct to a walking cast or healing footwear. In the patient with bilateral plantar foot ulcers, a walking cast may be applied to one foot and healing footwear to the opposite foot. In this case, crutches will improve balance and optimize pressure reduction in the feet.

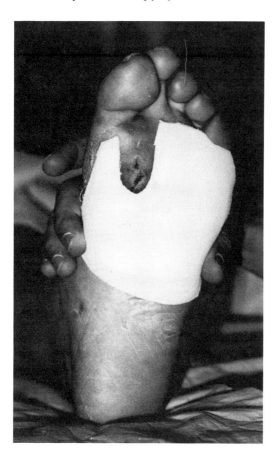

Fig. 6-15.   Felted foam technique for superficial wounds.

Interim Footwear

Most plantar ulcerations will completely heal with use of one of the three pressure reduction techniques. When an ulcer has closed, a critical phase in the healing process begins. Newly healed ulcers are extremely fragile; only a minimal amount of stress is necessary to cause reulceration. This vulnerability is due to the thinness of the new epithelium and the scarring that forms during wound healing. Stresses on the bottom of the foot that would ordinarily be dissipated in the normal, mobile soft tissues become concentrated in the adherent scar.[4]

Interim footwear is required at the time of healing for patients who have been treated with bedrest or walking casts. These devices must be readily available to protect the newly healed ulcer. Any delay in providing protective footwear to the patient is likely to result in reulceration. Soft molded plastazote sandals are recommended for interim use because they can be made in just a few hours at a relatively low cost (Fig. 6-17).

The interim sandal has a molded footbed and a rigid rocker sole. Medium

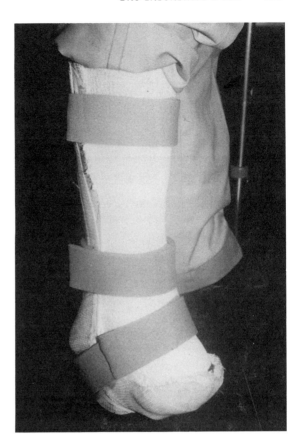

Fig. 6-16. Walking splint.

and firm plastazote material (Ali Med, Boston) is used to form the footbed. The sides of the sandal are bound with $\frac{1}{4}$-inch-thick rigid plastazote. Cotton webbing with velcro attachments is used for the straps, and the sole is made of crepe. Before the sole is attached, the base of the sandal is ground off from the MTHs distally. This initializes the shape of the rocker bottom sole design. A rigid cast boot can be modified for use as interim footwear if construction of a plastazote sandal is not possible. Plastazote ($\frac{1}{2}$-inch thick) is molded to form the foot bed, and crepe is cemented to the sole and sanded into a rocker design.

The patient is cautioned to progress slowly in walking for the first 3 weeks after the ulcer is closed. The use of partial weightbearing crutches may be advisable during this period. The patient or therapist must inspect the skin carefully after the patient walks for areas of redness or increase in temperature. Redness and warmth identify areas of tissue inflammation.[12] The development of neuropathic fractures (Charcot foot) must be considered at this time if the foot was immobilized by a cast or bedrest.[49] Signs of foot swelling, redness, and warmth should be evaluated by x-ray films to rule out neuropathic fracture. Failure of early diagnosis of these fractures results in severe deformities.

Several weeks of walking in interim footwear should result in maturation

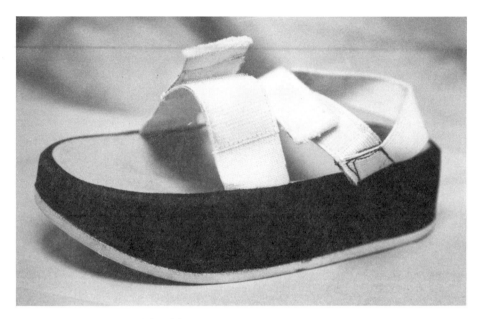

Fig. 6-17.   Molded plastazote sandal.

of healed ulcer site, and the patient may be ready to be fitted with definitive footwear. Individuals who have been treated with healing footwear are also fitted with definitive footwear when the newly healed ulcer has had time to mature.

Definitive Footwear

Definitive footwear is the final level in the management scheme for plantar ulcerations. Seven principles are commonly used in fabricating footwear for the insensitive foot.[4,50–55] These principles are designed to decrease plantar foot pressures.

Fabrication Principles

1. *Softness:* Soft elastic materials store energy and dampen the impact of forces over space and time. In the shoe, soft insole and soling materials may be used to reduce pressures on the bottom of the foot.

2. *Total contact:* Pressure equals force divided by area. An effective way of reducing pressure is to spread the forces out over a greater area. This may be achieved in the shoe by molding the insole to the bottom of the foot.

3. *Relief and build-up:* Total contact fit will not completely ensure even distribution of pressures on the bottom of the foot, since the tissues of the foot

are not of uniform firmness. Bony areas are much harder than soft tissue areas. To redistribute pressure further, the molded insole can be relieved or hollowed under hard bony areas and built up under soft tissue areas.

4. *Frictionless interface:* Friction or shearing occurs on the surface of the foot during walking. This can be reduced by covering the insole of the shoe with a smooth surface. Leather and nylon material are suited to this purpose.

5. *Rigidity:* Shear forces on the foot may be minimized by reducing movement within the shoe. This can be achieved by making the sole of the shoe rigid or by reinforcing a boot to eliminate ankle and subtalar joint movement.

6. *Rockering:* Most plantar foot ulcerations occur over the MTHs. In these cases, it is important to shift the stress off the ball of the foot during walking. This may be achieved by the rocker sole design.

7. *Balancing:* Alignment abnormalities frequently occur in the foot. These abnormalities result in abnormal pressure patterns on the bottom of the foot. Balanced orthotics may be used to reduce the abnormal pressures.

Footwear Selection Guidelines

General guidelines for the selection of footwear is based on the risk categories previously described in this chapter (Table 6-2).

Properly Fitting Shoes

Patients who have retained protective sensation (category 0) on the bottom of the foot do not need special footwear. Properly fitting shoes are the only recommendations for these patients.

Nonmolded Inserts

Nonmolded inserts are used for patients who have lost protective sensation but who have never developed plantar ulcerations (catagory 1). Spenco and PPT (poron) are good materials for making nonmolded insoles. These materials are soft, elastic, and extremely durable. PPT and Spenco may also be purchased with frictionless nylon coverings. Medium plastazote alone, commonly used as a shoe insert, is a poor choice because it readily bottoms-out unless backed by another material.

Extra-Depth Shoes

Whenever insoles are added to a shoe, there is a danger that a standard shoe may not have adequate space to accommodate the foot. Therefore, extra-depth shoes should routinely be used when fitting patients are fitted with either

Table 6.2. Footwear Selection Guidelines
Based on Risk Category

Category	Footwear
0	Proper fitting shoes
1	Nonmolded insoles Extra-depth shoes
2	Molded insoles Extra-depth rocker shoes
3	Molded insoles Extra-depth or custom-made rocker shoes
4	Fixed ankle boot Short leg walker Molded insoles Extra-depth rocker shoes

nonmolded or molded insoles. A good alternative to extra-depth shoes is a jogging shoe. Jogging shoes are manufactured with removable inserts, and custom-molded inserts can easily be fitted in their place. A transmetatarsal extra-depth boot is also available for the shortened foot (Prono Twist, Hackensack, NJ).

Molded Inserts

Patients who have a history of plantar ulcerations are fitted with molded insoles that spread plantar pressures on the foot. Soft thermoplastic materials are used on recently healed lesions but do not hold up over time. Firm pelite is an excellent thermoplastic material for most molded insoles. Extra-firm materials, such as Aliplast XPE, are used in molding balanced orthotics. Reliefs for bony prominent areas can be made by modifying a positive model of the foot. A filler material is applied to the model over the area of prominence and extending well distally. This will provide a corresponding relief in the orthotic as well as allow for elongation of the foot during walking. Molded orthotics are covered with leather, PPT, or Spenco to reduce surface friction and increase elastic properties at the tissue/device interface.

Rigid/Rocker Sole Modification

Most ulcerations in the insensitive foot occur at the metatarsal heads, and the rocker sole is effective in reducing pressure in this area of the foot.[53,56] Wedge crepe extra-depth shoes are readily modified into a rocker design. An ideal rocker slopes at an angle of about 45° and alleviates all contact of the distal sole during propulsion. The height of the sole necessary to achieve an ideal slope is minimized by bending up the toe of the shoe initially. The most effective rocker placement is just behind the MTHs. There is a tradeoff in rocker placement, however. The further back the rocker is placed, the higher the rocker needs to be made to maintain toe clearance with the floor. High rockers make the patient's gait unstable and have an obtrusive appearance. Although somewhat less effective in reducing pressure, rockers with slopes of about 30° that incorporate a curved radius are more readily accepted by some patients.

Among the most common sites of ulceration is the plantar surface of the great toe. A common cause of these ulcerations is limitation of great toe extension. The plantar surface of the toe is subjected to increased pressure during walking when motion is restricted. A rigid, sole modification is a method of accommodating for limited great toe after extension. The plantar surface of the great toe is protected from increased pressure by preventing the shoe from bending during heel-off. Additional rockering of the sole provides a smooth transition during walking. Because jogging shoes are popular footwear, they should be used for rigid, rocker sole modification whenever possible.

Custom Footwear

Extra-depth shoes meet the needs of most patients. Patients with shortened or abnormally shaped feet may require custom-made shoes, available by mail order at reasonable prices. When custom-made shoes are ordered by mail a semiweightbearing cast of the foot is needed. The specific modifications desired, such as additional room distal to the toes or extra-depth spacing to provide room for customized insoles should be requested from the vendor. These shoes are usually made rigid but may not be available with a rocker sole modification. Modification of the sole and orthotics are best done on site, where adjustments can be made on the patient.

The shortened foot is a particular problem in shoe fitting. Our best results have been obtained by fitting such patients with molded insoles and short rocker sole boots. The short boot minimizes distal foot pressures at heel-off and optimizes the spread of forces over the greatest area. A standard-length shoe with a toe filler commonly used for these patients produces a greater torque on the foot during walking as compared with a shortened shoe and results in greater plantar stress (Fig. 6-18). The disadvantage of short footwear is reduction in stability.

The Charcot foot is the endstage deformity in the insensitive foot. Progressive neuropathic fracturing can render the foot severely unstable and deformed. Severe Charcot deformities may require amputation. An active Charcot process requires long-term immobilization or surgery followed by long-term immobilization for healing to occur.[49] Early Charcot fractures are immobilized for 4 to 6 months in a walking cast followed by approximately 6 months in a fixed ankle brace (FAB) or short leg walking splint (Fig. 6-19). These devices fit the foot and leg snugly and minimize joint movement. Resumption of activity must be carefully controlled by monitoring the temperature and volume of the

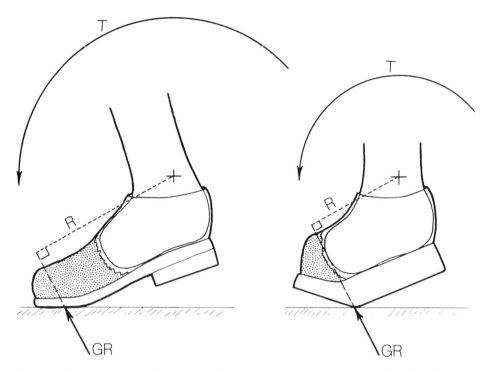

Fig. 6-18. Comparison of the torque [torque (T) = ground reaction force (GR) times perpendicular distance from the axis of rotation R)] acting on a short foot walking in a long shoe vs. a short rocker shoe.

foot and ankle. Patients are progressed to a rocker shoe with a molded insole when the temperature difference between the feet is less than 1°C. Other authors have recommended the extended use of a patella tendon bearing (PTB) brace after plaster immobilization.[34]

Assessment of Pressure

Despite our best efforts in fabricating and modifying footwear, ideal fit cannot be assured. Patients with an impaired pain warning system will be unable to identify areas of high pressure in their footwear. Two methods of evaluating pressure inside the shoe include the Harris footprint mat (Smiths Industries Medical Systems, Downs Surgical Division, 301 Gough Rd., Markham Ontario L3R4Y8) and the microcapsule slipper-socks (Slipper Sock Project, GWLHDC, Carville, LA).[2] These qualitative tests provide information on the peak pressure distribution inside footwear during walking and can identify potentially dangerous areas of high stress before injury occurs.

The slipper-sock is made of a polyurethane foam bonded to cotton. Pressure-sensitive microcapsules are impregnated into the cells of the polyure-

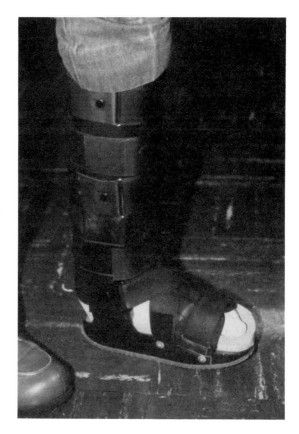

Fig. 6-19. Short-leg walker (3D Orthopedic, Dallas TX).

thane. The capsules contain a liquid blue dye and are graded to break at high stress levels on the foot. The socks are fitted to the foot, and the patient is instructed to walk 50 steps, after which areas of high shear and pressure can be identified by dark-blue staining.

The present state of the art of pressure transducers limits their clinical usefulness. Though quantitative and highly reliable under bench testing conditions, pressure transducers are subject to foot/device interface variability, making measurements between soft or molded orthotic materials questionable. Pressure transducers are best used for evaluating shoe and sole designs in which the interface between the foot and the device is controlled and unmolded.[57]

AUTHOR'S NOTE

This chapter was written in the authors' private capacity. No official support or endorsement by the United States Department of Health and Human Services is intended or should be inferred.

REFERENCES

1. Hall CO, Brand PW: The etiology of the neuropathic plantar ulcer. J Am Podiatry Med Assoc 69:173, 1979
2. Brand PW: The insensitive foot (including leprosy). In Jahss MH (ed): Disorders of the Foot. Vol. 2. WB Saunders, Philadelphia, 1982
3. Naafs B, Pearson JMH, Wheate HW: Reversal reaction, the prevention of permanent nerve damage, comparison of long and short term steroid treatment. Int J Lepr 47:7, 1979
4. Brand PW: The diabetic foot. p. 829. In Ellenberg M, Rifkin H (eds): Diabetes Mellitus, Theory and Practice. 3rd Ed. Medical Examination Publishing, New York, 1983
5. Eliasson SG: Neuropathy and the diabetic foot. p. 61. In Levin ME, O'Neal LW (eds): The Diabetic Foot. 3rd Ed. CV Mosby St. Louis, 1983
6. Swift TR, Hackett ER, Shipley DE, Miner KM: The peroneal and tibial nerves in lepromatous leprosy, clinical and electrophysiological observations. Int J Lepr 41:25, 1973
7. Sabin TD, Ebner JD: Patterns of sensory loss in lepromatous leprosy. Int J Lepr 37:239, 1969
8. Sabin TD: Temperature-linked sensory loss. Arch Neurol 20:257, 1969
9. Lawton JH: Repair of tendons and soft tissues. p. 129. In Marcus SA, Block BH (eds): American College of Foot Complications in Foot Surgery, Prevention and Management. 2nd Ed. Williams & Wilkins, Baltimore, 1984
10. Daniels C, Worthingham C: Muscle Testing, Techniques of Manual Examination. 3rd Ed. WB Saunders, Philadelphia, 1972
11. Medical Research Council: Aids to the Investigation of Peripheral Nerve Injuries. Her Majesty's Stationery Office, London, 1943
12. Bergtholdt HT, Brand PW: Temperature assessment and plantar inflammation. Lepr Rev 47:211, 1976
13. Harris JR, Brand PW: Patterns of disintegration of the tarsus in the anaesthetic foot. J Bone Joint Surg [Br] 48:4, 1966
14. Williams PL, Warwick R: Gray's Anatomy. 36th British Ed. Churchill Livingstone, London, 1980
15. Levin ME: Medical evaluation and treatment. p. 1. In Levin ME, O'Neal LW (eds): The Diabetic Foot. 3rd Ed. CV Mosby, St. Louis, 1983
16. Ross WF: Etiology and treatment of plantar ulcers. Lepr Rev 33:25, 1962
17. Price EW: Plantar Ulcers. p. 373. In McDowell F, Enna CD (eds): Surgical Rehabilitation in Leprosy. Williams & Wilkins, Baltimore, 1974
18. Ctercteko GC, Dhanendran M, Hutton WC, LeQuesne LE: Vertical forces acting on the feet of diabetic patients with neuropathic ulceration. Br J Surg 68:608, 1981
19. Sabato S, Yosipovitch Z, Simkin A, Sheskin J: Plantar trophic ulcers in patients with leprosy. Int Orthop 6:203, 1982
20. Sims DS, Birke JA: Reliability of Semmes-Weinstein monofilaments in Hansen's disease. J Am Podiatry Med Assoc (in review)
21. Birke JA, Sims DS: Plantar sensory thresholds in the ulcerative foot. Lepr Rev 57:261, 1986
22. Bell JA: Sensibility evaluation. p. 273. In Hunter JM, Schneider LH, Mackin EJ, Bell JA (eds): Rehabilitation of the Hand. CV Mosby, St. Louis, 1978

23. Coughlin MS: Mallet toes, hammer toes, claw toes and corns, Causes and treatment of lesser-toe deformities. Postgrad Med 75:191, 1984

24. Jahss MH (ed): Disorders of the Foot. Vol. 2. WB Saunders, Philadelphia, 1982

25. Edwards CA: Orthopedic Shoe Technology. Precision Printing, Muncie, 1981

26. Raines JK, Darling RC, Buth J, et al: Vascular laboratory criteria for the management of peripheral vascular disease of the lower extremities. Surgery 79:21, 1975

27. Wagner W: A classification and treatment program for diabetic, neuropathic and dysvascular foot problems. AAOS Instructional Course Lecture, Vol. 28, 1979

28. Williamson JR, Kilo C, Crespin SR: Vascular disease. p. 85. In Levin ME, O'Neal LW (eds): The Diabetic Foot. CV Mosby, St.Louis, 1983

29. Birke JA, Sims DS, Theriot SM: Your Feet, Self-Inspection, A Guide for Patients With Insensitive Feet (videotape). Produced by the Training Branch, Gillis W. Long Hansen's Disease Center, 1983

30. Boeker MJ, Leu MM: A study of the effects of hydration and emollients on the feet of the aged. J Am Podiatry Med Assoc 68:402, 1978

31. Birke JA, Sims DS, Theriot SM: Your feet, Skin Care, A Guide for Patients With Insensitive Feet (videotape). Produced by the Training Branch, Gillis W. Long Hansen's Disease Center, 1983

32. Sims DS, Birke JA, Theriot SM: Your Feet, Footwear Selection, A Guide for Patients With Insensitive Feet (videotape). Produced by the Training Branch, Gillis W. Long Hansen's Disease Center, 1983

33. Lang-Stevenson AI, Sharrard WJW, Betts RP, Duckworth T: Neuropathic ulcers of the foot. J Bone Joint Surg [Br] 76:438, 1985

34. Fritschi EP: Surgical Reconstruction And Rehabilitation In Leprosy. The Directory for Southern Asia Leprosy Mission, New Delhi, 1986

35. Jones RO: Ulceration in the neuroptrothic foot of Hansen's disease. J Am Podiatry Med Assoc 72:299, 1982

36. Peacock EE, Van Winkle W: Wound Repair. 2nd Ed. WB Saunders, Philadelphia, 1976

37. Srinivasan H, Mukherjee SM: Trophic ulcers in leprosy III. Lepr Rev 36:186, 1964

38. Anderson JG: Plantar ulcers in leprosy. Lepr Rev 32:16, 1961

39. Pollard JP, Le Quesne LP: Method of healing diabetic forefoot ulcers. Br Med J 286:436, 1983

40. Soderberg G: Follow-up of application of plaster-of-paris casts for non-infected plantar ulcers in field conditions. Lepr Rev 41:184, 1970

41. Coleman WC, Brand PW, Birke JA: The total contact cast. J Am Podiatry Med Assoc 74:548, 1984

42. Angel JC: The mechanism of the healing cast. Orthopedic Seminars, University of Southern California, Department of Orthopedics, Rancho Los Amigos Hospital 4:17, 1973–1974

43. Mooney V, Wagner FW: Neurocirculatory disorders of the foot. Clin Orthop Rel Res 122:53, 1977

44. Birke JA, Sims DS, Buford WL: Walking casts: effect on plantar foot pressures. J Rehabil Res Dev 22:18, 1985

45. Pollard JP, Le Quesne LP, Tappin JW: Forces under the foot. J Biomed Eng 5:37, 1983

46. Helm PA, Walker SC, Pullium G: Total contact casting in diabetic patients with neuropathic foot ulcerations. Arch Phys Med Rehabil 65:691, 1984

47. Enna CD, Brand PW, Reed JK, Welch D: Orthotic care of the denervated foot in Hansen's disease. Orthot Prosthet 30:33, 1976
48. Frykberg RG: Podiatric problems in diabetes. p. 45. In Kosak GP, Hoar CS, Rowbotham JL, et al (eds): Management of Diabetic Foot Problems. WB Saunders, Philadelphia, 1984
49. Warren G: Tarsal bone disintegration in leprosy. J Bone Joint Surg [Br] 53:688, 1971
50. Hampton GH: Therapeutic footwear for the insensitive foot. Phys Ther 59:23, 1979
51. Ross WF: Footwear and the prevention of ulcers in leprosy. Lepr Rev 33:202, 1962
52. Ward D: Footwear in leprosy. Lepr Rev 33:94, 1962
53. Bauman JH, Girling JP, Brand PW: Plantar pressures and trophic ulceration. J Bone Joint Surg [Br] 45:652, 1963
54. Berger N, Edelstein JE, Fishman S, Sprigner WP: Lower-Limb Prosthetics. New York University Medical Center, 1980
55. Root ML, Orien WP, Weed JH: Normal And Abnormal Function Of The Foot. Clinical Biomechanics, Vol. II. 1st Ed. Clinical Biomechanics, Los Angeles, 1977
56. Coleman WC: The relief of forefoot pressures using outer shoe sole modifications. Proceedings of the International Conference on Biomechanics and Kinesiology of Hand and Foot, Madras, India, December, 1985
57. Patterson RP, Fisher SV: The accuracy of electrical transducers for the measurement of pressure applied to the skin. IEEE Trans Biomed Eng 26:450, 1979

7 | Skin and Toenail Problems

Charles L. McGarvey III

The following chapter was written to aid the clinical physical therapist in assessment and treatment of common skin and toenail lesions of the lower extremities. Depending on the clinical setting, the physical therapist may be called on to assist the dermatologist, podiatrist, or general surgeon in the treatment of cutaneous lesions involving the lower leg. These treatments traditionally have consisted of hydrotherapy, wound debridement, and dressing changes.[1] Very often, it is the physical therapist who follows the patient on a daily basis, allowing the opportunity to observe acute changes in the status of the lesion. Being knowledgeable and alert to tissue changes enables the therapist to communicate new information to the referring physician, who in turn may alter the treatment plan accordingly.

TERMINOLOGY

As with many forms of specialization, specific terminology is often established to assist the clinician in correctly describing different processes and pathological conditions. Correct use of these terms identifies the physical therapist as an informed health care provider of those services. Some of the more commonly used terms are listed in Appendix 1 at the end of the chapter and lesions of the skin and toenail are shown in Figure 7-1.

ANATOMY OF THE NORMAL SKIN AND TOENAIL

This section identifies general facts about normal skin and its layers. Emphasis is placed on the components of each layer of the skin and how they relate to some of the more common lesions seen in the clinical environment.

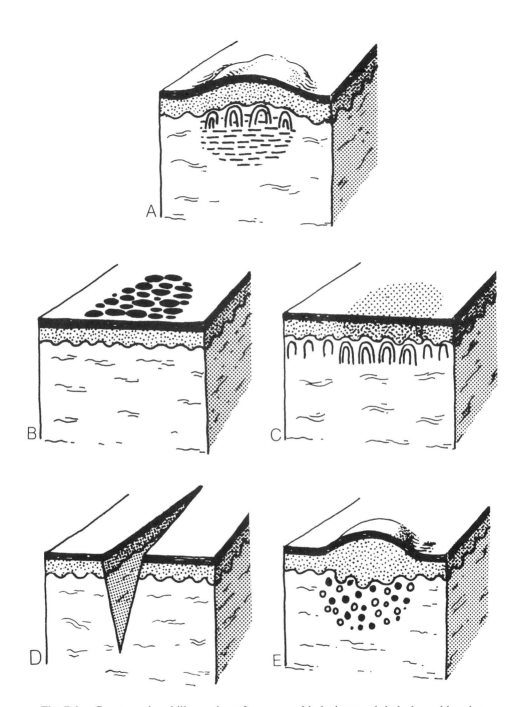

Fig. 7-1. Cross-sectional illustration of common skin lesions and their dermal involvement. (**A**) Hives (urticaria), (**B**) scales (squames), (**C**) spot (macule), (**D**) perioral fissures (rhagades), (**E**) pimple (papule). (*Figure continues.*)

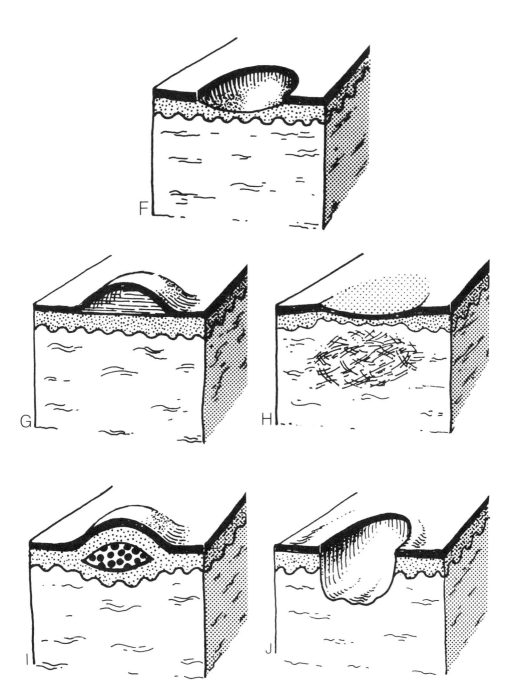

Fig. 7-1 (*continued*). (**F**) erosion (excoriation), (**G**) blister (vesicle), (**H**) scar (cicatrix), (**I**) pustule, (**J**) ulcer. (Rassner G, Kahn G: Atlas of Dermatology with Differential Diagnosis. 2nd. Ed. Urban and Schwarzenberg, Baltimore, 1983.)

Unfortunately, less is generally known about the toenail; however, the latter portion of this section describes its formation and function.

The skin is the largest organ of the human body. Histiologically, its embryonic roots are ectodermal in origin.[2] In the average man, the skin comprises approximately 4.5 kg of total body weight as compared with 3.1 kg in the average woman.[3] When the surface area of both extremities is considered, the skin covering both legs comprises approximately 36 percent of the total surface area of the body,[4] approximately the size of a 9 × 12 rug.[3] Most authors cite the following as the basic functions of the skin.[1-5]

Protection from external stimuli
Assistance in glandular and metabolic function
Thermoregulation
Sensation
Communication and expression
Special functions of certain regions

Authors differ slightly in classification of skin layers. Some authors refer to the skin as a two-layered structure, the epidermis and dermis, beneath which lies the subcutaneous or fatty layer.[1,4,5] Others describe the skin as a contiguous three-layer structure consisting of the epidermis, dermis, and hypodermis.[3] For the purpose of this chapter, I prefer use of the latter form (Fig. 7-2).

The epidermis is the outermost layer of skin, varying in thickness from between 0.2 to 1.2 mm—roughly the thickness of a sheet of paper.[3] It can be further subdivided into five layers, beginning from the deepest to the most superficial:

Basal (stratum germinativum),
Prickle (stratum sponosum),
Granular (stratus granulosum),
Lucid (stratus lucidum),
Horny (stratum corneum),

The first four layers (basal through lucid) represent the living portion of the epidermis; the last layer (horny) is considered a dead end-product.[1]

The epidermis is comprised of two main cell types, keratinocytes and melanocytes. Keratinocytes comprise approximately 90 to 95 percent of the total cell population whereas melanocytes make up the remaining 5 to 10 percent.[2] The principle function of keratinocytes is to produce keratin, a fibrous protein necessary for the production of the horny layer of the epidermis. The melanocytes are responsible for the production of melanin, the pigment that provides skin color. Both keratinocytes and melanocytes have their origins in the deepest layer (basal) of the epidermis and, with maturation (approximately 26 to 42 days), eventually are sloughed with the horny layer.[2] This process is called desquamation.

Although the epidermis lacks a true vascular supply, it receives its nutri-

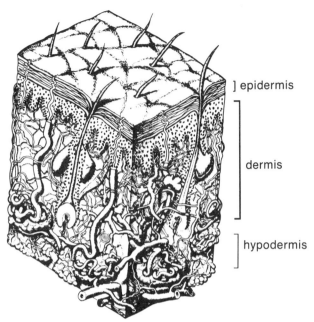

Fig. 7-2. Cross-sectional illustration of the three layers of skin, epidermis (top), dermis (middle) and hypodermis (bottom) and their respective components. (Courtesy of White Laboratories, Kenilworth, New Jersey.)

] epidermis

dermis

] hypodermis

tion through a process of tissue diffusion whereby, during capillary exchange, fluid enters the interstitial matrix in sufficient quantity to provide the epidermis with adequate sustenance.[4]

Among the functions of the epidermis the two most important appear to be protection from noxious stimuli and provision of a suitable environment for other skin appendages. Specifically, the protection of the horny layer serves to provide a physical barrier against the ingress of harmful toxins while functioning to retard the egress of necessary body fluids. In addition, through the process of pigmentation, the skin is protected against harmful doses of ultraviolet light. The epidermis also provides the necessary tissue state required for the terminal deposit of sensory fibers, eccrine, appocrine, and subcutaneous glands.[3]

Abnormal functioning of the epidermis can result in such conditions as hyperkeratosis, a hypertrophy of the horny layer, as is seen in the production of corns and calluses. Dyskeratosis, an imperfect cornification, also creates the possibility of infection and loss of body fluids. Overproduction of melanin causes tanning, excesses of which can lead to such abnormalities as skin carcinoma. A loss of pigmentation is usually manifested by a condition known as vitiligo.

Below the epidermis lies the second layer of skin, the dermis, sometimes referred to as corium. This layer, comprised of connective tissue, blood vessels, and nerves, makes up the bulk of the total skin structure.[3] It varies in thickness according to the body part and cannot be accurately measured because there is no true line of demarcation.[4] It is subdivided into two principle layers, a papillary (superficial dermal/epidermal junction) and a reticular layer (deep dermal/epidermal junction). Most important is the reticular layer and its components, containing the arterial and venule loops, autonomic and peripheral nerve branches, lymphatic capillaries and channels and, in some cases, a glomus body. A glomus body is a type of arteriovenous shunt often found in the tips of fingers, toes, and under nails.[1] This special vascular body, when stimulated, produces a marked increase in blood flow through the skin.

The cell types most often associated with the dermis are fibroblasts, histiocytes, and mast cells.[2,4] The fibroblasts are the principle cells responsible for the production of collagen, elastic fibers, and intracellular ground substance. Histiocytes are responsible for the formation of reticular fibers and phagocitization of bacteria. Most cells operate in a heparinlike fashion to interfere with blood coagulation when necessary.

In discussing fiber types, it should be recognized that collagen, (type I) is the tough resistant fibrous protein that makes up approximately 95 percent of the dermis, roughly one-quarter of human total protein mass.[1,3] Histologically, elastic fibers are those structures identified as being entwined among collagen bundles. Immature collagen (type III) is often identified as reticular fibers. The ground substance is the gel-like amorphous material containing proteins, enzymes, and mucopolysaccharides that is of great importance to the sustenance of the fiber types previously described.

The most important feature of the dermis is its blood supply,[4] which is actually in excess of the metabolic needs of the dermis, its principle function being thermal regulation of total body temperature.[3] The glomus body previously described lies in close proximity to these structures.

The nerve supply consists of sensory and autonomic branches. Sensory branches include hair follicles, fine nerve endings, and special nerve endings (i.e., Meissner's for touch and Vater-Pacini for pressure). The autonomic branches originate from the sympathetic system and supply the blood vessels, eccrine, and apocrine glands. Other appendages located in the dermis include the shaft of the hair follicle, the ductal portion of the eccrine (sweat) and apocrine (scent) gland, and the lobule and duct of the subaceous (sebum-producing) gland.

The functions of the dermis are not only numerous but also extremely important for the viability of the organ as a whole. Nutrition, support of the epidermis, thermoregulation, elasticity, and tissue repair (scarring) are among the main functions affecting the body's ability to react to environmental changes and differing climates.

Therefore, lesions involving the second layer of skin may interfere with the "heart" of skin function. Acute or chronic cellular changes due to direct trauma, bacteria, viruses, fungi, or neoplasm can create infiltrations of foreign cells and ultimately destroy the structure of that area of the skin. The changes manifested by this tissue destruction may appear as scars, atrophic skin, abscesses, ulcers, warts, or tumors.

The deepest layer, the hypodermis, is located inferior to the dermis and superior to the fascial plane. It is comprised of closely packed lipocytes that vary in thickness according to the body part. Its main function is that of insula-

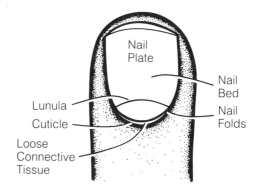

Fig. 7-3. Top view of the external landmarks of the toenail. (Modified from Beaven D, Brooks S: Color Atlas of the Nail in Clinical Diagnosis. Wolfe Medical Publications, London, 1984.)

tion, protecting the body from excessive external heat and heat loss when exposed to varying climates. It also aids in supporting the subcutaneous artery and vein, deep hair follicles, and certain sweat glands.

Toenail

Obviously located on the dorsal surface of the distal phalanx of each toe is the structure known as the toenail. Considered the longest sheet of keratin in the body, it is resistant to the attack of most parasites and decomposing micro-organisms.[2,6]

The toenail is subdivided into four major areas: nail plate, nail bed, lunula, and nail folds (Fig. 7-3). The nail plate, which is formed from an invagination of epidermis located under the posterior nail fold of each digit, consists of three distinct layers: dorsal portion, intermediate portion, and ventral portion. (Fig. 7-4). The dorsal portion is derived from the root of the proximal nail fold; the intermediate portion, which makes up the bulk of the nail, originates from the floor of the same region of the nail fold. The ventral portion, the most inferior aspect, arises from the distal part of the nail bed.[4]

The nail bed is simply an extension of the epidermis that is contiguous with the nail plate and extends to the point of the free margin of the nail. The translucency of the nail plate allows easy inspection of the normally pink nail bed. With trauma to either the nail or nailbed, however, this translucency is often lost and a semiwhite opaqueness is substituted. The lunula is identified as the semiwhite, crescent-shaped structure located at the proximal nail plate.

Growth of the toenail in the healthy, young adult is approximately 1 mm per month or one-third to one-half the rate of fingernails.[1,4] Approximately 1 year is required for total toenail replacement following mechanical trauma to the toenail matrix. In youth toenails grow quite rapidly during maturation, but slow down significantly with adulthood.[4] Toenail thickness also appears to differ between sexes, being slightly thicker in males.[6]

Historically, animals of various orders used their claws and in some cases,

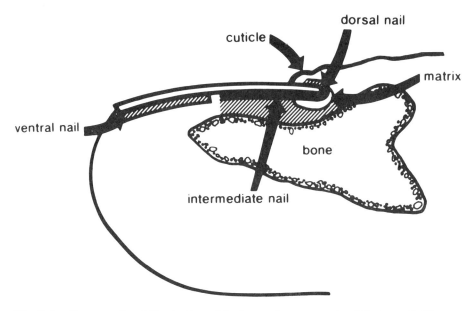

Fig. 7-4. Cross-sectional illustration of the internal components of the toenail. (Beaven D, Brooks S: Color Atlas of the Nail in Clinical Diagnosis. Wolfe Medical Publications, London, 1984.)

nails, to assist in their struggle for existence. These appendages were often used in their search for food, construction of homes and, ultimately, as a weapon in situations of combat. Higher primates such as humans, however, did not have the capability of nail retraction and have not used their nails in any significant offensive or defensive manner. Instead, humans have made use of these structures to assist in performance of certain fine motor tasks such as scraping or scratching. When polished or pointed, these structures have also been used to improve appearance.

The main importance of the nail to the clinician is its ability to reflect certain changes in the internal or external environment of the individual. For example, growth arrest lines, called also Beau's lines, are transverse lines that extend from the medial to the lateral edge of the nail plate. These lines, if noted on all nails, are indicative of a significant previous illness.[4,6] An absent lunula has been postulated to be compatible with certain chromosomal abnormalities, such as monosomia 4 and trisomy 21.6. Thickening, yellowing, and loss of nail integrity are often classified as classic signs for local fungal infection, circulation impairment, metabolic, or nutritional disorders. These signs, if detected early, may assist in early diagnosis and ultimately in early treatment, preventing what might prove to be a chronic disorder.

The two most common toenail disorders associated with younger and middle-aged groups are ingrown toenails and onychomycosis, respectively.[6] In the elderly, onychogryphosis (abnormal toenail growth) and peripheral vascular disease are most common.[6]

Clinical Evaluation and Documentation

In an attempt to be consistent with current methods practiced by many physical therapists today, the following section is presented in a subjective, objective, assessment, and plan (SOAP) note format. This format should not only present the information in a logical sequence but also can be used as a reference by the clinician to evaluate several skin lesions.

Problem

Initially, the patient may be referred to the physical therapy department with a proven diagnosis and specific recommendation for treatment. On the other hand, in a department that employs physical therapists with expertise in skin lesions, the patient may be referred for further examination and/or second opinion to assist the physician in ruling out a diagnosis. In either situation, a comprehensive interview with the patient will help establish personal and family history, present complaints, and the onset of signs and symptoms, all of which are critical to the establishment of baseline information.

Subjective

The first series of questions investigates the complaint. What was the date of onset? Was there an injury to the skin/toenail? Has there been a history, either personal or familial, of the same problem? Has the lesion received any previous personal or professional treatment? Is there any pain, loss of sensation, or loss of function related to activities of daily living (ADL). In the patient's opinion, is the lesion getting better or worse? Other questions related to present and past medical problems, occupation, medications, and living environment will assist the therapist not only in treatment, but also with recommendation of home programs designed to prevent reoccurrence of the same problem. Examples of such questions may be: Is the patient diabetic and currently on medication? If medication has been prescribed, what type and dosage is used and is the patient currently following directions for its use? Is the patient presently employed and doing a job that requires physical exposure or potential trauma to the legs? Ask the patient to describe the home environment and whether extracurricular activities involve potential for trauma. Would the patient have the necessary facilities to accomplish a safe and effective home program of wound care? In summary, the type of lesion and principal complaints generally dictate the questions asked of the patient. Ultimately, documentation of these answers will assist the therapist in determining the effectiveness of the treatment program.

Objective

Under inspection, a thorough description of the lesion, identifying location, size, depth, skin changes, color, odor, and sensation is essential. Location, identified as a certain distance from an anatomical landmark, is primary. Length, width, and depth measurements of lesions should be recorded in centimeters. Skin changes indicating abnormal hair patterns, texture, and color are important and should be noted. Color of the lesion and notation of any exudate can be useful in determining the pathological process occurring. Certain odors are often compatible with specific microbial invasion, such as *Pseudomonas aeruginosum.* Sensory examination, as discussed in a separate chapter in this text (see Ch. 6) is absolutely essential to appropriate therapeutic management of the problem. An example of documentation required to describe a vascular lesion of the lower leg may read as follows:

> Inspection: There is a single, oval, partial-thickness lesion located 4 cm superior to the medial malleolus of the right lower extremity. This lesion measures 4 cm × 3 cm and is approximately 1 cm in depth. The bed of this lesion appears dark red with necrotic exudate and has a foul-smelling, pungent odor. The borders of the lesion are irregular, and the surrounding skin appears tight, shiny, and devoid of hair. There is marked decrease to sharp/dull pinprick sensation in a stocking distribution of the entire right lower extremity from a point 10 cm superior to the medial malleolus to the toes.

Following an accurate description of the lesion, additional information related to the presence of edema, skin temperature, arterial pulses, and gait characteristics can be very valuable. Girth of the extremity can be measured above or below the lesion, a certain distance from an accepted bony landmark. These circumferential measurements, taken in centimeters with a paper or pliable plastic tape measure, should be done of both affected and nonaffected lower extremities to establish presence of edema or atrophy of musculature. Recording of skin temperature, also taken bilaterally, is often quickly accomplished through use of the back of one's hand to determine gross differences in temperature. More sophisticated methods of temperature monitoring make use of handheld skin thermistors, and determinations can be made even more accurately through the use of an infrared thermography unit. Palpation of arterial pulses can often give a gross appreciation of the presence of arterial pressure in the lower leg but are not significant for the status of venous return. Capillary refill time is a manual method often used to assess gross venous function clinically. The dorsalis pedis pulse can be normally palpated between the extensor hallicus longus and extensor digitorum longus tendons on the dorsum of the foot. It is absent 12 to 15 percent of the time and provides a secondary source of blood supply to the foot.[4] The main blood supply to the foot is derived from the posterior tibial artery, which is normally palpated between the tendons of the flexor digitorum longus and flexor hallicus longus, just posterior to the medial malleolus. The popliteal artery, often difficult to palpate, lies deep and to the center of the popliteal space. More refined methods using a blood pressure cuff or ultrasound Doppler can also determine the presence and strength of pulses of the lower leg. Documentation of the presence of these pulses in both legs can be advantageous. Abnormal gait characteristics during ambulation should also be noted. A description of the patient's ambulatory status is often of benefit to other health care professionals; often it is not known whether the patient is capable of ambulating in a safe and effective manner.

Finally, any limitations related to joint motion, muscle strength, and general function of the extremity above and below the lesion require documentation. Goniometry and manual muscle testing are methods used to quantify those deficits. Once recorded, these data are later used to determine whether changes have occurred in the musculoskeletal function of the extremity. Other areas that merit mention include a description and preference of footwear, a description of overall skin hygiene, and a brief statement regarding the state of behavior. Part or all of these factors may have a direct effect on the level of compliance exhibited by the patient during the future treatment program.

Assessment

The assessment portion of the examination is not generally used to present a diagnosis of the lesion. It serves instead to describe the current state of the lesion according to the subjective and objective data collected. An important statement can be made regarding the characteristics of the lesion (i.e., vascular, metabolic, or traumatic) and will often aid the referring physician in proper identification of a specific disease process. The assessment portion of the initial note should also contain a listing of short-term goals for the patient. Often noted are goals of improved healing, range of motion (ROM), strength, and ambulation. Concurrently, one would anticipate a reduction in levels of pain, fatigue, and edema.

Plan

The plan should describe, in detail, the use, frequency, and intensity of those physical therapy modalities used to effect a change in the original problem. This change can be measured objectively through achievement of the previously stated short-term goals. Accuracy in description of these therapeutic procedures is imperative. Unidentified changes in a patient's treatment program carried out by a substituting therapist could result in dire consequences. The lack of appropriate instruction or misinformation could not only be detrimental to the acute care of the patient but could prolong total rehabilitation time. Water temperature of hydrotherapy units, amount and concentration of solution placed in the water, medication placed on the wound, treatment time, and frequency of visits are examples of necessary information. This portion of the note is also an excellent area in which to list future recommendations regarding changing of specific modalities, frequency of visits, and use of ambulatory aids. In summary, it is imperative that these sections not only be legible but concise, complete, and reflective of the patient's current status and treatment.

COMMON SKIN DISORDERS

The purpose of this section is to present information related to common skin and toenail disorders commonly seen in the clinical environment. The section is divided into four main areas of classification: traumatic, microbiological, ulcerative, and toenail lesions. Each area is then further subdivided to include a brief description of clinical appearance, incidence, pathology, and recommended treatments for common lesions.

Trauma

Corns

Two common types of corns are often encountered by the clinician: hard corns and soft corns. Both are examples of hyperkeratized tissue produced as a direct result of two compressive forces acting on the skin. They differ primarily in location and, to some extent, in treatment. Hard corns appear generally as circumscribed, superficial lesions approximately 1 to 3 cm in diameter with a callused periphery and a firm seedlike core. They are usually located on the plantar aspect of the foot below such bony prominences as the metatarsal heads (MTHs) and also on the dorsum of the interphalangeal (IP) joints of the toes. Soft corns are similar in size but are found on the lateral aspect of the third or fourth proximal phalanx of the toe. They often appear as soft, thick, raised calluses with either a hard core or ulcerated center. Hard corns are generally the result of abnormal compressive stress between bone and the walking surface, whereas soft corns are caused by a direct force exerted on the skin by the bones of the two toes. The incidence of hard corns is somewhat greater than soft corns, with hard corns being characteristic of persons who walk great distances in improper footwear. Also implicated as a cause of hard corns are bony deformities and poor foot biomechanics. Soft corns on the other hand may be the result of toe deformities such as those that occur in rheumatoid arthritis or as a result of wearing shoes with a very narrow or pointed toebox. The treatment of hard and soft corns involves the same three basic objectives. The first objective is removal of the painful lesion by first softening the tissue with a warm, antiseptic bath and then carefully paring the lesion with a #10 scalpel blade. Once the top layer of keratinized tissue has been removed and is flush with the peripheral skin, careful curettage of the "seed" corn can be accomplished with a #15 scalpel blade. This procedure requires skill gained only through repeated practice and experience and should not be attempted by the novice. Detailed instruction by a competent clinician and practice with a scalpel using a paraffin bar should be completed prior to any clinical procedure. Although considered a noninvasive technique that is relatively bloodless, it should be practiced only on healthy individuals with no prior history of diabetes or circulatory insufficiency. The more complicated cases of patients with a history of diabetes or peripheral vascular disease should be referred directly to a local podiatrist or surgeon. The second objective is to prevent the recurrence of the same compressive forces responsible for the original lesion. Felt padding, metatarsal pads/bars, and custom-molded orthoses are all effective in reducing the stresses that cause hard corns. Lamb's wool or felt pads placed between the affected toes is beneficial in the temporary treatment of soft corns. Surgery may be necessary for bony correction of severely affected joints to permanently eradicate the problem. Finally, education of the patient about the causes of these lesions and recommendation regarding changes in footwear and possibly about work habits are often very beneficial.

Calluses

Calluses are also a form of hyperkeratized epidermal tissue formed as a result of shearing and torsion forces placed on the plantar aspect of the foot. These forces generally occur either with high velocity or repetitive stress over a short time, or with chronic abnormal weight shifting in an improper shoe. Also responsible are bony abnormalities that create deviations in biomechanical forces in the foot. The location of a callus is similar to that of a hard corn, as they are often found under the bony prominences of the feet. In contrast to the hard corn, however, calluses are usually larger and have no hard nucleus. The thickness of a callus is generally uniform, and although it is somewhat bothersome it usually is not painful. Patients with hard corns often complain of feeling as though they are "stepping on a small stone," whereas patients with calluses seldom complain of pain but of something thick and leathery on the bottom of their foot. The mechanism of callus formation is actually the body's normal response in reacting to an abnormal stimulus by producing a thicker resilient barrier. Treatment of these lesions should be at best conservative. If calluses are discovered early, light abrasion with a pumice stone followed by periodic application of an emollient will usually suffice. If, however, the callus has grown to such a size that it is not only prominent but may be causing a change in the biomechanical function of the foot, the softening and paring procedures previously described should be initiated to decrease the size of the callus.

Blisters

Blisters, or vesicles, are small fluid-filled sacs found at anatomic sites of the foot that are reacting to abnormal stress. These lesions characteristically require high torsion or shearing forces as a result of intimate contact with either the shoe or some other element of the sock/shoe component. Blisters form as a result of the disruption of the appendages between the first and second layer of skin. This form of disruption is so traumatic that the cellular damage to the epidermal–dermal junction causes a denaturatation of cellular proteins, the result of which is a loss of continuity of the epidermis and of proteases resulting in fluid accumulation.

Blisters most commonly occur in the young athlete who is beginning training and in persons who perfer the look of a new shoe over comfort or fit. Blisters may also occur as a result of wearing a new pair of well-fitted shoes for too long on the first few days after purchase.

Treatment of this lesion varies according to whether it has undergone spontaneous rupture or whether it has remained closed. The broken blister requires immediate attention in the form of a warm, antiseptic bath, application of an appropriate antibacterial ointment, and protective bandaging. The closed blister, in the opinion of many, should be left alone, as the fluid contained inside the vesicle is sterile and therefore should be protected. Any invasive procedure to drain this fluid invites the possibility of future microbial invasion and subsequent invasion. In time, the blister will rupture spontaneously, revealing granulation tissue that has formed in anticipation of the sloughing of the epidermal layer. This method of closed blister management requires a few days to evolve and unfortunately does not always fit the "time schedule" of the current generation. Subsequently, many patients opt to have these lesions drained and treated with antibacterial ointments and protective bandaging. The use of tincture of benzoin compound is often recommended for prevention of future blister formations. Benzoin is a resin-like compound that when combined with tannic acid and isopropyl alcohol initiates an astringent and antiseptic action on the skin. It is commonly considered a skin toughener.

Open Wounds

Open wounds incurred as a result of a direct blow, thermal injury, laceration, or gunshot wound are examples of traumatic injury. Because of the various mechanisms of injury, it would be difficult to discuss every possible effect on tissue pathology and clinical appearance. Rather, the descriptions should begin simply by identifying the wound as a superficial, partial- or full-thickness lesion. These degrees of tissue involvement are based on the same criteria used to describe depth of burns. Bleeding is very seldom a problem with a superficial wound but is often a major concern with partial- or full-thickness lesions. The primary difference between partial- and full-thickness lesions is the loss of deep pain sensation. A patient with a partial-thickness lesion retains the ability to discriminate pain, as in the pulling of a hair follicle or a needle prick; a patient with a full-thickness lesion is unable to perceive such stimuli.

Treatment, whether the wound is superficial or full-thickness, begins with a thorough cleansing of the wound and surrounding skin with hydrotherapy and an effective antiseptic solution. The lesion may then require mechanical debridement of necrotic tissue, which if not removed will retard production of new granulation tissue and eventual reepithelialization. Debridement should be attempted only with the approval of the physician and patient and carried out with instruments appropriate for the type of lesion. Sharp sterile scissors, hemostats, scalpel, and a steady but quick hand are the necessary instruments for safe and effective debridement of most wounds. Following debridement, application of an absorbent, nonadherent dressing to the wound is the last procedure accomplished prior to transportation of the patient. Some physicians prefer an adherent dressing as these dressings have the tendency to debride necrotic tissue when removed on the following day. These dressings should be removed with great care by the physical therapist, according to the patient's tolerance. Preliminary soaking in the hydrotherapy tank is often used to assist in removal of the more stubborn dressings. At no time should the turbines be engaged during this procedure. Daily hydrotherapy, debridement, and dressing changes are effective in facilitating granulation tissue, controlling infection, and promoting wound closure.

Microbiological Lesions

Fungal Infections

Often cited as the most common fungal infection of the feet is tinea pedis, universally known as "athlete's foot."[7-11] This particular fungal infection is usually caused by one of three microbial organisms: *Trichophyton mentagrophye, Trichophyton rubrum,* or *Epidermophyton floccosum,* all of which have been cultured from the normal flora of asymptomatic skin. As with most fungi, these organisms proliferate in warm, moist, dark environments. Certain persons are more prone than others to these infections owing to their particular habits or vocations, in particular individuals who wear their shoes for a prolonged period of time and undergo repeated stresses to the feet through aggressive walking and running. These stresses ultimately create skin lesions (i.e., blisters) that break down the skin's primary, external defense mechanisms and allow fungal microbes to invade.

During the acute stage of tinea pedis, *T. mentagrophyte* and *T. rubrum* are the usual organisms cultured. Symptoms consist of pruritus usually between the toes of one foot. Clinical inspection of these areas reveals macerated tissue between the toe webs and often the presence of vesicles containing yellow, serous fluid. As initial treatment, the patient is instructed to use foot baths containing a prescribed antiseptic solution for 20 minutes twice a day. Following the bath, proper drying is required prior to donning clean, dry socks. White cotton socks are generally preferred to dark synthetic styles. Open shoes or sandals are recommended as footgear for the next few weeks.

In the chronic stage, symptoms remain generally the same except that itching is more widespread, involving the sole and heel in a moccasinlike distribution. Vesicles are again evident but are much larger. Treatment during this stage is often more aggressive. Again the patient is instructed in a home program of warm soaks containing an antiseptic solution. This procedure is followed by complete drying of the feet and generous application of an antifungal solution containing either tolnaftate or miconazole agents. Griseofulvin is an oral, systemic medication that is not fungicidal but fungistatic. It is usually prescribed by a physician for chronic fungal infections, but because of the long treatment time (usually 1 year) and the drug's possible side effects on the gastrointestinal system, it is usually not the preferred treatment.

Following infection, probably the most effective long-term treatment of this condition is habitual prevention. Too often, following the remission of an acute episode of tinea pedis, the patient discontinues newly acquired hygenic habits and loyal application of antifungal medication. A few months later, the patient suffers an exacerbation of the same problem requiring a resumption of the previous aggressive treatment. Prevention, in the sense of compliance with good foot hygiene, frequent changing of socks, and periodic application of antifungal solutions to the asymptomatic foot is recommended on a daily basis for the patient's lifetime.

Bacterial Infections

Patients with an open wound of the lower leg or foot are often referred to the physical therapy department for primary wound care. Procedures include cleaning the wound with hydrotherapy, followed by cutaneous debridement of necrotic tissue, and finally by application of an appropriate dressing. The types of bacterial infections that classically occur in these lesions can be classified according to two categories: primary and secondary infections. Primary infections originate in the skin whereas secondary infections are usually a consequence of a preexisting lesion.[3] Examples of primary lesions include impetigo, folliculitis, and erysipelas. Secondary infections, such as infected ulcers, intertrigo, and erythrasma are the more common bacterial lesions encountered by the physical therapist. Historically, microbiologists and other researchers have studied the natural flora of the skin extensively.[13-19] Unfortunately, a remarkable diversity of opinion exists regarding the predominant organisms and the skin's ability to fight microbial invasion.[14-17] The ongoing debate is possibly best summarized in a statement by Friedman et al in their article describing bacterial flora of vascular ulcers. They state: "[T]he nature of bacterial flora is determined by host factors and by the interaction of microorganisms."[18] Staphlococci is the name of a family of microorganisms (i.e., *Staphylococcus aureus, S. albus, S. epidermidis*) that are among the most common causes of localized suppurative infections. Streptococci is the family name of a strain of bacteria containing four groups: pyrogenic, viridans, enterocccos, and lactic. These organisms are considered natural flora of the upper respiratory and intestinal tract.[20] *Escherichia coli,* and *Proteus mirabilis* are other common micrococci isolated from wound cultures in predominant numbers.

Clinically, infected wounds have a series of objective findings. Purulent drainage combined with erythema, an increase in skin temperature, and often a pungent odor are characteristic signs noted by the clinician. One of the more classical odors, seldom forgotten by the clinician, is that of the microorganism *Pseudomonas aeruginosa,* often cultured in extensive open wounds due to burns. Management of an infected, open wound requires the cooperation of physician and many health care providers, including the physical therapist. Initially, the physician obtains a culture of the wound and sends the specimen immediately to the microbiology/pathology laboratory for analysis. The laboratory report identifies the predominant organism and suggests the most effective antibacterial agent to control its spread. Common antibiotic drugs prescribed by the physician include ampicillin, penicillin, tetracycline, polymyxin B, and streptomycin.

Local wound management begins with referral to physical therapy. Hydrotherapy, using an appropriate antiseptic solution aids in cleansing and debriding the cavity of the wound. Two of the more common antiseptic solutions currently used are concentrations of povodone-iodine and sodium hypochlorite. Water temperatures are maintained between 22.4 and 22.6°C, and duration of treatment is usually no longer than 20 minutes. Further debridement of the wound can be accomplished either mechanically or chemically. Common methods of mechanical debridement include careful removal of adherent dressings, selected scraping and cutting of necrotic tissue, or use of hydrophilic pellets (Debrisan) combined with high-pressure water (Waterpik) to remove adherent exudate. Chemical debridement involves use of topical enzymatic ointments (Travase, Collagenase), which are purported to assist in removal of necrotic tissue by interfering with the polypeptide bonds that secure protein-laden areas of eschar. Use of these enzymatic debriders early in the course of eschar removal is sometimes recommended.

Following achievement of adequate debridement, a thin layer of a broad-spectrum, topical antibacterial ointment (Bacitracin, Neosporin) may be placed either on the dressing or carefully on the wound with a sterile tongue depressor. Finally, a clean bandage of gauze padding applied over the wound site and secured with a gauze wrap (Kerlix, Kling) allows wound drainage and protection. Further examples of preferred dressing techniques include wet-to-dry saline, acetic-acid soaks, dry dressings, and Unna's paste boot.

The objective of a double-barreled approach (local and systemic) to wound management of an infected lesion is facilitation of healing by secondary intention.

Viral Infections

One of the most common viral infections of the skin are verrucae, epidermal tumors caused by a papillomavirus and more commonly known as warts. Approximately 70 percent of verrucae diagnosed occur around the fingers and hands and are referred to as common warts. Roughly 24 percent of the remaining verrucae occur on the feet and are diagnosed as plantar warts.[19] These plantar warts require an incubation period of approximately 4 months, which makes identification of the innoculation mechanism quite difficult. These lesions characteristically occur in young children and adults, with peak incidence noted between the ages of 12 to 16 years. Females appear to have a higher incidence.

One of the most popular environmental factors historically associated with the occurrence of these lesions is a personal history of barefoot walking around public bath houses, gymnasiums, and health spas.[3] The actual process of innoculation has been postulated to be similar to the mechanism responsible for fungal infection. A break in the epidermis due to trauma allows invasion of the microorganisms into the skin matrix, thereby providing an avenue for viral infection. Plantar warts are generally classified according to size and configuration. Single warts are the most common lesions reported and appear as callused masses 1 to 2 cm in diameter located on the plantar surface of the foot. Mother-daughter satellite warts are a small group (fewer than 10) of single warts that appear clustered around a larger 2- to 3-cm "mother" formation. Mosaic warts, least common, are a collection (more than 20) of plantar warts occupying a large area on the plantar surface of the foot. Occasionally, plantar warts are identified between the toewebs and are subsequently misdiagnosed as tinea pedis.

Clinically, single plantar warts display the same characteristic appearance as hard corns. Several distinguishing factors can assist the clinician in differentiating between the two lesions, however. The first of these factors is the age of the patient. Plantar warts generally occur in the pubescent patient population, whereas hard corns are primarily noted in middle-aged and elderly populations. A second factor involves the location of the lesion. Hard corns are the direct result of abnormal pressure occurring typically over a bony prominence. Plantar warts can be identified at any point along the plantar surface of the foot because they grow in response to the innoculation of the papovavirus and do not require a pressure stimulus. Plantar warts are extremely sensitive to squeezing, whereas hard corns are more sensitive to direct pressure. Finally, once the callous cap is removed by careful paring, the appearance of the nucleus of the hard corn and plantar wart differ remarkably. The hard corn has a homogeneous core that can be removed easily without bleeding by the proper curettage technique. Conversely, the core of the plantar wart often displays a collection of small red and black dots. These dots represent the tips of capillary loops, some viable and some thrombosed, that supply the blood necessary for wart formation. As the wart matures, the core develops a cauliflower-like appearance that is easily identified. Curettage of this lesion often results in profuse bleeding with potential spread of the virus.

Following diagnosis of the lesion as a plantar wart, some physicians choose the more conservative approaches to treatment. One method consists of no treatment, in anticipation of spontaneous regression of the wart. One author has suggested that 30 percent of these lesions will regress spontaneously over a period of 3 to 6 months.[3] Other authors agree, but suggest a slightly longer period of 6 to 8 months.[12] Another conservative approach includes use of a 40 percent salicylic acid plaster left in contact with the wart for approximately 4 days. Following removal of the plaster, the white, macerated tissue is carefully pared to skin level and reexamined in 2 weeks. If the wart persists, the process is repeated a second and sometimes a third time. A third conservative approach to treatment of plantar warts has been the use of ultrasound as described by a few authors.[21-24] The general procedure followed by physical therapists in the administration of this treatment includes softening of the hyperkeratotic tissue by prior application of 40 percent salicylic acid plaster or hydrotherapy, and gentle paring of the hyperkeratotic tissue with a #10 scalpel blade to a point at which capillary tips are visible but not bleeding.

Administration of Ultrasound (Underwater)

The use of underwater ultrasound is preferred because of the water's unique transmission qualities and resultant patient comfort during the treatment period. Recommended levels of intensity range between 1.0 and 1.5 W/cm^2, for a period of 10 to 15 minutes.[21-24] The face of the transducer should be held stationary over the wart at a distance of approximately 1 inch. Occasional intolerance to the intensity may be relieved by increasing the distance between transducer and skin to 2 inches or by decreasing the power output. Frequency of treatments range between 2 to 15 patient visits over a 6- to 8-week period.[21-23]

For the persistent wart, wart excision and tissue destruction are among the next objectives of treatment attempted by the physician. Minor surgery, cryosurgery, electrosurgery, and laser surgery are procedures presently practiced by physicians to remove chronic verrucae. Minimal incision surgery consists of injection of a local anesthetic at the periphery of the wart followed by curettage using either a #15 scalpel blade or small curette. Cryosurgical procedures include use of carbon dioxide ($-78°C$) nitrous oxide ($-88°C$) or liquid nitrogen ($-190°C$) applied with special applicators directly to the wart. Electrosurgery requires an apparatus capable of producing waveforms between 50 and 500,000 cps at 250-1,800 V. the transformer produces bursts of high-frequency current necessary for coagulation, dessication, or fulguration of the wart. All these procedures result in tissue destruction with eventual necrosis. This necrotic tissue will ultimately form a line of demarcation, develop into a firm eschar, and slough, leaving a small area of scarring. In some cases, thick scarring may result, leading to a more lasting problem for the patient. Overall, these procedures are often painful and require a certain period of convalescence prior to full weightbearing on the affected site. Failure of these methods risks recurrence of the original lesion and possible formation of additional verrucae.

More recent treatment procedures advertised by podiatrists include use of laser therapy. This modality is used in the treatment of multiple foot lesions, including plantar warts, and is purported to result in less residual scarring.

Ulcers

Ulcerations of the lower extremities represent some of the more common referrals to the physical therapy department for open wound management. The reason for these referrals often represents the physician's attempt at conservative management of an existing, chronic lesion.

Various assessment techniques are used by the referring physician in differential diagnosis of chronic ulcerations. Examples of some of these testing procedures include the following:

Doppler examination of arterial and venous systems
Impedance plethysmography
Photoplethysmography
Ambulatory venous pressure
Venography
Arteriography
Oscillography
Thermography
Radionucleotide studies

Lower extremity ulcers involving the lower leg, foot, or toes may be due to a variety of internal or external causes and are often classified according to the pathological disease process (Table 7-1). Traditional physical therapy methods have included use of hydrotherapy, debridement, occlusive dressings and, in some cases, iontophoresis. Today, in addition to these traditional methods of management, the physical therapist has added newer methods of wound management including:

Eschar removal using proteolytic enzyme debriders
Use of hyperbaric oxygen
Exudate removal using hydrophilic pellets and high-pressure water
Application of total contact plaster casts
Fabrication of custom-molded foot orthotics
Modification of shoe structure
Patient education of disease processes and methods of prevention

The more common types of ulcerations referred to the physical therapy department are listed under the following categories:

Trauma: ischemic ulceration caused by external pressure. (low pressure over prolonged time) Example: decubitus ulcer.

Table 7-1. Classification of Ulcers of the Leg According to Causal Mechanism

I. External	a) Macroglobulinemia
A. Primary	b) Cryoglobulinemia
1. Trauma	C. Metabolic
2. Decubitus (trophic) ulcers	1. Diabetes mellitus
3. Neurotic excoriations; factitious	2. Gout
B. Secondary to a predisposing lesion	D. Autoimmune diseases
1. Burns (thermal and chemical)	1. Necrotizing angiitides
2. Radiodermatitis	2. Lupus erythematosus
3. Neoplasms	3. Scleroderma
II. Internal	4. Rheumatoid arthritis
A. Vascular diseases	5. Polyarteritis nodosa
1. Arterial	6. Pyoderma gangrenosum
a) Arteriosclerotic	E. Granulomas
b) Hypertensive ischemic	1. Microbiological
c) Thromboangiitis obliterans	a) Syphilis
d) Livedo reticularis	b) Erythema induratum
2. Venous	c) Atypical mycobacterial
a) Stasis	d) Leprosy
b) Thrombophlebitis	e) Deep fungal infections
B. Blood dyscrasias	2. Drugs
1. Anemias (heritable)	a) Halides
a) Sickle cell	III. Miscellaneous
b) Thalassemia	A. Acrodermatitis chronica atrophicans
c) Congenital hemolytic	B. Atrophie blanche
2. Dysproteinemia	

(Samitz M, Dana A: Cutaneous Lesions of the Lower Extremities. p. 154. JB Lippincott, Philadelphia, 1971.)

Vascular: ischemic ulceration caused by internal vascular dysfunction. Examples: venous stasis ulcer and arteriosclerotic ulcer.

Metabolic: neurotrophic ulceration caused by loss of sensation. Example: diabetic ulcer.

Trauma

Decubitus ulcers represent an ischemic response to abnormal, prolonged pressure over a bony prominence. In the lower extremity, they occur principally over the lateral malleoli, the lateral aspect of the fifth MTH, and the posterior heel. Geriatric patients and patients who are confined to a bed for prolonged periods of time tend to develop these chronic lesions. In the early stages of decubitus development, there is often a well-circumscribed area of redness over the bony prominence. If this area of pressure is not relieved, it will progress eventually to a full-thickness, necrotic ulceration that will require a long time and great effort to achieve complete healing. Physicians are keenly aware of the early signs of decubitus ulcer formation but often it is the nurse or physical therapist who initially discovers these early signs of abnormal pressure. Careful inspection of bony prominences of the lower extremities during bedside exercise programs assists in identification of a potential problem.

Early pressure relief can be achieved through several methods. Repositioning of the extremities every 2 hours is a traditional approach practiced by nurses; owing to the numerous other responsibilities required of nurses, however, this approach is often unrealistic. Positioning of the extremities with foam blocks, intravenous (IV) bags, blankets, or multipodis boots (L'nard Associates, Inc. 12087 62nd Street North Largo, FL 33541) are also used extensively at many institutions. Other techniques involve use of a specially designed bed in which air, water, or sand is constantly redistributed in an attempt to counteract these pressures. Whichever method is used, the objectives remain the same: early identification of a potential problem followed by use of pressure-relieving methods to prevent decubitus formation.

Unsuccessful attempts at pressure relief can result in decubitus formation. In the early stages of decubitus development, only a slight erythema may be noted over bony prominences. In the latter stages, a full-thickness ulceration develops, appearing as a circumscribed area of necrotic tissue that is leathery and very adherent to underlying tissue. Infection and osteomyelitis are sometimes complicating factors involved in more progressive lesions. Physical therapists have used proteolytic enzyme debriders, hydrotherapy, hyperbaric oxygen, and even iontophoresis to remove eschar and promote formation of granulation tissue of decubitus ulcers.

Vascular

Venous stasis ulcers are among the most common vascular lesions treated by physical therapists. These ulcers are located almost exclusively over the distal-medial aspect of the lower leg, just superior to the medial melleolus. Physiologically, they occur as a result of valvular incompetency and loss of vessel elasticity of the superficial and deep venous system.[25,26] Primarily affected are the perforating veins which serve as the communicating system between the deep and superficial veins.[27]

Initial clinical signs of venous stasis include dependent edema of the lower extremity, which if left untreated produces an area of hyperpigmentation over the distal-medial lower leg. Associated symptoms include pruritis, leading to scratching and excoriation of the involved area.[28] This process results in the development of a partial thickness ulceration, often located just superior to the medial malleolus. The lesion, if not infected, is generally not painful. The base of the ulcer is often pink with healthy granulation tissue, but because of venous insufficiency and resultant edema, wound healing becomes a chronic problem.

Early educational intervention during the initial stages of venous stasis can prove effective in prevention of ulceration. Emphasizing the detrimental effects of prolonged standing together with recommendations for frequent elevation of both lower extremities is very helpful. Encouragement to wear pressure gradient stockings on a daily basis is also strongly advised. Instruction in daily lower extremity exercise to assist in venous return should also be suggested to these patients.

For patients who are referred to the physical therapy department with an existing venous stasis ulcer, the principles of open wound management previously discussed should be initiated immediately. Hydrotherapy followed by mechanical debridement of necrotic tissue and the application of a clean, moist dressing is generally recommended until a base of viable, granulation tissue is established. Next, an occlusive dressing is applied directly over the ulcer in combination with some form of pressure gradient support. Recommendations include the application of an Ace bandage in a figure-eight fashion or the fitting of a properly sized antiembolic stocking.

Historically, a commercially prepared bandage (Dome Paste Unna Boot, Dome Division, Miles Laboratories 400 Morgan Lane West Haven, CT 06576) has been used quite extensively and proven effective in promoting wound closure by secondary intention.[28] This procedure requires a certain expertise in application and repeated removal and reapplication every 7 to 10 days until complete healing has been achieved. It has the advantage of allowing the patient to remain ambulatory, thus facilitating muscle contraction and venous return. Other forms of occlusive dressings that are presently being used in management of venous stasis ulcers are referred to as oxygen-permeable (Op-Site) and oxygen-impermeable hydrocolloid (HC) dressings (Duo-derm). Clinical reports indicate that these dressings assist in promotion of granulation tissue and reepithelialization by providing a moist wound environment.[29]

Resistant venous stasis ulcers may ultimately require surgical intervention. Reconstructive venous valve surgery, axillary vein transfer, vein stripping, and possible skin grafting are procedures that accomplish primary wound closure.[26,27] Regardless of whether conservative or surgical procedures are practiced, these patients will continue to require external, pressure gradient support of both lower extremities together with encouragement of home programs emphasizing elevation and exercise of their legs.

Arteriosclerotic Ulcers

Arteriosclerotic ulcers represent an ischemic response of soft tissue to an underlying occlusive arterial disease.[30] This occlusion interferes with the normal blood flow responsible for providing necessary oxygenation and nutrition of distal tissue. The precipitating mechanism is usually some form of external trauma to the anterior/distal aspect of the lower leg or foot, causing a break in the skin. Ordinarily, this break would heal by secondary intention but, because of the underlying occlusive disease, the injury progresses to a point of delayed healing and eventual ulceration.

Examination of the area will often reveal a pale, cold extremity with diminished or absent arterial pulses. The ulcer often appears as a deep cavitation with a yellow, gray necrotic base. These ulcers are characteristically very painful and may be located at any point along the lower leg or foot. Primary sites of ulceration are often noted over the distal toes, heels, and lateral aspect of the lower leg.

Hypertensive ulcers represent an ischemic response of soft tissue to underlying occlusive arteriolar disease. These ulcers are primarily seen in women with longstanding essential hypertension in their fifth through seventh decade of life.[31] These lesions are also seen in patients diagnosed with certain connective tissue diseases such as rheumatoid arthritis and suspected lupus erythematosus. The suspected cause of the ischemia is the development of small atheromatous emboli that result in the compromised blood flow of the arterioles. In contrast to the arterialsclerotic ulcer, examination of the patient with a hypertensive ulcer reveals normal skin color and arterial pulses. The hypertensive ulcer, however, is similar in appearance and is often located along the postero-lateral aspect of the lower leg. As are arterial sclerotic ulcers, these ulcers are very painful.

Physical therapy of arterial/arteriolar ulcers requires careful removal of adherent eschar through the combined use of hydrotherapy, proteolytic enzymes, and mechanical debridement. Once the eschar has been removed, attempts at localized vasodilatation can be accomplished under controlled conditions. Hyperbaric oxygen has also been used with favorable results.[32] Contraindications in the treatment of arterial ulcers include elevation of the lower extremities for prolonged periods or the use of occlusive dressing because such procedures could promote further vascular compromise.

Medically, attempts are made to control diastolic hypertension through the use of oral vasodilators. Surgically, resistant ulcerations may require sympathectomy, percutaneous transluminal balloon dilatation or arterial reconstruction in an attempt to reestablish adequate arterial blood flow.[33]

Metabolic

Chronic metabolic imbalances in the human body often result in major neurocirculatory changes. One of these changes involves the progressive development of peripheral neuropathies involving the hands and feet. Specifically, these individuals develop impaired cutaneous sensation and lose their ability not only to distinguish but to react to certain noxious external stimuli.

The patient with diabetes mellitus in poor control often displays such characteristic neuropathic changes, developing decreased peripheral sensation as a result of deficiencies of diffusion across the pathologically thickened membranes of capillary and postcapillary venule beds.[33] Diabetic ulcers of the foot are among the most common lesions indirectly caused by the neurotrophic changes that occur in peripheral neuropathies. The foot of the diabetic patient becomes "insensitive" to those daily, repetitive forces, "which if not adjusted to anatomically, can summate to form an ulceration."[34] These "painless" ulcers usually occur over the plantar aspect of the metatarsal heads (MTHs) and are the result of a combination of impaired cutaneous sensation and compressive loading over bony prominences. Unfortunately, these ulcers remain undetected by the patient until they have developed into full-thickness lesions. Because of this late detection, the ulcers are often further complicated by microbial infection and in some cases develop osteomyelitis. Inability to establish homeostasis of the metabolic state and failure of topical wound care can result in amputation of the affected limb.

Physical therapists working with diabetic patients need to exercise extreme care in several areas of clinical practice. The therapist should review the patient's chart daily to monitor glucose level changes. A diabetic patient "not in control" of the diabetic state will not respond favorably to local wound care.

The temperature of the water in the hydrotherapy tank should never rise above 22.4°C. At no time should the therapist apply adhesive tape to the skin during application of a dressing. The use of astringents such as isopropyl alcohol for skin or wound cleansing should be strictly avoided.

Traditionally, physical therapists have been involved with topical wound management of diabetic ulcers. Hydrotherapy, irrigation, and packing of mal perforans ulcers and application of bulky, absorbant, protective dressings have been procedures practiced in the past. Currently, some therapists have been actively involved in the treatment of diabetic and other neuropathic ulcers with total-contact, plaster walking casts. Studies suggest that these cases are helpful in controlling edema, avoiding additional trauma, and allowing early ambulatory activity.[35]

If conservative management proves effective in wound healing, only part of the total problem has been solved. In the future, these patients continue to risk exacerbation of the same lesion. Use of a soft, custom-molded foot orthotic placed in extra-depth shoes will help prevent these recurrences. Education of the diabetic patient regarding the disease process and future care of the feet is imperative. Instruction emphasizing daily inspection of the plantar aspects of the feet, proper foot hygiene, and recommendations regarding proper footwear are essential. The diabetic patient is seldom fully cured, but rather is treated for a very fragile, metabolic disorder. Noncompliance or complacency regarding medical status can result in irreversible tissue destruction.

Toenail Lesions

Three of the more common toenail lesions seen clinically are ingrown toenails (onychocryptosis), fungal infected toenails (onychomycosis), and overgrown toenails (onychogryphosis). The degree to which physical therapists are involved in the treatment of these nail disorders varies considerably. Some physical therapists in the uniformed services have had the opportunity to participate directly in primary care of these patients by practicing such procedures as partial nail resection in the management of ingrown toenails. Other physical therapists are limited by either their knowledge, skills, or legal liability and usually refer these patients to podiatrists and orthopedic surgeons. I suggest that therapists interested in providing primary care for these disorders thoroughly review individual state regulations related to the practice of such services before initiating them.

Ingrown Toenails

European authors tend to use the term onychocryptosis to describe ingrowth of toenails whereas American authors seem to prefer the term paronychia.[36–38] Irrespective of terminology, ingrowth is one of the more painful and disabling disorders affecting the toenail.

Causes for this condition include congenital abnormalities and metabolic disorders but primarily trauma due to ill-fitting shoes. Ingrowing toenails characteristically involve the medial or lateral borders of the great toenail. In the early stages, an area of erythema is usually located along the border of the nail, which is made worse as a result of "bathroom surgery." This can progress to a point of ulceration between the toenail and adjacent skin, and eventually mimic the signs and symptoms that occur as a result of the body's response to a foreign body. Because of the abundance of microorganisms in this environment, these lesions are easily infected, causing associated symptoms of intense great toe pain.

Treatment in the early stages consists of identification and removal of the causative mechanism and topical treatment of the affected area. Warm soaks followed by a gentle cleansing of the area with a topical antiseptic solution is followed by application of a thin layer of antibacterial ointment placed between the nail and skin border.

Treatment in the latter stages in which the ingrown toenail reveals signs of infection can become complicated, and referral to other medical professionals should be considered. A few of the procedures practiced by physicians to accomplish ablation of this problem include partial or total toenail resection with phenolization to destroy the nail matrix. Those procedures require the proper clinical environment, anesthesia, and surgical instruments to accomplish the task of partial or total toenail removal. Graphic descriptions of these methods are clearly presented in the literature for those individuals interested in the techniques.[38,39]

Onychomycosis

Fungal infected toenails, although seldom symptomatic, present as chronic hyperkeratotic deformities of the nail plate. These toenails become yellow, thickened, and brittle with age and are often bothersome when shoes with shallow toeboxes are worn. Cosmetically, the appearance of these nails is probably the most disturbing. Although not generally considered a medical emergency, the potential for ulceration and gangrenous changes under these nails in an individual with a history of diabetes or peripheral vacular disease should be acutely recognized.

Trichophyton rubrum, Trichophyton interdigital, and *Trichophyton mentagrophytes* are dermatophytes isolated in the development of this order.[40] The actual mechanism of infection is not clearly understood, but these infections begin at the distal edge of the nail and progress posteriorly to the nail bed.[3] Conservative treatment of this condition involves careful trimming of the distal toenail to a point even with the free margin of the nail. Careful horizontal filing of the toenail can then be carried out manually to decrease the thickness of the nail plate. At times, stabilization of the toenail with the therapist's other hand is necessary to prevent excessive medial lateral movement of the nail. At no time should the patient experience pain during the filing procedure. More aggressive methods include use of topical fungicides such as miconazole tincture or systemic administration of griseofulvin.[41,42] Although effective, these methods require regular administration of the particular drug over time. Problems with compliance and patient cooperation become complicating factors in the resolution of this chronic nail deformity.

Onychogryphosis

Onychogryphosis is the term associated with overgrowth of toenails. These lesions are sometimes referred to clinically as "ram's horn deformities" and are often seen in the geriatric population. Factors associated with the development of these deformities include a history of blunt trauma to the toenail, onychomycosis, or omission of regular trimming of the toenails. Nutritional deficiencies have also been identified.[43] As previously noted with onychomycosis, these nail deformities are generally not painful unless subjected to some form of external pressure on the nail plate, which then creates a concomitant pressure on the nail bed. These pressures predispose the underlying tissue to subsequent trauma and can result in ulceration. Extreme overgrowth of these nails can result in significant curvatures that cause the nail's free edge to penetrate the skin of the same or adjacent toe.

Conservative treatment of these deformities involves the same careful trimming and filing procedures described for onychomycosis but, because of the patient's age and possible history of peripheral vascular disease, great care is strongly recommended. More aggressive techniques practiced by physicians involve complete removal of the toenail, with calculated consideration given to the possibility of nail matrix destruction by phenolization.

AUTHOR'S NOTE

This chapter was written in the author's private capacity. No official support or endorsement by the United States Department of Health and Human Services is intended or should be inferred.

REFERENCES

1. Sauer G: Manual of Skin Diseases. 4th Ed. JB Lippincott, Philadelphia, 1980
2. Lever W, Lever G: Histopathology of the Skin. 6th Ed. JB Lippincott, Philadelphia, 1983
3. Samitz M, Dana A: Cutaneous Lesions of the Lower Extremities. JB Lippincott, Philadelphia, 1977
4. Marples M: The Ecology of the Human Skin. Charles C. Thomas, Springfield, IL, 1965
5. Rassner G, Kahn G: Atlas of Dermatology with Differential Diagnosis. Urban and Schwarzenberg, Baltimore, 1983
6. Beavan D, Brooks S: Color Atlas of the Nail in Clinical Diagnosis. Year Book Medical Publishers, Chicago, 1984
7. Bonar L, Dreyer A: Studies on ringworm funguses with reference to public health problems. Am J Pub Health 22:909, 1932

8. Berberian D: Dermatophytoses of feet. Sources and methods of prevention of reinfection. Arch Dermatol Syphilol 38:367, 1938

9. Jamieson R: Ringworm of the feet. Shoes and slippers as a source of reinfection. Arch Dermatol Syphilol 44:837, 1941

10. Peck S, Botvinick I, Schwartz L: Dermatophytosis in industry. Arch Dermatol Syphilol 50:170, 1944

11. Baer R, Rosenthal S, Rogachefsky H, Litt J: Newer studies on the epidemiology of fungus infections of the feet. Am J Public Health 45:787, 1955

12. Adams I, Whiting M, Savin F, Branford W: Affections of the skin and tissues. pp 77. In Neale D (ed): Common Foot Disorders Diagnosis and Management. Churchill Livingstone, New York, 1981

13. Evans C, Smith W, Johnston E, Giblett E: Bacterial flora of the normal human skin. J Invest Dermatol 15:305, 1950

14. Arnold L, Gustafson C, Hull T, et al: The self disinfecting power of the skin as a defense against microbic invasion. Am J Hygiene 11:345, 1930

15. Pillsbury D, Rebell G: The bacterial flora of the skin. J Invest Dermatol 18:173, 1952

16. Rebell G, Pillsbury D, Saint Phalle M, Ginsburg D: Factors affecting the rapid disappearance of bacteria placed on the normal skin. J Invest Dermatol 14:247, 1950

17. Cenbleet T: Self-sterilizing powers of the skin. Arch Dermatol Syphilol 28:526, 1934

18. Friedman S, Gladstone J: The bacterial flora of peripheral vascular ulcers. Arch Dermatol 100:29, 1969

19. Roberts SOB, Rook A: Bacterial infections, p. 541. In Rook A, Wilkenson D, Ebling F (eds): Textbook of Dermatology Vol 2. Blackwell Scientific Publications, Oxford, 1979

20. Anonymous: Dorland's Illustrated Medical Dictionary, 25th ed. WB Saunders, Philadelphia, 1974

21. Kent H: Plantar wart treatment with ultrasound. Arch Phys Med Rehabil 40:15, 1959

22. Kent H: Warts and ultrasound. Arch Dermatol 100:79, 1969

23. Rowe R, Gray J: Ultrasound therapy of plantar warts. Arch Dermatol 82:1008, 1960

24. Cherup N, Urben J, Bender L: The treatment of plantar warts with ultrasound. Arch Phys Med Rehabil 44:602, 1963

25. Lofgren K: Stasis ulcer. Mayo Clin Proc 40:564, 1965

26. Raju S: Venous insufficiency of the lower limb and stasis ulceration. Changing concepts and management. Ann Surg 197:688, 1983

27. Cockett F, Dodd H: The Pathology and Surgery of the Veins of the Lower Limb. Churchill Livingstone, London, 1976

28. Beninson J: Stasis dermatitis and leg ulcers. Postgrad Med 524, 1964

29. Friedman S, Su W: Management of leg ulcers with hydrocolloid occlusive dressing. Arch Dermatol 120:1329, 1984

30. Hines E: The differential diagnosis of chronic ulcer of the leg. Circulation 27:989, 1963

31. Spittell J: Diagnosis and management of leg ulcers. Geriatrics 38:57, 1983

32. Heng M, Pilgrim J, Beck F: A simplified hyperbaric oxygen technique for leg ulcers. Arch Dermatol 120:640, 1984

33. Siperstein M: The relationships of carbohydrate derangements to the microangiopathies of diabetes. p. 81. In Cerasi E, Loft R (eds): Pathogenesis of Diabetes Mellitus. Wiley Interscience, New York, 1969

34. Brand P, Bauman H, Girling J: Plantar pressures and trophic ulceration. J Bone Joint Surg [Br] 45:652, 1963

35. Mooney V, Wagner F: Neurocirculatory disorders of the foot. Clin Orthop Rel Res 122:53, 1977

36. Murray W: Onychocrytosis: Principles of non-operative and operative care. Clin Orthop Rel Res 142:96, 1979
37. Stone O, Mullins J: Chronic paronychia in children. Clin Pediatr 7:104, 1968
38. Lee T: The office treatment of simple paronychias and ganglions. Med Times 109:49, 1981
39. Robb T, Murray W: Phenol cauterisation in the management of ingrowing toenails. Scot Med J 27:236, 1982
40. Meyer J, Grundmann H, Schnyder U: Onychomycosis (trichophyton mentagrophytes) A scanning electron microscopic observation. J Cutaneous Pathol 8:342, 1981
41. Bentley-Phillips B: The treatment of onychomycosis with miconazone tincture. S Afr Med J 62:57, 1982
42. Davies R, Everall J, Hamilton E: Mycological and clinical evaluation of griseofulvin for clinic onychomycosis. Br Med J 3:464, 1967
43. Adams I, Smidt L: Nail disorders. p 103. In Neale E (ed): Common Foot Disorders Diagnosis and Management. Churchill Livingstone, New York, 1981

APPENDIX 1

Characteristics of Skin Lesions

Abscess–A localized collection of pus in a cavity formed by disintegration of tissues.

Denudation–Removal of the epithelial covering from any surface by surgery, trauma, or pathological change.

Erosion–A gradual breakdown or very shallow ulceration of the skin that involves only the epidermis and heals without scarring.

Excoriation–Any superficial loss of substance such as that produced on the skin by scratching.

Fissures–Any cleft, line, or groove due to loss of continuity of the skin without any loss of substance.

Fistula–Any abnormal passage or communication, usually between two organs.

Macule–A discolored spot on the skin that is not elevated above the surface.

Nodule–A small boss (rounded eminence) or node that is solid and can be detected by touch.

Papule–A small circumscribed, superficial, solid elevation of the skin.

Scales–Thin compacted platelike areas of cornified epithelial cells on the surface of the body.

Scar–A mark remaining after the healing of a wound or other morbid process.

Sinus–An abnormal channel or fistula permitting the escape of pus.

Tumor–A new growth of tissue in which the multiplication of cells is uncontrolled and progressive; also called neoplasm.

Ulcer–A local defect or excavation of the surface of an organ or tissue produced by sloughing of inflammatory necrotic tissue.

Vesicle–A small (less than 1 cm in diameter) blister; a small circumscribed elevation of the epidermis containing a serous liquid.

Wheal–A smooth, slightly elevated area on the body surface that is redder or paler than the surrounding skin.

Dorland's Illustrated Medical Dictionary, 25th Ed. WB Saunders, Philadelphia, 1974.

8 | The Foot in Athletics

Thomas G. McPoil
Trudy Culotta McGarvey

The joints of the ankle and foot are frequently injured in sports activities. An understanding of the anatomic structure and the biomechanical functions of these joints is required if the physical therapist expects to rehabilitate successfully injuries occurring in this region. The purpose of this chapter is to discuss sports injuries of the foot and ankle frequently encountered in the physical therapy clinic. The chapter is divided into two parts: the first section covers acute injuries and the second portion deals with chronic or overuse injuries. Each injury is discussed in regard to etiology, symptoms, evaluative findings, and treatment. Although it is not the purpose of this chapter to discuss foot biomechanics and evaluative techniques, references to these areas are made when necessary to discuss specific injuries.

ACUTE INJURIES

Biomechanical Implications

Injuries to the ankle joint complex, especially those involving ligamentous structures (sprains) are the most frequent type of acute injury in athletics.[1] The ankle joint complex, as defined by Brunnstrom[2] comprises the talocrural joint (upper ankle joint) and the subtalar joint (lower ankle joint). Approximately 90 percent of all ankle complex sprains occur laterally, involving the fibular collateral ligaments.[3] The ligaments most often involved in a lateral sprain of the ankle joint complex are the anterior talofibular and the calcaneofibular ligaments.

The lateral sprain usually occurs while the athlete is recovering from a jump, pivoting, or cutting while running. In these types of activities, due to a plantarflexed and slightly supinated position of the ankle joint complex, the anterior talofibular ligament is nearly vertical to the line of stress and is best suited to resist inversion.[4] Inman[5] has stated that in plantarflexion the anterior talocrural ligament plays a major role in restricting talar tilt within the mortise. Thus, forced supination of the ankle joint complex, while in plantarflexion, will place the anterior talofibular ligament in a position in which it alone must resist the imposed force. At this point, the calcaneofibular ligament, because of its downward and backward course, is more horizontal and less susceptible to injury. If the imposed force is severe, the anterior talofibular ligament will be torn and increased supination will occur. With this increased supination, the calcaneofibular ligament moves anteriorly and assumes a more vertical position. Should the force be extreme, supination and dorsiflexion will continue, causing the calcaneofibular ligament to rupture. If the force creating the injury is severe enough to rupture the calcaneofibular ligament, marked instability of the ankle joint complex will occur since this is the only ligament providing support to both the upper and lower ankle joints.[4,6]

Another important consideration in biomechanical factors involving injuries to the ankle joint complex is the action of the triceps surae muscle group. Aside from its function as a plantarflexor of the talocrural joint, the insertion of the Achilles tendon in relation to the subtalar joint axis causes the calf muscles to act as supinators of the subtalar joint.[7] Flexibility in this muscle group is extremely important because a lack of normal range of motion (ROM) could predispose the ankle joint complex to a position of plantarflexion and supination. This is discussed further in the section on prevention of ankle injuries.

EVALUATION PROCEDURES

Field Evaluation Techniques

The following sections consist of evaluation techniques, both general and in the field. Although most injuries of the foot and ankle are not life threatening, it is the responsibility of the sports therapist to provide emergency aid if needed. The first and most critical step of the primary evaluation on the field consists of a general assessment of the athlete's consciousness and vital signs. An athlete who is unconscious but stable should be immediately transported to the emergency room on a spinal board. In this instance, a spinal fracture is assumed until it is medically ruled out.

On the field evaluation of a conscious, stable athlete continues with a rapid, superficial examination of the location and nature of the injury prior to removal from the playing environment. The following signs are indicative of a fracture:

1. Exposed bony fragments or presence of bony deformity
2. Splinting or guarding of the injured region
3. Immediate localized edema and ecchymosis

4. Localized bony point tenderness
5. Loss of neurovascular status

Proper immobilization is essential with any of these signs, and emergency care is indicated.

General

In keeping with the standards of the medical profession, evaluation of the foot and ankle should follow in a logical and organized manner. The subjective-objective-assessment-plan (SOAP) note affords this and is recognized universally. The first step is to identify the location of the problem accurately. Patients are asked their chief complaint.

The second step is to obtain an accurate history. This is easily performed by asking the patient the following questions: When did you first notice pain? Did you injure it in any way? If so, what happened or how did it happen? Did you hear anything snap, pop, or tear? Did you notice immediate pain or swelling or was it delayed? Do you have any numbness or tingling? Do you have any previous history of trauma or injury to this area? If so, what was your course of treatment and did your symptoms resolve? What particularly increases or decreases your pain?

The evaluation process continues with the objective portion of the SOAP note, beginning with a general inspection of the involved ankle and foot. Observe for gross bony deformities indicative of a fracture and the immediate need for x-ray studies and immobilization. Continue inspection of the foot and ankle by noting the presence of swelling, ecchymosis, erythema, effusion, and evidence of splinting of surrounding muscles, all of which are indicative of a soft tissue lesion. Inspect the skin for cuts, abrasions, blisters, and/or open areas. Palpate the general area for heat and evidence of muscle splinting.

The objective portion of the evaluation continues with observation of the standing posture. Note any abnormalities, and record passive and active ROM of the foot and ankle. Passive supination and pronation of the subtalar joint is of particular value since this motion stretches the lateral and medial collateral ligaments, respectively. The tibiofibular ligament is stretched with passive inversion and eversion of the heel. Following ROM tests, assess the strength of the muscles crossing the ankle and foot.

Also included in the objective portion of the evaluation is a check of the neurovascular status of the lower extremity. Based on the above findings, several special tests for ligamentous stability may be indicated and are addressed later in this chapter. The objective portion is concluded with specific ligamentous, muscular, and bony palpation.

The next section is your assessment of the problem. This should include short-term and long-term goals, as well as criteria for returning to athletic participation, if the patient is an athlete.

The treatment plan should include specific modalities for immediate symptomatic pain relief. This may constantly be changed based on your objective findings. Also included should be any type of immobilization for protection and exercises for rehabilitation.

SPECIFIC CONDITIONS

Toe

Turf Toe

Turf toe refers to great toe pain as a result of trauma from playing on an artificial surface. More accurately it involves a sprain, bursitis, or tendonitis of the first metatarsalphalangeal (MTP) joint. The first interphalangeal (IP) joint may or may not be involved. One consistent clinical picture of great toe pain and edema of the first MTP joint is evident. The injury usually is the result of a forced hyperextension of the first MTP joint occurring when an athlete steps quickly at high velocity and then cuts sharply, changing direction.[8] Causative factors include footgear inadequate to handle the varying degrees of pressure and friction or alternating play between natural grass and artificial turf.[9]

Turf toe is very disabling; treatment consists of ice, rest, antiinflammatories, and shoe modification. Great toe taping is helpful when the athlete returns to competition and can be done to prevent restriction of MTP joint abduction, flexion, or extension.

Foot

Blisters and Calluses

Blisters, usually the result of mechanical friction, begin with an exudate between the superficial skin layer and the underlying dermis. They most commonly are caused by friction from adhesive tape, improperly fitting shoes, and/or a wrinkle in the sock. Prevention is the best treatment, but once a blister has developed, treatment is essential to prevent infection.

Even though blisters are usually minor problems, the location can be debilitating. When they occur on a weightbearing surface the skin over the blister must be protected since this provides a natural environment for healing. Cleanse the blister and surrounding region with soap and water or an iodine solution and swab with alcohol. To relieve the pressure, a sterile hypodermic needle should be used to pierce through the skin so that gravity will assist in adequate drainage of the fluid.[10] To enhance healing further, an antibacterial ointment can be injected with a sterile hypodermic needle into the space between the superficial skin layer and the underlying dermis. A sterile dressing with additional antibacterial ointment should then be applied.

For the athlete to compete, additional padding and protection must be placed over the blistered region. To relieve pressure over the blister, felt do-nuts, foot pads with relief areas, felt, and/or soft padding may be used. If the blistered area will be covered by tape, vaseline applied to the donut or padding is helpful to eliminate further friction.

Calluses of the foot are secondary to a constant repetitive rubbing of a shoe over a bony prominence, which causes the piling up of keratin. The most common sites for callus are underneath the metatarsal heads (MTHs), over the dorsal aspect of the interphalangeal joint in claw toes, and over the os calsis.

The best treatment for calluses is to eliminate the abnormal friction or pressure. Preventing a muscular imbalance by use of orthotic, metatarsal pads, heel wedges, etc. will relieve the weight over the callus. Proper care of calluses by soaking, trimming with a callus razor, buffing with an emory board, and softening with lanolin, will enhance the tissue elasticity and may be beneficial with calluses.

Contusions

Contusions located on the dorsum of the foot are frequently caused by an external force. They occur as the result of someone or something landing directly on top of the foot. The complications of this type of trauma may include damage of the nerves, vascular supply, periosteum, tendons, and joints of the foot.[10] Dorsal foot contusions are extremely sensitive to palpation and may be ecchymotic, edematous, hemorrhagic, and painful with weightbearing.

Contusions of the plantar aspect of the foot occur underneath the MTHs or the heel. Anatomic factors of the foot and excessive weightbearing or pressure predisposes an athlete to this type of injury.

Instep bruises frequently occur in the athlete with an extremely high arch and tightness of the gastrocsoleus complex. The heel cord tightness decreases the amount of dorsiflexion available, and the elasticity of the forefoot is dimin-ished. Therefore, with weightbearing, the pressure is transmitted on to the MTHs. Severe contusions of the MTHs is common, especially underneath the first MTH because of the excessive stress against the sesamoids.

Heel bruises frequently occur in hurdlers, long or triple jumpers, and basketball players. Repetitive loading of the heel ruptures the fibrous septa between the skin and the undersurface of the calcaneus. This causes crushing of the skin by the calcaneus since the fibrous fat pad of the heel is effectively "milked out."[11] The subcutaneous tissue lying between the thick plantar skin and muscle becomes ecchymotic and reacts with inflammation, forming the characteristic "stone bruise."[10]

Bruises of the heel and MTHs may develop into chronic inflammation of the periosteum. Early recognition of the acute process and management is essential. Ice and a pressure bandage should be used initially in the first 24 hours to control the inflammation effectively in conjunction with nonweight-bearing ambulation. Contrast baths, ultrasound under water, active ROM of the foot and ankle, and weightbearing when it can be performed pain-free should follow. The athlete should return to activity with the protection of a heel cup or taping with a foam rubber pad. These should be used as a preventive aid to stabilize the surrounding tissue and diffuse the force of trauma.

Strains

In compliance with the subcommittee on Athletic Nomenclature of the American Medical Association (AMA) Committee on Sports Medicine, a clear distinction between a strain and a sprain must be accepted. Structurally, the difference is that the muscle–tendon unit involves a motor element whereas a ligament primarily stabilizes.[10] Therefore, reference to a strain includes damage of the weakest link of the muscle–tendon unit and its bony attachment whereas a sprain includes ligamentous involvement.[12] Acute strains and sprains refer to an overstress, and chronic strains are secondary to overuse.

Plantar fascia strains of the foot usually occur in early training sessions in sports that require running. The plantar fascia is a broad dense band of connective tissue attaching to the under surface of the calcaneus and running the length of the sole of the foot. It functions to assist in maintaining stability of the foot and securing the longitudinal arch.

In normal standing, weightbearing is primarily on the heel and tension of the plantar fascia is minimal. The fascia tension is greatly increased with running however, since the weight is shifted onto the ball of the foot and forceful extension of the toes occurs to complete the pushoff phase. This powerful thrusting of the ball of the foot in running may cause tearing of the plantar fascia at its origin, causing an inflammatory response.

Initially, the athlete usually has localized tenderness on the plantar surface of the heel anterior to the calcaneal tubercles. Plantar fascia strains must be treated immediately to prevent the complication of a developing chronic longitudinal arch strain and a sprain of the spring ligament. Treatment consists of rest, ice, arch supports, taping, and exercises.

Fractures and Dislocations

Fractures of the foot are rare in athletics. The most vulnerable region of the foot, however, is the anterior region consisting of the metatarsals and phalanges. The most common fracture of the foot is the avulsion of the tendon of the peroneus brevis muscle from the base of the fifth metatarsal. This is sometimes referred to as a sprain-fracture since the mechanisms of injury are the same as for lateral ligament injury of the ankle and sprain occurs in conjunction.

Fractures of the foot and ankle classically present with pain, edema, localized tenderness, and increased pain with weightbearing. Diagnosis of fractures are confirmed by x-ray studies. Treatment is usually symptomatic for undisplaced fractures; ice, elevation, compression, and rest will decrease edema.

The form of immobilization depends on the area of the foot fractured and the condition of the surrounding structures. Plaster casts, posterior plaster splinting, taping, etc. are used to assure proper healing.

Ankle

The following information deals with the ankle, its injuries, and the importance of rehabilitation before the patient returns to athletic competition. The most common sports injury today is the ankle sprain. A sprain refers to damage of ligament fibers or its attachment from a violent force. Because the treatment of ligamentous injuries depends on the severity of trauma, evaluating the degree of injury is essential.

Sprains of the first degree are mild, easy to detect, and involve tearing of some of the ligamentous fibers without loss of stability.[8,10,12–14] Clinically, first-degree sprains evidence a minimum of edema, local tenderness, and pain. Therefore, treatment is usually symptomatic and consists of rest, ice, compression, and elevation. Ice will help break down the cycle of vessel spasm, reduce edema, and decrease pain but this will have no effect on the healing or strength of the ligament. Therefore, proper rehabilitative exercises and protective taping should be used.

Third-degree sprains are the most severe and cause total disruption of the ligament and loss of joint stability.[8,10,12–14] Clinically, the ankle is markedly edematous, hemorrhagic, tender, and painful, and abnormal motion is present on stress films. Treatment is controversial, but usually involves plaster immobilization for 6 to 8 weeks and/or surgical repair.

Ligamentous injuries that occur between these extremes are classified as second-degree sprains. These moderate sprains range from partial to almost complete avulsion of the ligament with some loss of function.[8,10,12–14]

Clinically, the ankle is moderately edematous, hemorrhagic, and painful, and local tenderness is present. Treatment is once again symptomatic, with nonweightbearing ambulation initially. Special emphasis should be placed on protection of the ankle from further trauma while promoting healing of the involved ligaments. Supportive dressings such as a posterior plaster splint, taping, an Unna boot, or a walking cast are essential.

Most ankle sprains occur as a result of an inversion stress with resulting lateral collateral ligament damage.[8,10,12–16]

Ankle joint instability correlates with the degree of ligamentous damage. Minimal instability occurs with a tear of the anterior talofibular ligament since it crosses the talocrural joint only. Marked instability of the ankle occurs with calcaneofibular ligament tears since it crosses both the subtalar and talocrural joint. Moreover, trauma to the calcaneofibular ligament is secondary to complete rupture of the anterior talofibular ligament.

Medial collateral ligament or deltoid ligament sprains are not as common. They usually occur as a result of a forceful eversion-external rotation stress. The pathomechanics, however, involve a high-velocity forced interal rotation of the tibia over a fixed usually dorsiflexed weightbearing foot. This causes the talus to be violently pushed against the lateral malleolus, stressing the deltoid ligament. This eversion force, depending on the severity, may also cause a fracture of the lower fibula or Pott's fracture. The same force may separate the fibula from the tibia by rupturing the tibiofibular ligament and widening the ankle mortise.

In addition to the standard evaluation of the foot and ankle, the following specific ankle joint stability stress tests are essential. In identifying the location and the severity of the injury, the anterior drawer test of the ankle identifies the integrity of the anterior talofibular ligament. The test is performed by placing one hand on the anterior aspect of the lower tibia and grasping the calcaneus with the palm of the other hand, and applying direct opposing forces.[17] If the talus subluxes anteriorly, the test is positive and indicates complete rupture and instability of the anterior talofibular ligament.

If the anterior drawer test is positive, a second stress test must be performed to check the lateral stability of the ankle. To check the integrity of the calcaneofibular ligament, the calcaneus is inverted. If the talus gaps and rocks in the ankle mortise, instability is present. The tilting of the talus within the mortise approximately 6 to 12° on an anterior-posterior view of an x-ray film is indicative of an isolated anterior talofibular ligament tear.[15] If on the same view, however, the talus opens between 12 and 30° laterally, the calcaneofibular ligament is also ruptured. Therefore, stress radiographs are essential in the clinical diagnosis of lateral collateral ligament sprains.

Achilles Tendon Injuries

A rupture of the Achilles tendon usually occurs with a violent contraction of the gastrocsoleus against resistance. The most frequent location for complete rupture is 1 to 2 inches above the tendoachilles insertion into the os calcis.[8,10,11,13] A sudden sharp pain and immediate loss of function is common with a rupture.

On physical examination, there is painful weightbearing, edema, ecchymosis, and tenderness over the tendoachilles. A defect or gap along the course of the Achilles tendon is usually palpable. Some active plantarflexion of the foot may be available, however. This is secondary to the normal function of the posterior tibialis, peroneals, and flexor muscles of the foot and ankle. Therefore, a special test to confirm the function of the tendoachilles—the Thompson test—should be performed. The patient kneels on a level surface with the feet hanging off the edge. The examiner then squeezes the patient's calf at its widest point; an involuntary plantarflexion of the foot is normal. Lack of plantarflexion with the Thompson test is indicative of a complete rupture of the Achilles tendon.

Even though conservative management of a complete rupture of the Achilles tendon is sometimes advocated, most authorities conclude that surgical repair is the treatment of choice for athletes.

Achilles tendinitis is an inflammation of the Achilles tendon and its surrounding synovium. This can be an acute or chronic condition and frequently occurs in athletes whose sports require running. Predisposing factors are very important in Achilles tendinitis: The primary factor is tightness of the gastrocsoleus complex. Other factors include tibia vara, cavus foot, subtalar varus, and forefoot varus.

The inflammatory response of the Achilles tendon results from trauma usually secondary to a lack of elasticity. Microtrauma or tiny tears of the Achilles tendon occur in sports requiring quick bursts of speed or may be the result of repetitive overuse. Clinically, the Achilles tendon is tender on palpation, edematous, and painful; crepitus may be felt with active motion. Resisted plantarflexion and passive stretching of the gastrocsoleus complex are uncomfortable.

Acute Achilles tendinitis treatment includes symptomatic relief with rest, ice, elevation, and protective taping, with the use of a heel lift to decrease the tension on the tendon. Active gastrocsoleus stretching is initiated when the patient is asymptomatic, and orthotics may be indicated if biomechanical abnormalities exist.

Most cases of acute Achilles tendinitis respond to conservative means. If the symptoms persist for 6 to 8 weeks, however, adhesions may form in the tendoachilles. Athletes with such adhesions will not only be unable to participate in sports, but will also have severe pain with ambulation, especially in climbing stairs. Therefore, chronic Achilles tendinitis requires immobilization in a short leg cast for approximately 4 weeks. Surgical repair is rare but may be necessary if the athlete is still symptomatic after removal of the short-leg cast or if symptoms recur with return to athletic competition.

Rehabilitation Considerations

Treatment

The rehabilitation process begins on the day of the injury with the ultimate goals of normal ROM, strength, and function of the foot and ankle. Functional criteria for returning to sports must follow the laws of specificity and be individualized based on the severity of the injury and the demands of the sport. Maintenance of an athlete's overall physical condition is vital and must be included in rehabilitation.

Rehabilitation of a foot and/or an ankle injury includes various types of modalities, exercises, and external supports. The usual progression of exercise begins with passive ROM, followed by active assisted and active ROM, and ends with resisted ROM exercises. Initially, the athlete may be nonweight-bearing; in this instance, swimming is an excellent mode for specific and overall conditioning. Once pain-free ROM is attained, strengthening is initiated. This can effectively be done using isometric, isotonic, and isokinetic exercises for the foot and ankle. The importance of eccentrically loading the foot and ankle with ambulation backwards, step ups and step downs backwards on a stool, and then progression to stairs should not be overlooked in the rehabilitation process. This is generally followed with jogging, running, figure-eights, cutting maneuvers, and activities specific to the sport performed pain-free. The athlete than returns to athletic competition with some type of preventive external support to the foot and/or ankle.

Prevention

The physical therapist's interaction with the athlete must go beyond evaluation with treatment and include preventive measures to reduce the risk of injury. In the past decade, preseason screening has proved an excellent tool for this purpose. In addition, recommendations regarding footwear, stretching, and prophylactic taping measures should be made available to the athlete.

Because the ankle joint complex is the area most frequently sprained during sports participation,[18] our discussion on prevention focuses on measures to prevent these injuries.

Stretching. McCluskey et al,[18] were one of the first groups to report the beneficial effects of calf muscle stretching to reduce ankle injuries. From their studies, they recommended that any athlete with less than 10° of dorsiflexion be placed on a stretching regimen. Ten degrees of dorsiflexion with the knee extended and the subtalar joint in a neutral position is the amount necessary for normal walking.[19] James[20] suggests that at least 15° of talocrural joint dorsiflexion is required in running. In considering the previously discussed point that the calf muscles are plantarflexors as well as supinators, it can be hypothesized that limited flexibility could predispose the ankle joint complex to a position leading to a lateral sprain.

Although dorsiflexion ROM is undoubtedly important, most techniques only emphasize maintaining the knee extended and ignore foot position. If the athlete's foot or lower extremity alignment causes the subtalar joint to pronate, increased mobility is created in the midtarsal joint. Thus, when calf muscle stretching is attempted while the subtalar joint is pronated, as tension develops in the Achilles tendon, if limitations in talocrural joint ROM exist, the mobile midfoot pronates or flattens. Only if the subtalar joint is maintained in a neutral position can an effective stretch be given specifically to the talocrural joint. To ensure that the subtalar joint is maintained in neutral, the athlete should either stretch in the orthotic device or place a lift (i.e., rolled washcloth or plywood) under the medial aspect of the foot to maintain a neutral position during stretching (Fig. 8-1). The athlete, maintaining the knee extended with a quadriceps set, may then perform the stretch.

Shoe considerations. For athletes with a previous history of ankle sprains, the high-top shoe appears to provide greater protection to the ankle joint complex than does the low-cut shoe. Garrett and Regua[21] reported, in a study

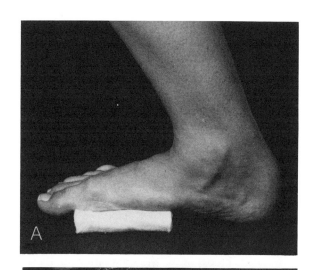

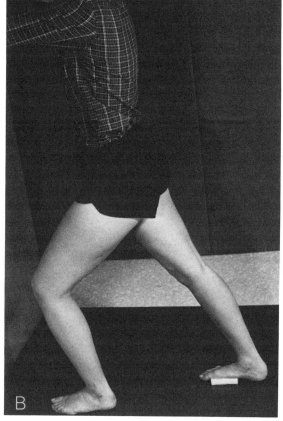

Fig. 8-1. Calf muscle stretching technique: (**A**) Lift placed under medial aspect of foot; (**B**) athlete performing stretch with knee extended.

involving more than 1,000 intramural athletes, that individuals using high-top shoes suffered fewer sprains than did athletes wearing low-cut shoes.

Preseason screening considerations.   The physical therapist, in performing a preseason screening examination, can evaluate several factors that could predispose the athlete to an ankle complex injury.

The athlete should demonstrate between 10 and 15° of talocrural joint dorsiflexion with the knee extended and the subtalar joint in neutral. Thus, modifications in ROM requirements may have to be made depending on the clientele being screened.

Certain foot types have also been shown to increase the athlete's chances of spraining the ankle joint complex. Weil et al,[16] reported that forefoot valgus and uncompensated rearfoot varus deformities play a role in the etiology of lateral sprains in basketball players. Schoenhaus and Jay[22] have also reported that the forefoot valgus foot type can lead to lateral sprains owing to a supinatory rock created during the contact phase of walking. The physical therapist can easily incorporate the evaluation of these foot types into the preseason screening.

Adhesive strapping.   For the past 20 years, the effectiveness of adhesive taping for the prevention of ankle and foot injuries has been controversial. Although numerous arguments have been made, the primary reason for questioning effectiveness has centered on research demonstrating that adhesive tape loses 50 to 60 percent of its supportive strength after 10 to 20 minutes of exercise. For an excellent review of the literature, the reader is referred to the manuscript by Metcalf and Denegar.[23] It must be assumed, however, from the available research that adhesive strapping, even after stretching with activity, can effectively restrict the *end* ROM (where injury occurs) and subsequently prevent injury.

Several important principles should be adhered to when applying tape to the athlete. These include:

1.   The anatomic joint to be supported should be appropriately positioned prior to the application of the tape. The athlete should also be instructed not to move from that position until the taping procedure is completed. In example, the ankle joint complex, being taped for an inversion sprain, should be positioned with the talocrural joint in neutral and the subtalar joint in slight eversion.

2.   When the athlete is taped, each piece of tape should overlap the previous strip by approximately $\frac{1}{4}$ to $\frac{1}{2}$ inch. This prevents tape separation with subsequent skin irritation and also increases the strength of the taping procedure.

3.   The clinician applying the tape must allow it to fit the natural shape of the anatomical structure, especially when applying linen nonelastic adhesive tape. Care must also be taken to apply the tape at angles that allow it to adapt to the normal body contours. Failure to do so will result in wrinkles and/or gaps in the tape, which can lead to dermal irritation.

4.   When maximum support is necessary, the adhesive tape should be

applied directly to the skin. It should be assumed that when foam or gauze prewraps are used, movement between the skin and taping base may occur.

Careful preparation of the athlete prior to the application of adhesive tape is extremely important to prevent possible skin irritation and to increase the support for the taping procedure. The steps for preparing the athlete for taping should include the following:

1. The skin should be cleansed with soap and water and then thoroughly dried. This removes perspiration and skin oils which prevent the tape from adhering properly to the skin surface.
2. All hair should be removed from the area to be taped. This prevents possible irritation to the hair follicle.
3. A commercial skin toughener (containing benzoin and resin) should be applied to the skin to offer protection as well as improved tape adherence.
4. To counteract skin breakdown secondary to the application of adhesive tape, especially in the Achilles tendon and instep areas, gauze pads or an underwrap of polyester/urethane foam should be used. The latter material is a thin, porous, lightweight substance that snugly fits the contours of the body, and foam prewraps are commonly used because of these important qualities.

Foot strapping techniques. As is discussed in the following section on overuse injuries, many of the foot problems treated by the physical therapist are secondary to abnormal pronation. Two techniques for taping the foot to prevent abnormal pronation are presented.

1. Low Dye taping technique. The low Dye taping technique was designed by Ralph Dye, D.P.M., in an attempt to provide functional mechanical support to the joints of the feet.[24]

Supplies:

1. Tape adherent
2. 1 or $1\frac{1}{2}$-inch tape (cloth)

Position of patient:

Leg completely extended with the talocrural joint in neutral and the subtalar joint slightly supinated.

Procedure:

1. A strip of 1 or $1\frac{1}{2}$-inch cloth tape is applied just proximal to the lateral aspect of the fifth MTH, wrapped around the posterior aspect of the calcaneus and attached just proximal to the medial aspect of the first MTH (Fig. 8-2).
2. Two more strips of tape are applied in the same direction and, on completion, the three strips of tape are contoured into the medial longitudinal arch.

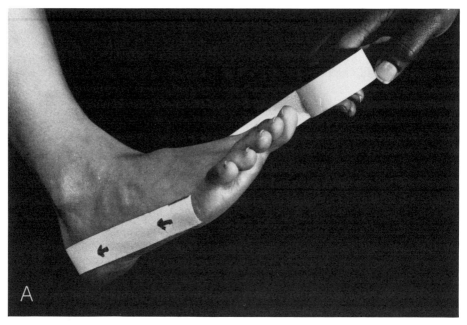

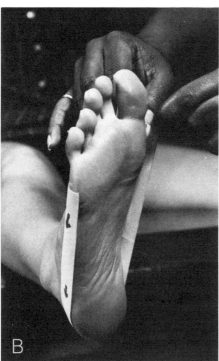

Fig. 8-2. Low Dye taping procedure: **(A)** tape applied to the fifth metatarsal head and wrapped around heel; **(B)** tape attached to the medial aspect of the first metatarsal head.

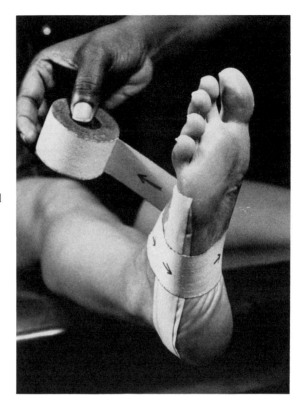

Fig. 8-3. Medial longitudinal arch support strip.

3. A longitudinal strip is now placed just distal to the prominence of the anterior tibial tendon on the dorsum of the foot. It is started on the lateral side of foot, brought around under the medial longitudinal arch, and then to the top of the instep (Fig. 8-3).

4. Two more strips are added in the same direction, overlapping approximately ½ inch. These strips give support to the medial longitudinal arch (Fig. 8-4).

2. Cross X technique

Supplies: Same as low Dye

Position of patient: Same as low Dye

Procedure:

1. A strip of tape is placed on the medial aspect of the first MTH and is taken posteriorly around the heel and then brought back, crossing over the plantar surface of the arch, and is attached on the plantar aspect of the first MTH (Fig. 8-5).

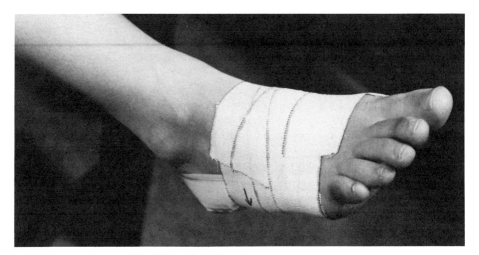

Fig. 8-4. Completed low Dye procedure.

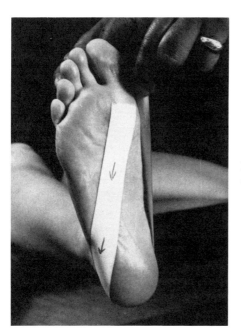

Fig. 8-5. Cross-X taping technique: medial tape strip.

2. The second strip starts at the lateral aspect of the fifth MTH and is taken around the posterior aspect of the calcaneus, across the plantar surface of the foot, and attached on the plantar surface of the fifth MTH (Fig. 8-6).

3. Four more strips of tape are applied, two in each direction (Fig. 8-7).

4. Three to four longitudinal strips are now applied as described in steps 3 and 4 of the low Dye technique (Fig. 8-8).

3. Ankle joint taping techniques. Numerous taping procedures have been reported for providing stability to the ankle joint complex. Several investiga-

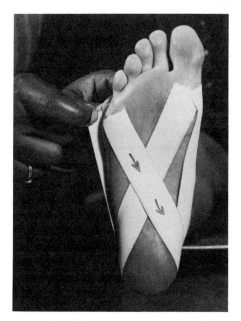

Fig. 8-6. Cross-X taping technique: lateral tape strip.

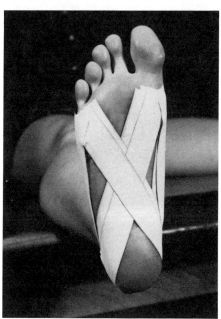

Fig. 8-7. Completion of the three cross Xs.

tions have reported on the effectiveness of the Gibney basketweave taping procedure with heel locks.[25-28] The basketweave portion of the procedure is designed to support the talocrural joint; the heel locks provide stability to the subtalar joint.

The application of a Gibney basketweave with heel locks is described for preventing the inversion sprain.

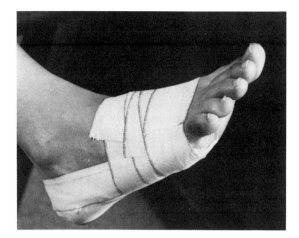

Fig. 8-8. Completed cross-X taping procedure with medial longitudinal arch lifts.

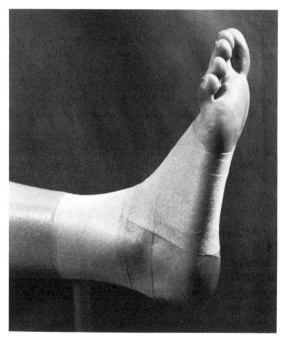

Fig. 8-9. Application of foam prewrap.

Supplies:

1. Tape adherent
2. Foam prewrap
3. 1½-inch cloth tape

Position of Patient:

Long sitting with knee extended and the talocrural joint neutral; subtalar joint slightly everted (if taping to prevent inversion sprain).

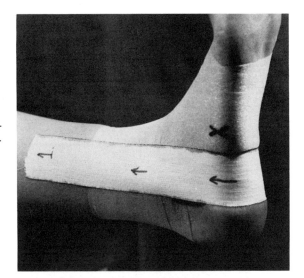

Fig. 8-10. Gibney basket-weave: application of first stirrup.

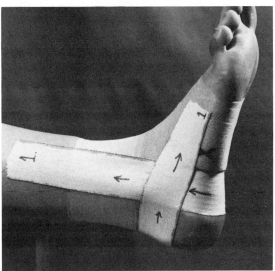

Fig. 8-11. Gibney basket-weave: application of first horizontal tie-down.

Procedure:

1. Tape adherent is applied and allowed to dry.

2. Foam prewrap is applied in a figure-eight direction around the upper portion of the forefoot and approximately 4 inches above the medial malleolus (Fig. 8-9).

3. The first stirrup is applied starting on the medial aspect of the leg (approximately 6 inches above the medial malleolus) and is pulled around the plantar surface of the calcaneus and then pulled snugly to the lateral side. (Fig. 8-10).

4. A horizontal tie-down strip is then applied starting 3 inches anterior and

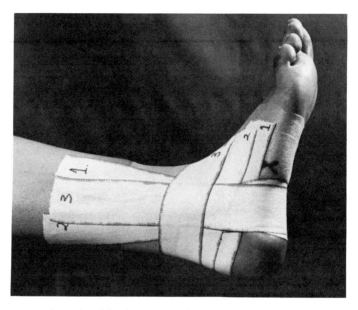

Fig. 8-12.   Completed basketweave of three stirrups and three tie-downs.

1 inch distal to the medial malleolus; it is taken posterior behind the calcaneus and attached in front of the lateral malleolus (approximately 4 inches) (Fig. 8-11).

5. Steps 3 and 4 are repeated twice more with an overlap of $\frac{1}{2}$ inch between strips (Fig. 8-12).

6. The first heel lock is started 4 to 5 inches above the medial malleolus on the anterior aspect of the lower leg. It is then brought down the medial aspect of the leg behind the calcaneus, across the lateral aspect of the calcaneus, back under the plantar surface of the foot, and finally is attached at the point where it started (Fig. 8-13).

7. The same procedure is followed in the opposite direction to apply the lateral heel lock. Two heel locks in each direction are normally applied.

8. Because all the forces applied with the tape have been from a medial to lateral direction in an attempt to prevent the inversion sprain, two arch lifts are applied to support the medial longitudinal arch (see Fig. 8-3). A figure-eight can be applied as well to provide additional support. The completed strapping procedure is shown in Fig. 8-14.

To prevent dermal irritation, particularly when the tape is applied directly to the skin, an appropriate method of tape removal must be used. Tape is commonly removed with scissors or tape cutters. For the ankle, removal should start on the plantar surface of the foot and proceed up the medial aspect of the leg. The plantar approach is used because the tissue in that area is more tolerant than the dorsum of the foot. Once cut, the tape should be removed by being pulled parallel to the skin while traction is applied in the opposite direction. The

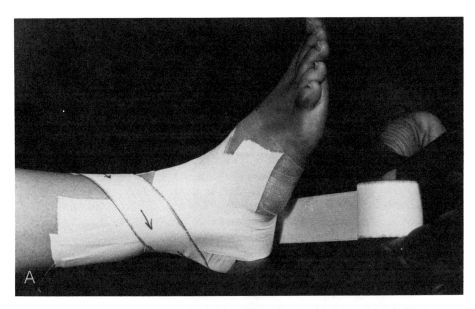

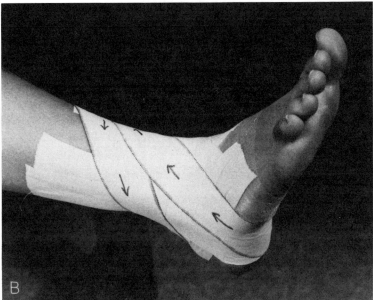

Fig. 8-13. (**A** and **B**) Application of medial heel lock.

tape should never be removed by pulling perpendicular to the skin. It is important that commercial tape removers be used to prevent buildup of adhesive residue and skin tougheners, which can also cause dermal irritation. If a commercial tape remover is used, the dermal areas to which this substance has been applied must be thoroughly cleansed with soap and water to prevent additional

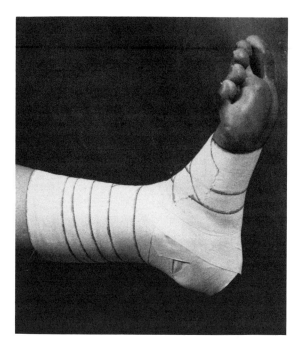

Fig. 8-14. Completed Gibney basketweave taping procedure with heel-locks.

irritation. Tape should always be removed after each practice or athletic event. To prevent possible dermal irritation, adhesive tape should never be left on the skin for more than 24 hours without being removed.

CHRONIC OR OVERUSE INJURIES

General Implications

Abnormal pronation of the subtalar joint is often described as a common cause of overuse injuries. Lutter[29] states that the most important factor in the production of running injuries, not only in the foot but throughout the entire lower extremity, is excessive pronation. Magazine articles have heightened the athlete's awareness of excessive pronation as a cause of foot injury. This is evident in the clinic, where athletic clients may request an orthotic device to treat an injury that they feel is caused by "excessive pronation." The therapist must remember, however, that although the patient may be complaining of some type of foot injury and although an abnormal degree of pronation is present, the etiology of the pronation may not necessarily be from the joints of the foot. Root et al,[19] in presenting numerous causes for pronation, lists only four deformities that occur in the midtarsal and subtalar joints and lead to abnormal subtalar joint pronation. The remaining factors occur throughout the lower extremity and include genu valgus and varum, tibia vara, internal and external torsional deformities of the tibia and femur, as well as soft tissue tightness reducing joint ROM. Thus, effective treatment procedures for overuse injuries associated with excessive pronation can only be initiated after a thorough evaluation of the entire lower extremity and not just the foot and ankle. For a complete overview of evaluative procedures, see Ch. 3.

The physical therapist should also be aware of the problems confronting athletes with a pes cavus or high arch foot type. These individuals have a relatively small weightbearing pattern and because of the limited amount of pronation have a reduction in shock absorption.[30,31] Individuals with a pes cavus foot type are susceptible to various conditions, including plantar fasciitis and heel pain as well as stress injuries in the proximal joints due to a reduction in shock absorption.[19,31] Although most of the conditions that we discuss are caused by abnormal pronation, the patient with a pes cavus foot type may require an orthotic device to decrease the strain on foot structures, especially owing to the high vault of the medial longitudinal arch. They should also be directed toward shoes designed to provide high shock absorption.

Specific Conditions

Forefoot

Metatarsalgia. Metatarsalgia is described as pain in the anterior segment of the foot. Often, with increased stress in the MTH region, sesamoiditis will occur as the sesamoids become inflamed. The symptoms include pain and tenderness of the plantar surface of the MTHs, development of callus under the prominent MTH, and increased pain during midstance and propulsion phases of walking. Usually the athlete cannot run. The etiology of metatarsalgia in the athlete is usually an alternation of normal biomechanics of the forefoot. This alteration is often secondary to abnormal subtalar joint pronation. The pes cavus foot type can develop pain in the metatarsal region, however, because of the high arch and increased stress on the forefoot. Treatment involves restoration of normal biomechanical function as well as relief of pressure on the symptomatic area to allow the inflammation to subside. If the symptoms have existed for a short time and abnormal pronation of the subtalar joint is the primary etiology, a functional orthotic device should be used. If the patient has been suffering from these symptoms for a long time, however, a metatarsal bar may have to be added to the running or athletic shoe to reduce the symptoms. Once the inflammation has subsided, only the orthotic device is required to maintain normal mechanical functioning. Individuals with the pes cavus foot types suffering from metatarsalgia respond well to an orthotic device that gives total contact to the medial longitudinal arch. Preventing collapse of the arch will reduce the stress on the MTHs.

Hallux abducto valgus. Hallux abducto valgus (HAV) is a deformity of the forefoot caused by a progressive subluxation of the first metatarsal-phalangeal joint. Initially, lateral displacement of the proximal phalanx of the hallux occurs as abnormal subtalar joint pronation creates a hypermobile first ray. Further progression leads to a metatarsus primus adductus, with continued abduction of the hallux on the first MTH. Eventually, the hallux will press into the medial aspect of the second toe.

The etiology of the HAV deformity in the athlete has been linked to abnormal subtalar joint pronation,[32] along with the degree of forefoot adductus that exists. Root et al,[19] state that a foot type with a forefoot adductus of greater than 15° in the presence of abnormal subtalar joint pronation will tend to develop a HAV deformity.

Footwear has been shown not to be a primary cause of the HAV deformity.[33] The importance of good shoes must be emphasized, however, to the athlete who selects conservative management. Poorly fitting shoes have been shown to accelerate the rate of progression of a HAV in the presence of abnormal subtalar joint pronation.[19]

Symptoms of the athlete with HAV are varied. Chronic ingrown nails on the lateral border of the hallux are common secondary to pressure exerted by the second toe.[32] This problem is accentuated by wearing shoes with a narrow forefoot. Often the patient may complain of tenderness and neuritis over the bunion. This is caused by compression of the cutaneous nerves in this region by the forepart of the shoe. The instability of the first ray also causes increased weightbearing on the second and third MTHs. This excessive pressure leads to metatarsalgia symptoms as well as callus development under the lesser MTHs.

Management of HAV can be either surgical or conservative. Numerous surgical procedures have been reported for the correction of the HAV deformity. Surgery corrects only the deformity, however, and does not address the faulty biomechanics that caused the initial HAV deformity. The abnormal pronatory forces must be controlled postoperatively with good footwear and, if required, orthotic devices. Conservative management includes proper footwear and orthotic devices to control abnormal subtalar joint pronation if a forefoot and/or rearfoot imbalance exists. Use of orthotic devices limits the progression of HAV.[32] The athlete with a HAV deformity should be advised to wear shoes with as much room in the forefoot as possible to accommodate increased width. The shoe should also have a reinforced heel counter to give additional rearfoot control in an attempt to reduce excessive pronation.

Morton's toe. Morton's toe is described as a short first metatarsal bone.[34] This hereditary foot type is quite common in athletes and with continued activity can become extremely disabling.[24] In this condition, normal forefoot balance is disturbed due to the shortened first metatarsal, which causes abnormal subtalar joint pronation. Abnormal subtalar joint pronation creates hypermobility of the first ray during forefoot loading. This increases the amount of weight borne by the second metatarsal, causing symptoms similar to metatarsalgia (i.e., plantar pain and callus).[1] This deformity can usually be recognized clinically because the second toe is longer than the hallux. Treatment involves a rigid orthotic with an extension under the first metatarsal to the end of the hallux.

Toe Deformities

Hallux limitus. Hallux limitus is described as a restriction in first MTP extension. Walking on level ground requires approximately 65° of extension at the first MTP joint. Hallux rigidus is a term used to describe ankylosis of the first MTP joint.[1]

The etiology for hallux limitus/rigidus is any condition that prevents the first MTP from moving below the transverse plane of the lesser MTHs.[19] Common causes preventing normal first MTP movement in athletes include hypermobility of the first ray in conjunction with eversion of the rearfoot (secondary to subtalar joint pronation)[19]; a long first metatarsal bone[19]; and traumatic injury to the first MTP joint (i.e., hyperextension, severe crush injury).

The symptoms include pain in the first MTP joint, restricted first MTP joint extension, and increased out-toeing on the affected side. In severe cases, the athlete may complain of proximal pain at the cuneonavicular and talonavicular joints as these articulations attempt to compensate for the restricted ROM.

Conservative treatment in acute injuries include rest, ice, compression, and elevation. After 48 hours, joint mobilization can be initiated with lower grades to reduce pain, followed by stretch articulations as inflammation subsides. Propulsion phase must be prevented in these patients, as well as stair and incline ambulation, until inflammation subsides. This can be accomplished using a standard postoperative shoe with a wooden rocker sole. In chronic conditions, when restriction of first MTP extension is less than 15°, a metatarsal bar can be extremely successful. In athletes with extreme limitations, however, surgery may be the only means of restoring normal function to the first MTP joint.[35]

Hammer toes and claw toes. Hammer toes refers to a deformity in which the proximal interphalangeal (IP) joint is flexed.[36] This condition often results from wearing shoes that do not fit properly. A claw toe deformity, in which the MTP joint is extended and the proximal IP joint is flexed, often results from a weakness or imbalance of the foot intrinsic muscles.[36] Athletes with hammer or claw toes often complain of pain secondary to callus or corns on the dorsal aspect of the toes. In most cases, pain is caused by pressure on the dorsum of the flexed joints because of a shallow toe box in the shoe. Conservative treatment for these patients is prescription of shoes with a deep toe box. Although several athletic shoes do come with extra-depth toe boxes, styles and last shapes are limited. One method to increase the toe box in a standard shoe is to remove the insole and cut away the material distal to the MTHs. This allows continued cushioning to the level of the MTHs while providing increased depth in the toe box. In addition, especially for athletes suffering from claw toes, muscle strengthening exercises for foot intrinsics should be given (i.e., towel rolling, picking up marbles or rolls of tape with toes).[36] With severe deformities, surgery may be necessary to provide complete relief.

Rearfoot Conditions

Retrocalcaneal bursitis. Athletes suffering from retrocalcaneal bursitis can have involvement of the deep bursa, positioned between the Achilles tendon and calcaneus, or the superficial bursa, lying between skin and Achilles tendon.[37] The etiology, especially for deep bursa irritation, is excessive compensatory subtalar joint pronation.[37] Often the posterior aspect of the runner's shoe, if poorly padded, will create irritation to the superficial bursa.[36] The symptoms include pain, swelling, and inflammation over the posterior aspect of the calcaneus. Initial treatment includes ice as well as antiinflammatory medication.[38] If excessive pronation is believed to be contributing to the etiology, functional orthotics should be prescribed and used once initial symptoms subside. Newer models of running and sport shoes have well-padded Achilles tendon extensions to reduce superficial bursa irritation. Persons with such irritation also benefit from rigid counters in their shoes to reduce excessive subtalar joint pronation. In chronic severe conditions, surgery may be necessary to remove the irritating tissue or calcaneal bone spurs secondary to prolonged inflammation.

Plantar fasciitis. Plantar fasciitis is one of the most common causes of heel pain in runners.[38] The chronic or overuse type of plantar fasciitis usually results from abnormal pronation of the subtalar joint creating microtears in the plantar fascia. The medial aspect of the plantar fascia is most often affected at its insertion on the medial tuberosity of the plantar surface of the calcaneus. Continued inflammation of this area of the calcaneus, secondary to plantar fasciitis, will cause formation of a heel spur.[38]

Symptoms include pain with initial steps after a period of nonweightbearing, as in first arising in morning, followed by a reduction in symptoms after 30 to 45 minutes of daily activity. However, after 2 to 3 hours the pain will begin to intensify as activities continue throughout the day. This type of patterning is often reported by a jogger, who notes that the pain, although severe at the start of the run, diminished during the run only to recur toward the end or after completion of the workout.

Palpation is an important diagnostic tool because pain should be elicited with pressure over the anteromedial aspect on the plantar surface of the calcaneus. Pain that is reported with palpation directly under the plantar surface of the calcaneus usually indicates a heel contusion and *not* plantar fasciitis. Additional assistance in confirming diagnosis can be obtained from the subjective portion of the examination. Often the athlete with plantar fasciitis will report that symptoms occurred with a rapid and major adjustment in the training schedule.

Treatment for the chronic type of plantar fasciitis requires correction of the underlying mechanical abnormalities causing the abnormal pronation of the subtalar joint. To provide symptom relief, antiinflammatory drugs can be used, as can various other modalities (i.e., ultrasound, ice massage). Cross-friction massage in conjunction with slow, passive stretching of the plantar fascia can be effective following ice massage to the painful region. Correction of the mechanical factors causing abnormal pronation requires a functional orthotic device. Even if an osseous imbalance does not exist in the foot, athletes suffering from plantar fasciitis respond well to a semirigid or commercial foot orthosis. This acts to prevent collapse of the medial longitudinal arch and reduce the stress on the medial band of the plantar fascia. Clients with a pes cavus foot type and subsequent high vault to the medial longitudinal arch respond very well to an orthotic device fabricated to provide total contact in the medial arch. If treatment for plantar fasciitis is continually unsuccessful, possible entrapment of the medial calcaneal branch of the tibial nerve should be considered.[38]

Cuboid syndrome. Cuboid syndrome, which describes a partial subluxation of the cuboid secondary to abnormal pronation, occurs in approximately 4 percent of athletes complaining of plantar foot pain.[1] Cuboid syndrome often occurs early in the season as the athlete attempts to run farther than normal or over uneven terrain.[39] Increased speed workout as well as a sudden twisting of the foot can also lead to symptoms. The etiology is abnormal subtalar joint pronation, which creates cuboid hypermobility. Normal foot function provides for a stable cuboid to act as fulcrum for the peroneus longus tendon as it travels to its insertion on the first ray. If the cuboid is unstable, however, secondary to abnormal subtalar joint pronation, contraction of the peroneus longus will cause a displacement of the cuboid.

The symptoms include pain on the lateral aspect of the foot over the calcaneocuboid joint as well as at the fourth and fifth cuboideometatarsal articulations. The athlete will often complain of pain in the area of the cuboid during walking.[39] Diagnosis, however, is often hampered by referred pain, which tends to make the athlete report generalized foot discomfort.

Treatment centers on manipulation of the cuboid to restore proper alignment of the calcaneocuboid joint. The manipulation procedure has been described in detail by Newell and Woodle.[39] Once proper alignment of the cuboid has been established, pain in most cases is markedly decreased with palpation of the calcaneocuboid joint. Ice should be used to reduce any inflammation secondary to the procedure. To prevent recurrence, an adhesive strapping technique or a functional orthotic device should be prescribed to prevent abnormal subtalar joint pronation. In addition, footwear offering good rearfoot control should be recommended.

Lower Leg

Shin splints. Shin splints is a general term applied to a complex of conditions that lead to pain and irritation to the shin region of the lower leg.[40] Shin splints can occur in any sport and is often associated with the untrained or unconditioned athlete, a change in event or playing surface, an increase in jumping activities, a change in footwear, as well as a rapid, major adjustment in training schedule.[24] Due to these factors, shin splints is considered an overuse type of injury in which microtrauma occurs to musculotendinous structures and the perosteum in lower leg. In general, shin splints is categorized as affecting the anterior or medial aspects of the lower leg. Because the etiology and treatment varies for these two regions, each is considered separately.

Anterior shin splints is usually due to an imbalance between the anterior muscle group and the calf muscles. In the untrained runner, poor running techniques may cause the athlete to overuse the anterior muscle group to prevent foot slap after heel strike. In addition, the untrained runner may not have the required 10 to 15° of dorsiflexion, indicating a lack of flexibility in the posterior muscle group. Decreased flexibility in the calf muscles will cause the novice runner to overuse the anterior group of muscles to assist in toe clearance during swing, especially while running uphill. Trained runners who engage in uphill running or increased sprinting associated with speed-interval training are also apt to overuse the anterior muscle group. In addition, anterior shin splints are common with sudden changes in playing surface (i.e., from grass to artificial turf surfaces.)[36]

The symptoms for anterior shin splints include pain and tenderness along the lateral border and distal half of the medial crest of the tibia. Pain increases with active dorsiflexion as well as with passive stretching of the dorsiflexors of the ankle.[36]

The treatment consists of ice to decrease inflammation along with an elastic wrap for compression to the region. Once inflammation subsides, treatment emphasis is on calf muscle stretching as well as gradual resistive exercises to the anterior muscle group if weakness is noted. The athlete should not be allowed to resume activity until all symptoms have subsided, 10 to 15° of ankle dorsiflexion is attained, and normal strength of the anterior muscle group strength is attained. Resumption of activity must be gradual, with small increases in mileage.

Medial shin splints in most athletes is a posterior tibial tendonitis secondary to abnormal subtalar joint pronation. Thus, the athlete who excessively pronates will overuse the tibialis posterior as the muscle attempts to support the medial longitudinal arch. Runners who train on crowned roads and do not change street sides can also develop medial shin splints because the downside leg (leg farthest away from the crown) will tend to pronate.[36]

Symptoms include pain in the posterior medial compartment approximately 4 to 6 inches proximal to the medial malleolus. Pain is often increased with resisted plantarflexion and inversion movements.

Initial treatment includes the same procedures described for anterior shin splints to decrease inflammation. Successful treatment of medial shin splints requires adhesive strapping or functional orthotics, however, to prevent excessive pronation of the subtalar joint. In addition, once symptoms have subsided, resumption of activity must be gradual.

Two associated conditions of which the physical therapist should be aware when treating the athlete with shin splints have symptoms that can mimic both the anterior and medial types but present a greater danger to the client.

Anterior compartment syndrome is a serious complication following an injury to the lower leg. It often occurs after a blow or repeated blows to the shin but can also take place after a rigorous early training session, especially if the athlete is in poor physical condition.[1,36] In this condition, swelling occurs within the anterior fascial compartment, compressing the anterior tibial vein and artery as well as the deep peroneal nerve. Anterior compartment syndrome can be differentiated from shin splints in that symptoms *do not* improve with rest and ice application.[36] If the clinician suspects a possible anterior compartment compression, the athlete should be referred back to his or her own physician for reevaluation. Untreated anterior compartment syndrome can result in muscle eschemia and nerve paralysis (i.e., drop foot).[1]

Stress fractures of the tibia and fibula may also demonstrate the same symptoms as shin splints. Tibial stress fractures generally appear more in runners with pes cavus foot types, whereas fibular stress fractures often occur in pronated feet.[1,36] Differential diagnosis is difficult because roentgenograms are often negative 2 to 3 weeks after injury. Even after 2 weeks, all that is seen is a thin callus cloud over the site of injury. Subjectively, the athlete will complain of severe pain with activity, whereas rest causes relief. Bone percussion techniques can be used to distinguish between bone and soft tissue pain. One technique involves firmly tapping the fibula and tibia distally and proximally to the site of tenderness.[1] A sharp, stabbing sensation is often indicative of a stress fracture. A second technique involves striking the heel upward to elicit a sensation similar to that reported by the athlete.[1,36] If the therapist suspects a possible stress fracture, the athlete should be referred back to his or her own physician for further treatment.

FOOTWEAR

The importance of footwear in the management of overuse injuries cannot be overemphasized. Patients being treated for recently acquired overuse injuries can often be managed successfully with appropriate footwear along with modifications in training regimen. Even athletes who are fitted with foot orthoses require good footwear to provide a firm foundation for proper orthotic function.

With shoe styles and features being constantly changed by manufacturers, it is almost impossible for the physical therapist to keep abreast of current shoe models. Certain characteristics, however, can be suggested for specific foot types. For example, for added rearfoot control, a reinforced extended medial heel counter with a high posterior quarter might be recommended. An athlete with claw or hammer toes should have extra depth in the toe box. Athletes who are fitted with functional orthotics should have a "fully-boarded" shoe (fiberboard from heel to toe) to provide a firm base for the devices. These are just a few suggestions.

Finally, the therapist is strongly encouraged to make contact with several local athletic shoe suppliers to identify individuals with expertise in the features of the various shoe models. Therapists can then give retailers specific information about the necessary shoe features that will aid in the athlete's treatment program (i.e., shock absorption, curved vs straight last, rearfoot control, etc.).

REFERENCES

1. Arnheim DD: Modern Principles of Athletic Training. 6th Ed. Times Mirror/CV Mosby, St. Louis, 1985
2. Brunnstrom S: Clinical Kinesiology. 3rd Ed. FA Davis, Philadelphia, 1972
3. Landry ME: The common inversion sprain and its treatment in the athlete. J Am Podiatry Assoc 66:166, 1976
4. Rubin G, Witten M: The talar-tilt angle and the fibular collateral ligaments. J Bone Joint Surg [Am] 42:311, 1960
5. Inman VT: The Joints of the Ankle. Williams & Wilkins, Baltimore, 1976
6. Brantigan JW, Pedegana LR, Lippert FG: Instability of the subtalar joint. J Bone Joint Surg [Am] 59:321, 1977
7. Mann R, Inman VT: Phasic activity of intrinsic muscles of the foot. J Bone Joint Surg [Am] 46:469, 1964
8. Scott WN, Nisonson B, Nicholas JA: Principles of Sports Medicine. Williams & Wilkins, Baltimore, 1984
9. Doller J, Strother S: Turf toe. J Am Podiatry Assoc 69:687, 1979
10. O'Donoghue DH: Treatment of Injuries to Athletes. 4th Ed. WB Saunders, Philadelphia, 1984
11. Williams JG, Sperryn PN: Sports Medicine. 2nd Ed. Williams & Wilkins, Baltimore, 1976
12. Garrett WE: Strains and sprains in athletes. Postgrad Med 73:200, 1983
13. Ellison AE, Boland AL, DeHaven KE, et al: Athletic Training and Sports Medicine. American Academy of Orthopedic Surgeons, 1984
14. McCluskey GM, Blackburn TA, Lewis T: A treatment for ankle sprains. Am J Sports Med 4:158, 1976
15. Kaplan EG, Kaplan GS, Vaccari OA, et al: A triligamentous reconstruction for lateral ankle instability. J Foot Surg 23:240, 1984
16. Weil LS, Moore JW, Kratzer CD, et al: A biomechanical study of lateral ankle sprains in basketball. J Am Podiatry Assoc 69:687, 1979
17. Hoppenfeld S: Physical Examination of the Spine and Extremities. Appleton-Century-Crofts, New York, 1976
18. McCluskey GM, Blackburn TA, Lewis T: Prevention of ankle sprains. Am J Sports Med 4:151, 1976
19. Root ML, Orien WP, Weed JH: Normal and Abnormal Function of the Foot. Volume II. Clinical Biomechanics, Los Angeles, 1977
20. James SL: Chondromalacia of the patella in the adolescent. p. 205. In Kennedy JC (ed.): The Injured Adolescent Knee. Williams & Wilkins, Baltimore, 1979
21. Garrick JG, Requa RK: Role of external support in the prevention of ankle sprains. Med Sci Sports 5:100, 1973
22. Schoenhaus HD, Jay RM: Cavus deformities: conservative management. J Am Podiatry Assoc 70:235, 1980
23. Metcalf GR, Denegar CR: A critical review of ankle taping. Athletic Training 18:121, 1983
24. Hlavac HF: The Foot Book. World Publications, Mountain View, CA, 1977

25. Libera D: Ankle taping, wrapping, and injury prevention. Athletic Training 7:73, 1972

26. Bigley G, Karst RT: The measurable support given to the ankle joint by conventional methods of ankle taping. Master's Thesis: University of Wisconsin, Madison, 1959

27. Malina RM, Plagenz LB, Rarick GL: Effect of exercise upon the measurable supporting strength of cloth and tape ankle wraps. Res Q 34:158, 1963

28. Rarick GL, Bigley G, Karst R, et al: Measurable support of the ankle joint by conventional methods of taping. J Bone Joint Surg [Am] 44:1183, 1962

29. Lutter L: Injuries in the runner and jogger. Minn Med 63:45, 1980

30. Subotnick SI: The cavus foot. Phys Sports Med 8:53, 1980

31. Schuster RO: Foot types and the influence of environment on the foot of the long distance runner. Ann NY Acad Sci 301:881, 1977

32. Berman BL: Etiology and management of hallux valgus in athletes. Phys Sports Med 10:103, 1982

33. Clough JG, Marshall HJ: The etiology of hallux abducto valgus. J Am Podiatry Assoc 75:238, 1985

34. Morton DJL: Human Locomotion and Body Form. Williams & Wilkins, Baltimore, 1952

35. Calliet R: Foot and Ankle Pain. FA Davis, Philadelphia, 1972

36. Kulund DN: The Injured Athlete. JB Lippincott, Philadelphia, 1982

37. Roy S, Irvin I: Sports Medicine. Prentice-Hall, Englewood Cliffs, NJ, 1983

38. Brody DM: Running injuries. Ciba Clin Symp 32:1980

39. Newell SG, Woodle A: Cuboid syndrome. Phys Sports Med 9:71, 1981

40. Slocum DB: The shin splint syndrome. Am J Surg 114:875, 1967

9 | Physical Modalities for Foot Pain

Marie A. Schroeder

In attempts to control foot and ankle pain, a comprehensive approach including evaluation, treatment of causes, pain modulation, and prevention of recurrence is necessary. Physical modalities of heat, cold and electricity generally play an adjunctive role in therapy. Because few well-designed clinical studies exist in this area, especially in relation to foot and ankle pain, emphasis is placed on current pain theories and physiologic effects of modalities and their clinical implications. Perhaps interest in clinical research or new approaches to modality use will be stimulated.

PAIN THEORIES

The challenge of controlling pain is complicated by lack of agreement concerning a definition of pain. There is, however, widespread agreement as to what pain is not.

> No longer is pain considered a sensation, a "primary emotional experience" as is vision, hearing, touch, or smell. Instead, the complexity of the pain experience is recognized to include the physical perception of pain, suggestion, and the emotional state, expectations, personality, and cognitive view of the person experiencing it.[1]

Several theories have attempted to account for the nature of pain. The specificity theory assumes pain to be a specific modality, like vision or hearing. It proposes that free nerve endings in the periphery are specific pain receptors, transmitting impulses along A delta and C fibers and the lateral spinothalmic tract to a pain center in the thalamus. Perhaps the most important weaknesses in this theory are (1) the lack of identification of one type of receptor, fiber, or spinal pathway that when stimulated always and only produces sensations perceived as pain; and (2) surgical lesions made at almost every level of the peripheral and central nervous system (CNS) have frequently not been successful in abolishing pain.[1,2]

Based on Goldscheider's proposal that stimulus intensity and central summation are the critical determinants of pain, two kinds of theories, recognizing the concept of patterning of input and grouped under the general category of "pattern theory," have been suggested. Based on Nafe's suggestion that all cutaneous qualities are produced by spatiotemporal patterns of nerve impulses, the pattern theory of Weddell and Sinclair proposes that all fiber endings (apart from those innervating hair cells) are alike. Intense stimulation of nonspecific receptors evokes a pattern of impulses interpreted by the brain as pain, based on its intensity and frequency. This ignores, however, the physiologic evidence of receptor/fiber specialization.[1,2] Livingston, on the other hand, stresses central summation mechanisms while acknowledging physiologic specialization. Reverberating circuits in spinal interneurons result from intense pathologic stimulation, and otherwise non-noxious stimuli can trigger these circuits to generate abnormal volleys of impulses that are interpreted centrally as pain.[1,2] Similarly, Hebb and Gerard suggest that pain results from hypersynchronized firing in central cells.[2]

The input-controlling theory proposes that a rapidly conducting fiber system normally inhibits synaptic transmission in a more slowly conducting system, thereby modifying the input pattern and preventing summation from occurring. Under pathologic conditions, the slow system establishes dominance, resulting in protopathic sensation, diffuse burning pain, or hyperalgesia.[2]

Melzack and Wall's gate control theory proposes that neural mechanisms in the dorsal horns of the spinal cord act like a gate, modulating the flow of nerve impulses from peripheral fibers to the CNS. Large fiber input tends to close the gate, and small fiber input tends to open it. In addition, descending inhibition from the brain has profound influence on the gate.[2,3]

For pain to be perceived, central transmission (T) cells must be stimulated. The substantia gelatinosa (SG) acts as a gating mechanism, modulating afferent impulses before they influence T cells.[2] Impulses from mechanoreceptors traveling on large diameter A fibers close the gate, blocking activation of T cells. Nociceptor input traveling on small diameter A delta and C fibers opens the gate, and T cells are activated. Nociceptive input also directly stimulates T cells. T cells convey information to multiple pain control centers in the brain (Fig. 9-1).[1,2] Also, intense stimulation of small fibers activates areas in the brainstem to produce a tonic descending inhibitory response governing transmission through the dorsal gray matter, closing the gate and blocking further T cell transmission.[1,2] The central control trigger theory proposed later by Melzack and Casey implicates dorsal column transmission of large fiber input to activate central inhibitory mechanisms that cause a descending influence to modulate pain transmission neurons within the dorsal horn.[3a,4]

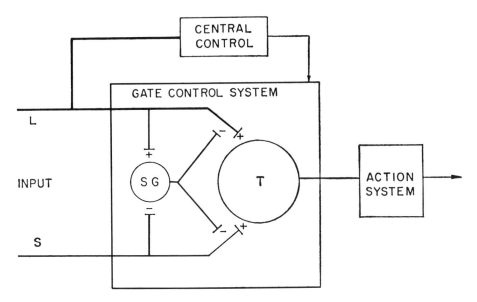

Fig. 9-1. Schematic diagram of the gate control theory of pain mechanisms: L, large-diameter fibers; S, small-diameter fibers. Fibers project to the substantia gelatinosa (SG) and first central transmission (T) cells. The inhibitory effect exerted by SG on the afferent fiber terminals is increased by activity in L fibers and decreased by activity in S fibers. The central control trigger is represented by a line running from the large fiber system to the control mechanisms; these mechanisms, in turn, project back to the gate control system. The T cells project to the entry cells of the action system. +, excitation; −, inhibition. (Melzack R, Wall PD: Pain mechanisms: a new theory. Science 150:971, © 1965 by the American Association for the Advancement of Science.)

Recent advances in pain research have revealed that endogenous opiates, naturally occurring substances that possess opiatelike properties, exist in the body. High concentrations of receptors for these substances have been isolated throughout the CNS, especially in areas associated with nociception: thalamus, limbic system, periaqueductal gray, and substantia gelatinosa. The endogenous opiates probably represent neuromodulators inhibiting the transmission of pain.[1,5] Areas of greatest opiate receptor density and major sites of morphine action correspond to the anatomic areas identified by Melzack and Wall as significant in presynaptic inhibition of pain, as well as the descending inhibitory mechanism.[1,2]

Independent peptidergic systems are recognized in the endogenous opiate system. Enkephalins are short-chain (5-amino acid) peptides, are relatively weak, and rapidly degrade (half-lives are less than 1 minute). Endorphins are long-chain peptides and are more resistant to enzymatic degradation. β-endorphin has a half-life of at least 2 to 3 hours. Other endorphins have been isolated.[5]

Substance P is an 11-amino acid chain peptide that acts as a neurotransmitter for noxious input. When present in high concentrations, substance P excites neurons sensitive to nociceptive stimuli promoting propagation of pain impulses. In low concentrations, however, it facilitates endorphin release, causing nociceptive inhibition. Substance P may, therefore, be a regulatory peptide.[5]

Serotonin is a naturally occurring amino acid that participates in temperature regulation, pain, sleep, mood, and appetite. Diminished levels of serotonin are associated with increased pain and depression. At CNS synapses, it may enhance release of pain-inhibiting endogenous opiates. In cases of peripheral trauma, however, serotonin is considered a pain-producing substance exciting tissue chemoreceptors.[5]

The amount of serotonin and the rate of synthesis in brain neurons are directly dependent on the amount of tryptophan (a serotonin precursor) in the diet. Tryptophan is also a precursor of niacin (vitamin B_3). Foods high in tryptophan are eggs, meat, poultry, and dairy products. A high-carbohydrate, low-protein diet will increase serotonin because ingestion of carbohydrates enhances transport of tryptophan into the CNS. Consequently, diet can play an important role in pain management.[5]

CLINICAL APPLICATIONS

The proposed pain theories have significant impact on clinical management of pain. Perhaps most important is the suggestion of the gate control theory that pain relief might be achieved by enhancement of normal physiologic activities instead of through disruption by irreversible lesions in the central or peripheral nervous systems.[3] Specifically, physical modalities can be used to enhance large diameter afferent activity (e.g., transcutaneous electrical nerve stimulation (TENS), heat/cold modalities).[3,6] Also, small fiber activation through brief intense TENS applied to trigger points probably increases input to the central biasing mechanism, which could close the gate and reduce pain.[3] Treatment outcome might better be predicted (e.g., patients with peripheral neuropathies characterized by loss of large afferent fibers may be worsened by TENS).[7] Decreasing sensory input through successive anesthetic blocks of trigger points, peripheral nerves, or sympathetic ganglia will diminish the input through the gate and cause cessation of activity in reverberating neural circuits. Therefore, increasing or decreasing input might have the same effect, permitting normal motor activities which tend to prevent the recurrence of abnormal central neural activity.[3]

Pharmacologic agents capable of stimulating or inhibiting the peripheral receptors, substantia gelatinosa, or brain stem may have significant impact on pain control.[2,6] For example, drugs that stimulate or inhibit the substantia gelatinosa are effective (i.e., halothane and barbiturates). Analgesics probably inhibit peripheral receptor transmission. In regard to inflammation, the cause of pain is not entirely understood. Bradykinin, a product of tissue breakdown, might be implicated in the pathogenesis of the pain associated with inflammation. Phenylbutazone and aspirin, both antiinflammatory medications, evidently antagonize its action at the receptors.[6]

PHYSICAL MODALITIES

Presently, experimental and clinical research, in the realm of the physiologic effects of local heat and cold application and use of electricity for pain relief, offer many equivocal findings. Information generally agreed upon will be presented. Frequently, the desired outcome of intervention with physical modalities is the same (e.g., pain relief). Mechanisms by which the various modalities might achieve these goals, when better understood, will afford a more efficient and effective therapeutic approach. This is especially true in the use of heat and cold in which physiologic effects are usually reciprocal. The information provided is limited to local applications.

THERAPEUTIC HEAT

Specific physiologic effects of heat are dependent on the mode of application, depth of penetration, and temperature increase. The specific heating modality used is usually chosen for its particular heating pattern, allowing peak temperatures to occur in the tissue to be treated.[8] Regardless of the mode of application, general physiologic effects of therapeutic heat include[1,8]:

1. Local blood flow increases.
2. Rate of tissue metabolism increases until an optimal temperature is reached. Beyond this temperature, metabolism slows until cell death occurs from denaturation of proteins.
3. Capillary permeability and rate of capillary filtration increase, allowing protein to escape into the interstitial space, leading to fluid retention.
4. Speed of skeletal muscle contraction increases until the optimal temperature for metabolism is reached.
5. Muscle tension decreases.
6. Muscle spasm is reduced.
7. Joint stiffness decreases.
8. Extensibility of collagen tissues increases.

Specific Physiologic Responses

Based on the physiologic effects of therapeutic heat, this modality can be used to alleviate foot and ankle pain. The clinical problems for which heat might be indicated include contractures, joint stiffness, muscle spasms, inflammation, trauma, arthritis, and pain.

Contractures

Rationale for treatment of contractures with local heat is based on the demonstration of increases of extensibility of collagen with temperatures within the therapeutic range (41 to 45°C). Increased extensibility of tendons has been reported following ultrasound exposure, due to the rise in tissue temperature. At normal temperatures, a tendon has essentially elastic behavior. At therapeutic temperatures of 45°C, however, viscous properties dominate and tension rapidly and significantly decreases. To achieve residual elongation, a load must be applied while the tissue temperature is in the therapeutic range. Clinically, stretch must be applied during or immediately following heat application to achieve elongation of the contracted tissue. Experiments have demonstrated that a load capable of producing the prescribed residual elongation alters the tendon strength less when applied at therapeutic temperatures than when applied at normal tissue temperatures.[8]

Joint Stiffness

Local heating reduces joint stiffness. Elastic, viscous, and frictional stiffness bear the same mutual relationships in the arthritic as in the normal joint. Patients with rheumatoid arthritis as well as some other connective tissue disorders exhibit significant increases in elastic stiffness of the joints as compared with normal subjects. Selective heating of joints to between 43 and 45°C has been demonstrated to decrease joint stiffness in rheumatoid patients. Subjective complaints generally correlate with objective measurements of stiffness. An exception exists when temperatures are lowered to the point of sensory impairment; stiffness can no longer be perceived despite objective measurements of increased joint stiffness.[8]

Muscle Spasm

Muscle spasms secondary to underlying skeletal, joint, or neuropathology can be reduced by application of heat. Objective evidence of the physiologic mechanisms producing this response is limited. With regard to the muscle spindle, the effect of temperature on primary and secondary afferents in a prestretched muscle under a tension of 100 pounds has been reported. Heating the spindle increases the firing rate of group I-A afferents as well as that of the secondary afferents exhibiting a high background discharge (Fig. 9-2).[9,10] Cooling depresses the rate of firing of both groups. Secondary afferents with a low initial discharge rate demonstrate depression or cessation of firing when heated; cooling activates firing. Most secondary afferents cease firing when heated. These secondary afferents respond more to tonic than phasic changes, whereas I-A primary afferents respond greater to phasic stretch. If muscle spasm is mostly a tonic phenomenon, this might explain the physiologic mecha-

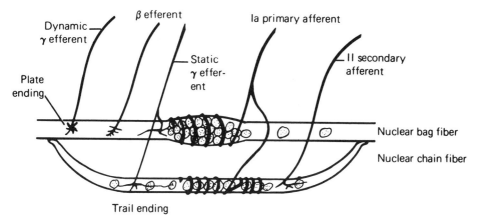

Fig. 9-2. Diagram of muscle spindle. (From Ganong, as modified from Stein RB: Peripheral Control of movement. Physiol Rev 54:215, 1974.)

nism involved. Golgi tendon organs reportedly increase their firing rate in response to heating within the therapeutic range. Because Golgi tendon organs exert an inhibitory effect on extrafusal muscle fibers, this might supplement the action of the secondary afferents in alleviating spasm.[8]

Superficial heat primarily raising skin temperature might also reduce muscle spasm. Stimulation of the skin of the neck region has been shown to decrease γ fiber activity resulting in decreased spindle excitability.[8]

Warming can also reduce sustained contractions that occur in tension syndromes by increasing blood flow. Prolonged muscle contraction results in ischemia and excessive accumulation of metabolic byproducts. This, in turn, contributes to pain and perpetuates abnormal muscle contraction, creating a pain cycle (Fig. 9-3).[11] Heating muscle tissue increases blood flow, allowing improved oxygen exchange and reduction in metabolites. Reducing ischemia alleviates pain, thus mitigating the need for guarding (spasm) (Fig. 9-4).[8,11]

Inflammation

Superficial heat localizes inflammation and accelerates abscess formation of superficial infections such as folliculitis, furuncles, carbuncles, and paronychia. This allows easy drainage of the abscess, spontaneously or surgically. Use of deep heat (e.g., diathermy, for promotion of abscess formation in deep tissues might be catastrophic).[8]

Heat can produce inflammatory reactions at higher temperatures. Temperature increases cause an increase in capillary permeability to protein and cell migration. If temperatures are high enough, proteins become denatured and polypeptides and histaminelike substances are produced. Vascular alterations are directly affected by heat but are also chemically mediated by the release of bradykinin and histaminelike substances which produce vasodilatation.[8]

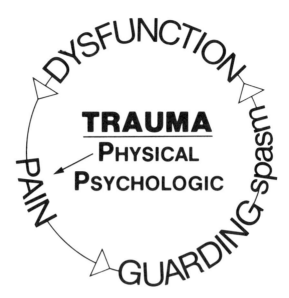

Fig. 9-3. Primary typical primary typical acute/chronic pain cycle. (Mannheimer JS, Lampe GN: Pain and TENS in pain management. p. 7. In Mannheimer JS, Lampe GN (eds): Clinical Transcutaneous Electrical Nerve Stimulation. FA Davis, Philadelphia, 1984.)

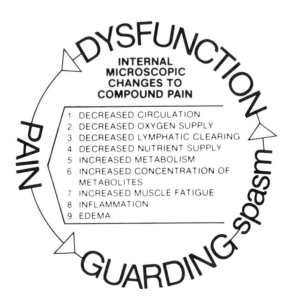

Fig. 9-4. Primary pain cycle and associated internal changes. Physical modalities are used to reverse these microscopic changes. (Mannheimer JS, Lampe GN: Pain and TENS in pain management. p. 7. In Mannheimer JS, Lampe GN (eds): Clinical Transcutaneous Electrical Nerve Stimulation. FA Davis, Philadelphia, 1984.)

Trauma

Superficial and deep heat have been frequently advocated for subacute and chronic stages of injury. Although usually recommended 24 to 48 hours following injury, a safer guideline is to avoid heat until active swelling has ceased.[12] The rationale used assumes that heat helps to resorb hematomas and swelling. Most studies, however, have reported equivocal findings or no difference when compared with no-treatment controls.[8]

Arthritis

In the rheumatoid joint, destructive enzyme activity frequently creates disabling pain. It has been speculated that if joint temperatures are raised high enough, destructive enzymes (e.g., collagenase) might be inactivated. Because vigorous heating can produce an inflammatory reaction by itself, this is probably unlikely. Mild heating has also been suspected of accelerating collagenase activity since increasing temperature facilitates the rate of chemical reaction. In vivo studies are not available to clarify these speculations.[8]

Pain

Heat application might directly alleviate pain by acting as a counterirritant as described by the gate control theory.[3,8] Other researchers offer limited support for this theory and rank heat third as compared with other counterirritants in relieving pain. Pain relief might also be explained in part through the action of endorphins. Limited physiologic data exist supporting this suggestion.[8]

Methods of Heat Application

Heating modalities can be categorized according to the predominant method of heat transfer (i.e., conduction, convection, or conversion) or according to their ability to heat superficial or deep tissues selectively (Table 9-1).[8]

Superficial Heat

Conduction. When a temperature gradient exists in a stationary medium, which may be a solid or a fluid, the term conduction is used to refer to the heat transfer that occurs across the medium. The mechanism of conduction is diffusion of energy from the more energetic to the less energetic particles of a substance due to random molecular motion.[13] Clinically, conduction is referred

Table 9-1. Heating Modalities Subdivided According to Primary Mode of Heat Transfer

Primary Mode of Heat Transfer	Modality	
Conduction	Hot packs	
	Paraffin bath	
	Fluidotherapy	Superficial heat
Convection	Hydrotherapy	
	Moist air	
Conversion	Radiant heat	
	Microwaves	
	Shortwaves	Deep heat
	Ultrasound	

(Lehmann JF, DeLateur BJ: Therapeutic heat. p. 404. In Lehmann JF (ed): Therapeutic Heat and Cold. 3rd Ed. © 1982 The Williams & Wilkins Co., Baltimore.)

to when this phenomenon occurs between two objects of different temperatures that are in contact. In the human body, the quantity of blood flow in addition to the temperature gradient will affect the rate of transfer. To raise tissue temperatures, heat must be transferred at a rate faster than it can be dissipated.[8]

Examples of conductive heat modalities include moist heat packs, paraffin, and recently marketed gel packs; depth of heat penetration is usually 1 cm or less.[8] Hot packs have been recommended for treating foot and ankle pain due to painful lower motor neuron neuritis and connective tissue diseases.[8,14,15] Hot packs, heating pads, and hot water bottles have been reported as effective in treating injuries after active swelling or inflammatory process has ceased, as well as for draining superficial infections. Most of these reports are offered as clinical observation.[12,16] Paraffin baths can be used to decrease joint stiffness in the rheumatoid foot or to treat subacute and chronic sprains and strains of the distal lower extremities.[8,12,15]

Convection. Convection refers to a heat transfer between a surface and a moving fluid when they are at different temperatures.[13] A fluid can be a gas or a liquid, a substance whose particles easily move and change their relative position.[17] The actual transfer of energy from the fluid to solid surfaces in contact with it occurs by means of conduction, but the energy is transported from one point in space to another primarily by displacement of the fluid. Hydrotherapy and fluidotherapy are examples of convective heating.[18] Heating through use of hydrotherapy has been suggested for foot and ankle pain due to intrinsic muscle trauma, connective tissue diseases, neuritis, tenosynovitis, contractures, suppurating wounds, decubitus ulcers, hematomas, early stages of peripheral vascular disease, varicose veins, subacute synovitis, strains, and sprains, especially of the plantar ligament and tarsal joint.[14-16] Fluidotherapy has been demonstrated to raise the temperature of joint capsules in the foot effectively.[19]

Thermal radiation. A body whose surface temperature is above absolute zero emits electromagnetic (primarily infrared) radiation. Radiation incident on a surface of another body can be reflected, transmitted into or through it, and/or absorbed. Absorbed radiation excites the body thermally and is referred to as radiant heating. Examples of radiant heat modalities are infrared and ultraviolet radiation.[18] In treating foot and ankle pain, radiant heat is occasionally used for open wounds, lesions resistant to healing and injuries for which the weight of a moist heat pack would be uncomfortable.[12] General indications include reflexogenic relief of muscle spasms due to underlying joint or skeletal pathology and treatment of rheumatic joints in which direct temperature elevation of the joint is contraindicated but relief of a secondary spasm is desired.[8]

Deep Heat

Conversion. Conversion is the mechanism of heat transport by which various forms of energy (e.g., mechanical, electrical, or electromagnetic) are transmitted into a body in which they appear primarily as heat; nonthermal energy is converted into thermal energy. Conversion includes all forms of diathermy and radiant heat.[18] Radiant heat is a form of superficial heat, however, and has already been discussed.

Diathermy includes three forms of energy: (1) high-frequency currents (short-wave), (2) electromagnetic radiation (microwaves), and (3) ultrasound (acoustic waves).[8] Shortwave diathermy conducts an alternating current from a generator, through a capacitor, through the person being treated to another capacitor, and back to the generator. Systemic ions in the body line up with the alternating polarity and create friction as they collide. Theoretically, capacitor-electrode heating will induce greatest power absorption in subcutaneous fat.[8] If the object to be heated is small and subcutaneous fat is negligible (e.g., ankles or feet), relatively uniform heating occurs.[8] Inductive applicators have demonstrated experimentally higher energy absorption in muscle (a deeper, high-water-content tissue). Shortwave diathermy has been recommended for treatment of pain due to muscle spasms, stiffness, contractures of joints with little soft tissue covering, and later stages of traumatic arthritis.[8] Heating proximal to a vascular occlusion has been recommended to effect reflex vasodilation in a distal area.[8,14] It can also be applied to the lumbar area to provoke reflex heating and dilation of extremity vessels.[14]

Microwaves are a form of electromagnetic radiation used to heat muscle selectively, since most of the energy is absorbed by tissues with high water content without undue heating of subcutaneous and cutaneous tissues. Recommendations for use include fibrous muscular contractures, secondary muscle spasm, and joints with thin soft-tissue covering.[8] The literature contains subjective reports of benefits in healing surgical and traumatic foot lesions.[20]

Ultrasound is a form of high-frequency acoustic vibration. The ultrasound wave is longitudinal, with alternating areas of compression and rarefaction that move forward and then backward along the line of propagation. The wave changes direction, and energy is transferred at each tissue interface, causing a localized rise in temperature. Absorption and velocity in collagen suspensions have been reported to be much greater than in suspensions of globular proteins. Therefore, joint capsules, scars, and tendons may be selectively heated. Joint temperatures have also been selectively raised as have larger nerve trunks imbedded in myofascial interfaces.[8]

When a peripheral nerve is exposed to ultrasound at intensities between 0.5 and 1.5 W/cm^2, conduction velocity decreases. At intensities below 0.5 or above 2.0 W/cm^2, conduction velocity increases. It is not clear why this occurs.[21]

Chemical effects of ultrasound, which are due at least in part to thermal effects, include increased enzyme activity, increased ion exchange rate, increased cell membrane permeability, and increased rate and volume of diffusion across cell membranes.[1]

The literature recommends use of ultrasound for foot pain due to plantar ligament and tarsal joint strain, Dupuytren's contracture of the feet (reportedly softens fibrous tissue but doesn't stop disease progression), bursitis (increases permeability of semipermeable membranes), neuritic pain in scar tissue, heel pain associated with ankylosing spondylitis or Reiter's syndrome, and varicose ulcers (reportedly aids tissue repair).[14-16] Underwater ultrasound and hydrosonic baths have been subjectively reported to benefit largely musculoskeletal foot pain.[22] Ultrasound decreases pain from plantar warts and can totally destroy such lesions; direct contact has been more effective than the underwater technique for this purpose.[23]

Phonophoresis. Phonophoresis is the use of ultrasound to drive molecules of a substance, usually an antiinflammatory and possibly an anesthetic medication, into tissues. These molecules become broken down into ionic compounds that are free to recombine into useful radicals for use in chemical reactions in the body. Phonophoresis is capable of driving molecules into tissues to depths up to 2 inches.[1,23]

Medications commonly used in phonophoresis include:[1,12,23]

1. One to 10 percent hydrocortisone cream, to decrease inflammation.
2. Two to 5 percent lidocaine ointment (Xylocaine), for anesthetic purposes.
3. Dexamethasone and 2 percent lidocaine gel, for antiinflammatory and anesthetic purposes.
4. Ten percent salicylate (Myoflex), also for antiinflammatory and analgesic purposes.
5. One to 4 percent iodine/salicylate (Iodex with methyl salicylate), for antiinflammatory and analgesic purposes when a sclerolytic agent is desired to enhance the salicylate effects.

Medications are chosen based on the quality, nature, and severity of pain. Usually a liquid or an ointment contains the desired ingredient and serves as the coupling agent.[21] Chemical sensitivities of the patient will dictate which medications should not be used.[1]

Specific subjective reports of benefits in treatment of foot pain include those in heel pain secondary to plantar fasciitis and in tenosynovitis.[14] Clinical research has shown ultrasound and phonophoresis as well as iontophoresis and ice massage to be equally effective in reducing shinsplint pain, but ultrasound has not been as effective in increasing active range of motion.[24]

General Contraindications to Heat Therapy

Because dosimetry of heat application is not exact, subjective feedback on the part of the patient to perceive pain during administration of heat modalities is necessary. Therefore, its use is generally contraindicated in an obtunded patient or over anesthetic areas. Heat should not be applied if active hemorrhage or swelling exists. Heat should not be applied to tissues lacking sufficient blood supply because ischemic necrosis might result from the inability to respond vascularly to increases in metabolism. It is contraindicated over malignant tumors (due to possible acceleration of tumor growth and formation of metastases) as well as during acute thrombophlebitis (due to increased risk of emboli). Caution is necessary when applying heat to patients with inadequate cardiac or respiratory reserves.[8]

Contraindications to Superficial Heat

In patients with foot and ankle pain, paraffin and fluidotherapy should not be used to treat open wounds. Radiant heat should not be used for patients who are light-sensitive, and caution should be taken with superficial heat of any kind for patients who are heat- or photosensitive.[8]

Contraindications to Deep Heat

Contraindications that should be considered when treating foot and ankle problems are the presence of metal implants, cardiac pacemakers, or other electronic packets for controlling electrophysiological orthoses. The exception is that ultrasound may be used safely with metal implants,[8] but my clinical experience has shown that ultrasound can be occasionally painful even with low intensities when used over metal implants. Ultrasound should not be used with modern plastic joint replacements, since no data exist showing whether the heat will destroy the plastic or damage surrounding tissues. Shortwave diathermy should be applied so that a significant rise in temperature does not occur in growth zones of bones in children. As long as the pain threshold is not exceeded in ultrasound application, growth disturbances are not observed.[8] Ultrasound is contraindicated for healing fractures because it may delay or prevent callus formation.[21]

THERAPEUTIC COLD

General Physiological Effects

The physiological effects of local cold application that are generally agreed on include:

1. Local vasoconstriction occurs. Subsequently, this causes a decrease in local blood flow, which in turn causes a reduction in local swelling and hemorrhage.[1,25-27]

2. With prolonged cold application, a secondary vasodilation occurs, referred to as the "hunting response," as a protective mechanism to maintain temperatures at a level adequate to prevent tissue damage.[1,16,25-27] Dilation of blood vessels is believed to occur largely in the muscle.[25]

3. Cellular metabolism becomes depressed, thereby reducing the oxygen requirements of the cell.[1,16,26,27]

4. Nerve conduction velocity in peripheral nerves slows in response to cooling.[1,25-27]

5. Peripheral receptors become less excitable.[1]

6. Muscle spasm and spasticity can be reduced.[1,25,27]

Specific Physiological Responses

Cryotherapy is the use of local cold applications for therapeutic reasons. Foot and ankle problems in which cryotherapy might be desirable for direct or indirect pain relief include: mechanical trauma, inflammation, muscle spasm, and spasticity.

Mechanical Trauma

Acute mechanical trauma is commonly treated with local cold applications in an attempt to effect vasoconstriction. This is achieved indirectly through a reflex vasoconstriction through the sympathetic fibers and can also be accomplished by direct cooling of the blood vessels, as documented in the literature.[25] Decreasing blood flow through damaged vessels reduces edema. Less histamine is released, and therefore less capillary breakdown occurs.[26] Histamine is responsible for vasodilation and exudate formation.[27] Immediate application of cold can minimize the severity of local cellular damage not only by restricting hemorrhage and edema, but also by reducing metabolic demands. Therefore, tissue viability can be preserved despite the temporary compromise in vascularity. Although it is generally assumed that edema is reduced with cooling and increased with heating, the effectiveness in reducing edema may depend on the type of cold application used (e.g., cold water vs cold packs).[25]

Pain occurring as a result of trauma can be reduced directly or indirectly through cold application. Cold directly affects sensory endings and pain fibers. Indirect pain relief is achieved by decreasing painful swelling and muscle spasm as well as the amount of histamine released.

Clinical researchers tend to judge the effectiveness of cold application for traumatic injuries through reports of symptomatic relief and time until return to functional activities.[26,28] Specifically, earlier return to function following ankle sprain injuries has been demonstrated with cryotherapy initiated within 36 hours as compared with cryotherapy initiated later than 36 hours and also as compared with heat administered within 1 hour, within 36 hours, or later than 36 hours after trauma.[26]

Inflammation

The method of application of cold to a body part may influence whether edema will increase or decrease. Experimentally produced inflammatory edema is not always reduced and sometimes is aggravated by cooling. The agent responsible for the inflammation seems to dictate the response. Heat always produces a different response, usually in the opposite direction of that resulting with cooling.[25]

Cold retards toxicity and spread of bacterial inflammatory reactions.[25] Cooling acute or subacute rheumatoid joints may inhibit collagenase activity, reducing cartilage destruction.[6,25] The impression that cooling may alleviate rheumatoid symptomatology is based mostly on subjective reports.

Pain from bursitis has been relieved by aspiration, thereby decreasing pressure. Therefore, cold is usually preferable to heat for acute bursitis because it may decrease swelling, indirectly relieving pain, although the exact mechanism by which this is achieved is not clear.[25]

Cold, especially in the form of coolant sprays such as fluoromethane or ethyl chloride, has been subjectively reported to relieve pain from trigger points, myofibrositis, and myofascial pain. These are believed to act as counterirritants, but more study is necessary in this area.[25]

Pain and stiffness can be reduced in the rheumatoid joint by application of cold. Pain relief is achieved by direct effects on the pain receptors and fibers. Stiffness, while objectively increased with cold application, can subjectively be reduced if the application is vigorous enough to decrease sensation.[25]

Spasticity and Muscle Spasm

Although cold reduces spasticity and muscle spasm, the exact mechanism of its action is not clear. It has been suggested that increased γ efferent discharge does not directly produce tension on a muscle, but causes increased sensory discharge of muscle spindles. This reflexly elicits muscle contraction through excitation of the α motor neurons.[27] Theoretically, change in discharge of the muscle spindle as a result of cooling could be due to an effect on extrafusal muscle, intrafusal fibers, or sensory endings. At least 10 minutes of cold application are necessary to cool muscle significantly. Some experiments support the idea that cold primarily affects the sensory wrappings in the spindles, probably as a result of changes in membrane stability. With the initial lowering of temperature, spindle sensitivity increases. Below 30°C, spindle sensitivity decreases with further lowering of muscle temperature.[25]

Cold applied long enough to produce a drop in muscle temperature has been shown to cause a decrease in the Achilles tendon reflex. Cooling the muscle has been suggested to produce a direct effect on the spindle and possibly also on the γ efferents, causing a reduction in spindle sensitivity, which may be the basis for reduction of muscle tone. Reportedly, cooling increases α motor neuron excitability, which may be the basis for use of ice massage for neuromuscular facilitation techniques.[25]

Superficial cold application may cause a reflex sympathetic influence on the muscle spindle prior to actual cooling of the muscle, causing a reduction in sensitivity and consequently reducing spasm or spasticity. This has not been directly demonstrated. To obtain prolonged and optimal reduction in spasticity, cooling the muscle is essential. Superficial cooling and its possible effects on skin enteroceptors and sympathetic stimulation are less well documented and clinically are reported to be less significant in functionally altering spasticity.[25]

Cold seems to affect peripheral nerves based upon myelination and fiber diameter. According to experiments with cats, cooling affects small medullated fibers first, then the large medullated fibers, and finally the unmedullated fibers. Smaller γ efferent fibers are more sensitive to cold than are larger α efferents. This information is, however, somewhat species dependent. Several studies are consistent in reporting that the sensory fibers important for motor learning [e.g., proprioceptive fibers that are myelinated large-diameter fibers] are relatively insensitive to cold (Table 9-2).[25]

Heat vs Cold in Regard to Muscle Tone

Therapeutic heat and cold clinically reduce muscle spasm and spasticity. To summarize what has been presented, key events during heating and cooling are reviewed.

Most secondary afferents in the muscle spindle respond more to tonic than phasic stretch and become less sensitive (i.e., rate of firing decreases) in response to heating. This is supplemented by an increased firing of Golgi tendon organs (also in response to heating), which exert an inhibitory effect on muscle tone. Because muscle spasm is considered largely a tonic phenomenon, these secondary afferents probably exert the main influence on muscle tone.[25]

Although cold initially increases muscle spindle sensitivity, muscle temperatures below 30°C cause a decrease in sensitivity. This response is probably due to changes in membrane stability of sensory wrappings and decreased γ efferent excitability.[25] Temperatures at both ends of the physiologic spectrum appear to cause a reduction in spindle sensitivity.

Table 9-2. Nerve Fiber Type, Function, Diameter and Conduction Velocity

Fiber Type	Function	Fiber Diameter (μm)	Conduction Velocity (ms)
A α	Proprioception, somatic motor	12–20	70–120
β	Touch, pressure	5–12	30–70
γ	Motor to muscle spindles	3–6	15–30
δ	Pain, temperature, touch	2–5	12–30
B	Preganglionic autonomic	< 3	3–15
C Dorsal root	Pain, reflex responses	0.4–1.2	0.5–2
Sympathetic	Postganglionic sympathetics	0.3–1.3	0.7–2.3

(Ganong WF: The Nervous System. 2nd Ed. Appleton & Lange, East Norwalk, 1979.)

Due to the complexity of the neural mechanism in spasticity, studies on hemiplegic patients have demonstrated increases, decreases, and no effect on the spasticity of the involved extremity in response to cooling.[25] Apparently, the factor or factors dictating resultant tone in response to heating or cooling are still unclear. Although heat can reduce spasticity, effects are short-lived due to rapid return to normal tissue temperatures as a result of the increased blood flow. This does not allow functional training in motor skills. The thermodynamics of cooling tissues maintains muscle temperatures below normal long enough to allow functional training. The prolonged results of heat used to reduce muscle spasm probably occur due to interruption of the pain cycle.[25]

Pain

Pain can be reduced by the direct effect of cold on the pain receptors and fibers. Peripheral receptors become less excitable following cold application. Cold also creates a competitive inhibition within the central nervous system.[25,27] Cold decreases nerve conduction velocities of peripheral nerves at a rate of 2.4 m/s/°C.[23] Pain perception and muscle contractibility diminish with cooling.[1]

Indirect pain relief might be achieved by reducing edema secondary to inflammation or trauma as well as by reducing spasm or spasticity. If the perception of pain is overcome, perhaps the pain cycle is broken and motor impulses causing muscle spasm cease.[27] The exact cause-and-effect relationship is apparently unclear.

Methods of Cold Application

Cold can be applied in three ways. Convective cooling, which is achieved by air movement over the skin, is not mentioned in the literature concerning foot and ankle pain. Evaporative cooling results when a substance applied to the skin uses thermal energy to evaporate; surface temperature is lowered.[1] The literature reports use of vapor-coolant spray (ethyl chloride or fluoromethane) for treatment of foot pain secondary to acute trauma such as traumatic tendinitis, contusion, strain, fibrositis, contractures of intrinsic foot muscles. It has also been used to treat trigger points causing foot pain, cramps due to mechanical causes, and neuritic pain in scar tissue.[14]

Conductive cooling occurs when a cold object is in contact with the body part to be cooled; heat transfers from the body part to the object. Examples of conductive cold applications are ice massage, cold-water immersion, and cold packs. Three types of cold packs can be used. Plastic bags or wet towels filled with cubed or shaved ice are inexpensive and frequently used, especially in the home. Chemical cold packs are available but are expensive and cannot be reused. Temperatures produced by mixing the chemical contents are not consistent, however, and if the pack should rupture, chemical burns can occur. Flexible gel cold packs are convenient and reusable.[12]

Conductive cooling is the most commonly reported method of cooling and the literature recommends it for treatment of acute trauma, such as ankle sprains, foot and ankle surgery, fractures, contusions, tendinitis, strains, and muscle spasms.[12,14,16,26,28] It has also been used for effective relief of foot and ankle pain due to connective tissue diseases, such as rheumatoid arthritis, for heel pain due to plantar fasciitis, as well as for cramps secondary to mechanical causes or trigger points.[14,15] Cold therapy is usually performed in conjunction with compression and elevation of the body part being treated and occasionally with intermittent compression devices. Contrast baths have been recommended for relieving foot pain due to arthritis and other connective tissue diseases, contusions, fractures, and chilblains.[15,16] Dependent positioning may, however, negate effectiveness if edema reduction is also intended.[29]

Adverse Effects

Cold is contraindicated in hypersensitivity syndromes, which can be grouped into three categories. In the first group, histamine or histaminelike substances are released in response to cold. This syndrome is responsive to treatment by desensitization to cold by cold-water immersion or subcutaneous administration of histamine. In the second category, hypersensitivity is the result of cold hemolysins and agglutinins. The third group of hypersensitivity syndromes result from the presence of cryoglobulins. These syndromes sometimes occur in patients with associated diseases, such as lupus erythematosus, atypical pneumonia, leukocytoclastic vasculitis, rheumatoid disease, progressive systemic sclerosis, or multiple myeloma. Raynaud's phenomenon may be manifested in the second and third categories.[25] Cold is contraindicated in Raymaud's disease and should be used cautiously with very young and elderly persons and with individuals who have peripheral vascular disease or other circulatory problems.[1] Overexposure can cause tissue damage and can occur with use of modalities capable of dropping the temperature below the freezing point and possibly with use of supercooled ice blocks for massage. Excessive evaporative cooling through improper use of ethyl chloride and chlorofluoro-methanes can produce frostbite. Residual injury due to frostbite depends on the length of time the tissue is frozen, the temperature during the frozen state, and the duration of thawing. Therefore, treatment time should be limited according to the type of cold modality used with regard to how vigorously it will cool.[25]

ELECTRICAL STIMULATION

Transcutaneous Electrical Nerve Stimulation (TENS)

The gate control theory of pain explains in part why peripheral electrical nerve stimulation may alleviate or abolish the perception of pain. In response to this proposition, direct stimulation of the dorsal column of the spinal cord was attempted. The need to predict which patients would respond favorably to dorsal column stimulation led to the development of a device for transcutaneous electrical stimulation of peripheral nerves. This means of stimulation apparently controlled the pain perception almost as well as the dorsal column implants. Consequently, TENS has become an integral part of pain management.[30]

TENS stimulates the nervous system by applying controlled, low-voltage electrical pulses through the skin by surface electrodes. Although indications for use of TENS seem almost limitless, it is not a panacea for resolution of all pain. TENS is best used as an adjunct to a comprehensive program of pain management including evaluation, treatment of causes, pain modulation, and prevention of recurrence. TENS is usually applied in conjunction with drug and other forms of therapy for pain relief.[11]

Although numerous studies claim effectiveness for TENS in various clinical manifestations of pain, scientifically valid data concerning the underlying neurophysiologic mechanisms are still scarce.[1,31] Recent literature has, however, delineated specific protocols for treatment of specific pathological conditions and effectiveness of TENS in pain associated with these conditions. More attention has been paid to specific electrode placement and stimulation characteristics allowing replication and comparison of studies on specific diagnostic groups of patients.[32]

Neurophysiologic Mechanisms

Many clinicians believe that the gate control theory accounts for the effects of TENS in controlling pain. Application of this theory proposes that large-diameter afferents can be selectively stimulated, in this case by small voltages from TENS devices, causing segmental stimulation of the dorsal horn of the spinal cord and effecting presynaptic inhibition (closing of the gate).[1,31] Limitations of this theory lie in observations that pain can be modulated in the absence of large-diameter axons. Melzack and Casey have suggested a modified theory, the central control trigger theory, which implicates the dorsal column transmission of large fiber input to activate the central inhibitory mechanisms that descend to modulate pain transmission neurons in the dorsal horn of the spinal cord. Another hypothesis is that TENS may produce an antidromic blocking of pain impulses. Although TENS is capable of reducing sympathetic tone, the role of the autonomic nervous system and its possible impact on pain modulation require further investigation.[31]

TENS has been implicated in pain modulation through the release of endogenous opiates from various sites throughout the CNS, particularly the periaqueductal gray in the brainstem. Further study is necessary to determine specific sites of TENS action as well as pharmacologic agents capable of antagonizing the effects of TENS.[31]

Stimulation Modes

Conventional TENS is the most commonly used mode. Electrical wave parameters include a pulse rate of 50 to 100 Hz (high rate), a pulse width of 40 to 75 μs (narrow width) and an intensity optimally to a level of comfort with a deep perception of paresthesia throughout the painful area. Onset of pain relief is rapid but relatively short-lived, although prolonged relief of pain is reported. This mode is designed to stimulate large myelinated afferent fibers selectively; muscle contraction or fasciculation should not be apparent.[33]

Acupuncturelike TENS uses a low pulse rate (1 to 4 Hz), wide pulse width (150 to 250 μs) and a strong intensity. Onset of pain relief is slow, necessitating at least 20 to 30 minutes of treatment time, with strong visible muscle contractions in segmentally related myotomes; effective relief of pain usually lasts for prolonged periods. This mode of TENS is usually not well tolerated in the area of pain. Despite the name (acupuncturelike TENS), stimulation does not have to be performed on acupuncture points.[33] Analgesia produced by acupuncturelike TENS has been observed to be reversible with administration of naloxone, implicating a release of endogenous opiates with this mode.[1,33]

Brief, intense TENS uses a pulse rate of 100 to 150 Hz (high), a pulse width of 150 to 250 μs (wide), and an intensity to tolerance, causing a tetanic contraction or nonrhythmic fasciculations. Treatment time of 5 to 15 minutes is recommended, and electrode placements close to the painful areas are suggested. Pain relief is of rapid onset but usually diminishes quickly. This mode is recommended for use with performance of gentle manual therapeutic techniques, suture removal, skin debridement, and possibly minor surgical procedures.[33]

Pulse-train (burst) TENS is achieved with a wide pulse width (100 to 200 μs), high intensity (to tolerance, producing strong, rhythmic contractions with a background paresthesia), and a combination train of pulses with high-frequency bursts with each low-rate pulse.[33]

Table 9-3. Specific Guidelines To Optimal Stimulation Site Selection

1. Delineate the nature, location, and structural source of pain.
2. Determine the spinal cord and segmental levels that innervate the involved structure (joint, muscle, peripheral nerve, etc.) or region of pain.
3. Use the illustrations and related tables for initial location of optimal stimulation sites (OSS) that are anatomically and/or physiologically related to the involved structure or area of pain.
4. Palpate for tenderness or scan for increased electrical conductance (decreased skin resistance) those OSS that exist within or adjacent to, or which innervate the area of pain.
5. The choice of OSS and electrode placement arrangements depends on the specific stimulation mode to be used as well as the pain distribution.
   a. When conventional, low-intensity pulse-train (burst) or brief, intense modes are used, electrode placement must ensure the perception of electrical paresthesia throughout the entire area of pain (use OSS at related spinal cord segments and over superficial aspects of the peripheral nerves that arise from them).
5. b. Strong, low-rate and high-intensity, pulse-train (burst) modes require muscle contraction of segmentally related myotomes, which may or may not be located away from the painful region (use OSS that are motor points and/or located over superficial aspects of mixed nerves innervating the painful region).
   c. It may be necessary to stimulate bilaterally in a criss-cross manner, contralaterally, or only proximal to the painful region in specific pain syndromes such as bilateral low back pain, postherpetic neuralgia, or peripheral nerve injury, respectively, to obtain greater benefit.
6. Electrodes of varying sizes and shapes may also need to be used.

(Mannheimer JS, Lampe GN: Electrode placement sites and their relationship. p. 249. In Mannheimer JS, Lampe GN (eds): Clinical Transcutaneous Electrical Nerve Stimulation. FA Davis, Philadelphia, 1984.)

Guidelines for Electrode Placement

For an area of the body to be an optimal site for TENS, several factors must be considered: The site should allow stimulation to be directed into the CNS; the area should be segmentally related to the pain-causing structure; the area should allow easy access for electrode placement, including total contact of the pad with the skin; and the anatomic landmark chosen should be distinctly located.[33] Specific guidelines for optimal stimulation site selection have been suggested by Mannheimer (Table 9-3).[34]

Factors Influencing Effectiveness of TENS

Attempting to control pain with TENS requires several considerations. Mannheimer and Lampe have suggested hindering, enhancing, and restoring factors that should provide the clinician with greater insight to the use of TENS for pain modulation (Table 9-4).[5]

If the patient is not capable of applying the TENS device, a family member or another available person must administer the device and therefore should be included in the educational aspects of the treatment program. Moreover, if the patient is unable to inform the therapist as to the effectiveness of TENS for pain relief, another person must be available to observe and report changes in the patient's behavior that might indicate a change in perception of pain.

Table 9-4. Factors Influencing the Effectiveness of TENS

Hindering	Enhancing	Restoring
Senility	Wean from medications	Tryptophan loading
Dependency	Tricyclics/tryptophan	Ice massage
"Cure syndrome"	D-phenylalanine	Change stimulation mode
↓ Manual dexterity	Stimulation close to area of	Change electrode placement
Visual impairment	pain (brief, intense)	sites
Unwillingness of patient to	Increased tolerance should	Reevaluate pain distribution;
evaluate alternate elec-	result from a gradual	it may have changed
trode placement sites after	progression to stronger	Modulate current parame-
initial failure with TENS	stimulation parameters	ters
↑ pain perception after	If stronger stimulation	
TENS	modes cannot be tolerated	
Diazepam	at the painful region, try	
Narcotics/addiction	stimulation in segmentally	
Corticosteroids	related, but not painful,	
Prolonged pain and stress	myotomes on ipsilateral,	
Poor posture and/or body	contralateral, or bilateral	
mechanics	regions	
	Pulse-train stimulation may	
	be tolerated better than	
	acupuncturelike stimula-	
	tion with equal effective-	
	ness	
	Do not stimulate over areas	
	of dry, scaly skin	
	Place electrodes over motor	
	points when using acu-	
	puncturelike, burst, or	
	pulse-train modes	
	Use self-adhering electrodes	
	Skin preparation may en-	
	hance electrode adherence	
	Patient should perceive	
	stimulation throughout the	
	area of pain with conven-	
	tional TENS	
	Placement of one electrode	
	at the proximal and distal	
	extent of pain (conven-	
	tional and brief, intense)	
	Evaluation of posture and	
	body mechanics	

TENS, transcutaneous electrical nerve stimulation.

(Mannheimer JS, Lampe GN: Factors that hinder, enhance, and restore the effectiveness of TENS: physiologic and theoretical considerations. p. 529. In Mannheimer JS, Lampe GN (eds): Clinical Transcutaneous Electrical Nerve Stimulation. FA Davis, Philadelphia, 1984.)

Conditions Responsive to TENS

Subjective reports of effectiveness of TENS with foot and ankle pain include: peripheral neuropathies (including frostbite), fractures, or sprains; postherpetic neuralgia; and various soft tissue and osseous surgical procedures.[33]

Contraindications and Precautions

TENS should not be used on a patient with a pacemaker, particularly a demand pacemaker. Stimulation is contraindicated over the carotid sinuses because this could cause a hypotensive response and/or cardiac arrest due to a vasovagal reflex. Precautions should be taken in cases of pregnancy, use around the eyes, internal use, epilepsy, other seizure disorders, cerebrovascular accident, transient ischemic attacks, anterior chest wall pain in cardiac patients, and incompetent patients.[35]

Iontophoresis

Iontophoresis is the use of direct (galvanic) current to drive chemical ions of like charge into the subcutaneous tissue. Ionizable compounds must be used, and the physiologic effect depends on the ion used.

Effective analgesic ions include:[1]

1. Lidocaine (Xylocaine): Five percent ointment. Administer under the positive pole. This is a fast-acting analgesic but results are short-lived.
2. Cortisol (Hydrocortisone): One percent cortisol demonstrates delayed onset of pain relief but has a prolonged effect due to antiinflammatory action. Administer under the positive pole.
3. Magnesium: Administer under the positive pole. This ion effects decreased muscle spasm by inhibiting muscle contraction and increases vasodilation because of inhibition of smooth muscle contraction in walls of the vasculature.
4. Iodine (Iodex ointment): Administer under the negative pole. This is a sclerolytic agent and is frequently combined with methyl salicylate (also a negative ion), an antiinflammatory agent.
5. Acetic acid/lithium: Acetic acid is administered under the negative pole, and lithium is administered under the positive pole. These ions are used for treatment of painful calcific deposits and gouty tophi through exchange of the deposits for chemicals administered. In the process of replacement iontophoreses, insoluble radicals in the deposits are replaced with the more soluble radicals: acetic acid (2 percent solution) for calcific deposits, and lithium (2 percent solution) for gouty tophi.

Because galvanic current is used, chemical changes under the electrodes, especially under the more irritating negative electrode, can irritate the skin. To avoid this, the negative electrode should be larger than the positive electrode, and the skin should be treated with an astringent and then cornstarch following treatment. The equipment and skin should be monitored frequently (every 3 to 5 minutes) to prevent complications.[1]

Treatment of postacute soft tissue injuries, tendinitis, strains, bursitis, tenosynovitis, and neuritic pain in scar tissue have been subjectively reported as indications for treatment.[12,14] Contraindications for the medications used and for electrical stimulation apply.[12]

AUTHOR'S NOTE

This chapter was written in the author's private capacity. No official support or endorsement by the United States Department of Health and Human Services is intended or should be inferred.

REFERENCES

1. Mirabelli L: Pain management. p. 600. In Umphred DA (ed): Neurological Rehabilitation. CV Mosby, St. Louis, 1985
2. Melzack R, Wall PD: Pain mechanisms: a new theory. Science 150:971, 1965
3. Melzack R: Myofascial trigger points: relation to acupuncture and mechanisms of pain. Arch Phys Med Rehabil 62:114, 1981
3a. Melzack R, Casey KL: Sensory, motivation and central control determinants of pain. p. 423. In Kenshalo DR (ed): The Skin Senses. Charles C Thomas, Springfield, Illinois, 1968
4. Wolf SL: Neurophysiologic mechanisms in pain modulation: relevance to TENS. p. 41. In Mannheimer JS, Lampe GN (eds): Clinical Transcutaneous Electrical Nerve Stimulation. FA Davis, Philadelphia, 1984
5. Mannheimer JS, Lampe GN: Factors that hinder, enhance, and restore the effectiveness of TENS: physiologic and theoretical considerations. p. 529. In Mannhiemer JS, Lampe GN (eds): Clinical Transcutaneous Electrical Nerve Stimulation. FA Davis, Philadelphia, 1984
6. Gerber L: Principles and their application in the rehabilitation of patients with rheumatic disease. p. 1849. In Kelley WN, et al (eds): Textbook of Rheumatology. WB Saunders, Philadelphia, 1981
7. Long DM, Campbell JN, Gucer G: Transcutaneous electrical stimulation for relief of chronic pain. p. 593. In Bonica JJ, et al (eds): Advances in Pain Research and Therapy. Vol. 3. Raven Press, New York, 1979
8. Lehmann JF, DeLateur BJ: Therapeutic heat. p. 404. In Lehmann JF (ed): Therapeutic Heat and Cold. 3rd Ed. Williams & Wilkins, Baltimore, 1982
9. Ganong WF: The Nervous System. 2nd Ed. Appleton & Lange, 1979
10. Stein RB: Peripheral control of movement. Physiol Rev 54:215, 1974
11. Mannheimer JS, Lampe GN: Pain and TENS in pain management. p. 7. In Mannheimer JS, Lampe GN (eds): Clinical Transcutaneous Electrical Nerve Stimulation. FA Davis, Philadelphia, 1984
12. Ellison AE, et al: Athletic Training and Sports Medicine. American Academy of Orthopaedic Surgeons, Chicago, 1984
13. Incropera FP, Dewitt DP: Fundamentals of Heat & Mass Transfer. 2nd Ed. John Wiley & Sons, New York, 1985
14. Mennell, JM: Foot Pain. Little, Brown, Boston, 1969

15. Bardwick PA, Swezey RL: Physical modalities for treating the foot affected by connective tissue diseases. Foot Ankle 3:41, 1982
16. Feldman RS, Hugar DW: Physical therapy: its use in podiatry. J Foot Surg 20:102, 1981
17. Roberson JA, Crowe CT: Engineering Fluid Mechanics, 2nd Ed. Houghton Mifflin, Boston, 1980
18. Sekins KM, Emery AF: Thermal science for physical medicine. p. 70. In Lehman JF (ed): Therapeutic Heat and Cold. 3rd Ed. Williams & Wilkins, Baltimore, 1982
19. Borrell RM, Parker R, Henley EJ, et al: Comparison of in vivo temperatures produced by hydrotherapy, paraffin wax treatment and fluidotherapy. Phys Ther 60(10):1273, 1980
20. Zulli LP: Pulsed high frequency electromagnetic energy for adjuvant care of foot lesions. J Am Podiatry Assoc 58(8):343, 1968
21. Griffin JE, Karselis TC: Physical Agents for Physical Therapists. Charles C Thomas, Springfield, 1978
22. Kaiser HS: A new method of applying ultrasonic therapy. J Am Podiatry Assoc 60(7):280, 1970
23. Antich TJ: Phonophoresis: the principles of the ultrasonic driving force and efficacy intreatment of common orthopaedic diagnoses. J Orthop Sports Phys Ther 4(2):99, 1982
24. Smith W, Winn F, Parette R: Comparative study using four modalities in shinsplint treatments. J Orthop Sports Phys Ther 8(2):77, 1986
25. Lehmann JF, DeLateur BJ: Cryotherapy. p. 563. In Lehmann JF (ed): Therapeutic Heat and Cold. Williams & Wilkins, Baltimore, 1982
26. Hocutt JE, et al: Cryotherapy in ankle sprains. Am J Sports Med 10:316, 1982
27. Olson JE, Stravino VD: A review of cryotherapy. Phys Ther 52:840, 1972
28. Hayden CA: Cryokinetics in an early treatment program. Phys Ther 44(11):990, 1964
29. Sims D: Effects of positioning on ankle edema. J Orthop Sports Phys Ther 8(1):30, 1986
30. Hymes A: Introduction: a review of the historical uses of electricity. p. 1. In Mannheimer JS, Lampe GN (eds): Clinical Transcutaneous Electrical Nerve Stimulation. FA Davis, Philadelphia, 1984
31. Wolf SL: Neurophysiologic mechanisms in pain modulation: relevance to TENS. p. 41. In Mannheimer JS, Lampe GN (eds): Clinical Transcutaneous Electrical Nerve Stimulation. FA Davis, Philadelphia, 1984
32. Gersh MR, Wolf SL: Applications of transcutaneous electrical nerve stimulation in the management of patients with pain: state-of-the-art update. Phys Ther 65(3):314, 1985
33. Mannheimer JS, Lampe GN: Electrode placement techniques. p. 331. In Mannheimer JS, Lampe GN (eds): Clinical Transcutaneous Electrical Nerve Stimulation. FA Davis, Philadelphia, 1984
34. Mannheimer JS, Lampe GN: Electrode placement sites and their relationship. p. 249. In Mannheimer JS, Lampe GN (eds): Clinical Transcutaneous Electrical Nerve Stimulation. FA Davis, Philadelphia, 1984
35. Lampe GN, Mannheimer JS: Some limitations of TENS. p. 57. In Mannheimer JS, Lampe GN (eds): Clinical Transcutaneous Electrical Nerve Stimulation. FA Davis, Philadelphia, 1984

10 | Therapeutic Exercise and Mobilization

Damien W. Howell

This chapter examines the use of therapeutic exercise as it relates to the foot and ankle. Only a brief discussion of general concepts and guidelines of therapeutic exercise is presented. For an in-depth discussion of the general concepts and guidelines of therapeutic exercise, the reader is referred to several excellent texts on the subject.[1,2] Particular emphasis is placed on certain aspects of therapeutic exercise that have not been adequately dealt with in other texts or on those aspects that have particular importance for the foot/ankle. The following specific concepts are discussed: closed kinetic chain exercises, eccentric exercise, identification of the stage of inflammation and relation of the stage to exercise and activity, stretching exercise, progression of exercise, mobilization, and maximization of patient involvement. Patient examples designed to illustrate the application of the above concepts will be presented.

An initial step in the development of an exercise program is to identify the functional demands that may be placed on the patient. Analysis of the potential demands should address the magnitude, directions, duration, velocities, and frequency of forces to which the foot/ankle will be subjected. Is the patient going to be using the foot/ankle primarily in a closed kinetic or open kinetic chain? Is the patient going to be subjected to high-velocity high-impact type forces, or is the patient going to be exposed to relatively low repetitive forces?

Specific initial limitations of the patient should be identified next.[3] What is the chief complaint of the patient? What is it that the person cannot presently do? Are there any contraindications to exercise? What surgery was done? Is there any limitation of range of motion (ROM)? What is the age of the patient and should other appropriate limitations be identified? Is an acute and/or chronic inflammatory process occurring, and is the inflammatory process pri-

257

marily in contractile tissue, noncontractile tissue, or both? Was the injury traumatic or insidious?

By elucidating the specific demands that the patient will face and identifying the limitations that the patient has, the therapist is guided toward designing an exercise program that is individualized for the patient.

SPECIFICITY/CLOSED KINETIC CHAIN

The application of a specific exercise elicits a specific physiologic adaptation or specific training response. Training responses are optimized when exercise programs are designed to meet the specific needs and capacities of the participants.[4] The more the exercise program can be designed to simulate the functional demands of the patient, the better the exercise therapy.[3,4]

Therapeutic exercise for the foot/ankle should be no different than for any other region on the body except that the exercises should be done in a weightbearing situation whenever possible. The typical specific functional demands of the foot and ankle most commonly occur during weightbearing (closed kinetic chain).[5] Joint motions and muscle actions are distinctly different when the foot is on the ground as compared with when the foot is not in contact with the ground.[5-7] Ground reaction forces can be very large and difficult to reproduce during nonweightbearing exercises.[8,9] Therefore, I believe that closed kinetic chain exercise is preferable exercise programs are designed for patients with disabilities of the foot and ankle.

Occasionally, however, open kinetic chain exercises are necessary (e.g., in the early stages of repair of an Achilles tendon rupture, ground reaction forces would be too much for the tendon). In this situation, open kinetic chain exercises such as curling towels with toes, picking up marbles or resistive exercises with surgical tubing may be more appropriate.[1,2]

ECCENTRIC EXERCISES

Careful analysis of the functional demands placed on the foot/ankle during weightbearing activities will reveal a significant amount of eccentric muscular contraction.[5] The use of eccentric types of exercises for management of problems around the foot/ankle has not been adequately explored.

Using data available from indirect measurements of muscle/tendon forces and mathematical calculations, Wilkie has proposed that a muscle tendon unit is subjected to the greatest amount of force during high-velocity eccentric types of muscle contraction.[10] Therefore, concentric and isometric tyes of muscle contraction may only result in a submaximal force being applied to the muscle tendon unit. Theoretically, a high-velocity eccentric contraction may generate more tension in the muscle tendon unit[11] (Fig. 10-1).

Considering the above information, one can begin to appreciate why the classical evaluation scheme for soft tissue injuries as proposed by Cyriax is

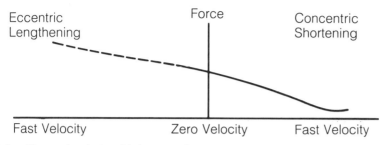

Fig. 10-1. Theoretic relationship between force, velocity, and type of muscle contraction.

often not sufficient to reproduce the chief complaint in patients with tendinitis.[12] I have found that patients with tendinitis often do not complain of symptomatic discomfort if asked to contract isometrically against manual resistance of the muscle at the midpoint of the available ROM. A manually resisted isometric contraction of a muscle at the midpoint in the available ROM probably does not result in enough force being applied to the muscle tendon unit to reproduce the chief complaint, whereas a high-velocity eccentric contraction may result in sufficient force being applied in the muscle tendon unit to reproduce the chief complaint.

This may explain the often-observed reproduction of the chief complaint in patients with tendinitis when the therapist suddenly removes a manually resisted isometric stimulus. There is a sudden co-contraction as the antagonist tries to readjust the carefully balanced forces of muscular contraction. The sudden co-contraction of the antagonist may result in an eccentric co-contraction of the agonist, and this occurs in a very short period of time. This high-velocity eccentric contraction may provide sufficient stimulus to the muscle tendon unit to elicit symptoms (e.g., after the resistance is suddenly released from a maximal isometric contraction of the toe flexors, it may result in the subject reflexly contracting the toe extensors). As the toe extensors are contracting to readjust the forces of muscle contraction, the toe flexors are eccentrically contracting at a high velocity.

I suggest that if a patient has possible tendinitis and the chief complaint cannot be reproduced with an isometric contraction the evaluation should be expanded. The patient should be carefully questioned to determine if symptoms that are elicited during functional-type activities occur during the periods of deceleration (eccentric contraction) (e.g., returning to a foot flat position from a toe raise may elicit the symptom in a patient who is suffering from tendinitis of a plantar flexor supinator muscle). Attention should be paid to whether the symptoms occur during the sudden removal of the resistance of an isometric test. Often the therapist may need to increase the magnitude of the stimulus by requesting that the patient perform eccentric contractions against greater forces or at a higher velocity. Forces of greater magnitude can be created by requesting that the patient perform weightbearing activities at a high velocity.

If one of the patient's limitations is identified as a chronic inflammation of a specific tendon, the task becomes one of designing an exercise program that is specific, progressive, and optimal. Curwin and Stanish[11] propose an exercise protocol for the management of patients with tendinitis that incorporates eccentric exercise. They provide some preliminary clinical data supporting the effectiveness of the exercise program.[11] The protocol calls for stretching the tendon, followed by eccentric strengthening exercise, followed by stretching, followed by cryotherapy. Curwin and Stanish suggest that the resistance or velocity of the eccentric exercises is either increased or decreased according to the presence or absence of symptoms. The goal is to have the activity or exercise be of sufficient magnitude to reproduce the chief complaint only during the last one-third of the repetitions or the last one-third of the duration of an exercise or activity. The rationale is that reproduction of the chief complaint can be used as an indicator to assure the therapist and patient that affected tissue (tendon) is being stimulated. If the exercise causes the symptom during the entire activity or exericse, however, the involved tissue is being stimulated excessively. No data or rationale was provided by Curwin and Stanish as to why the last one-third of an exercise program was chosen, as opposed to the last one-quarter or last one-half.

According to Curwin and Stanish, initially an eccentric resistance exercise should be applied to a muscle at a relatively constant velocity.[11] If symptoms occur before the last one-third of the exercise is achieved, the resistance is decreased; if symptoms do not occur by the time the last one-third of the exercise is reached, the resistance is increased. As the symptoms improve, the exercise is progressed by modifying the velocity in a similar manner.

Despite the limited amount of data supporting the effectiveness of using eccentric exercises, the logic of using eccentric exercises for patients with tendinitis around the foot/ankle appears sound and should be incorporated with closed kinetic chain type exercises.

INFLAMMATION AND EXERCISE

An inflammatory process can be a limiting factor in the type and amount of activity or exercise in which a person can participate. The following general classification scheme can be used when attempting to identify and manage a patient's musculoskeletal problem. A problem can be classified first as either primarily located in contractile tissue, noncontractile tissue, or both, and second as being either in the acute or chronic stage of inflammation.

Inflammation is a succession of changes that occur in living tissue when it is injured.[13] Inflammation occurs during the first of the three phases of wound healing, the cellular reaction phase.[14] The acute inflammatory process is rapid, and the course of repair is relatively short, whereas chronic inflammation progresses slowly, is of longer duration, and usually results in the formation of scar tissue.[13]

When the distinction between acute and chronic inflammation is based solely on time, it ignores the possibility that an acute inflammatory process can occur concurrently with a preexisting chronic inflammation. Many times the inflamed tissue is so deep that it is impossible for the clinician to observe any edema, erythema, or increase in temperature that is typically associated with acute inflammation. An expanded clinical criterion is needed if we are to differentiate between acute and chronic inflammation in our clinical decision process. The following section elaborates a clinical classification scheme for acute and chronic inflammation based on signs and symptoms.

I suggest that the clinician should interpret the occurrence of reproduction of the chief complaint to the end feel during passive ROM testing as a sign that can be used to distinguish between acute and chronic. Cyriax proposes that by relating when the chief complaint is elicited during passive ROM testing to the perception of end feel by the therapist an assessment can be made about the severity of the patient's problem.[12] Incorporating this concept with the concept of inflammation, the following expanded criteria for acute inflammation can be considered. During passive motion testing, the end feel is described as a muscle spasm, or as empty, and the patient will complain of increased pain or discomfort before end feel is reached. During the transition from the acute to the chronic phase of inflammation, the patient may complain of pain at the same time that end feel is reached by the therapist performing passive motion testing. The patient with acute inflammation will typically report that an injury occurred within the previous 72 hours. The patient will typically describe the pain or discomfort as unaffected by changes in position. The patient may have difficulty sleeping. The pain will be relatively constant as opposed to intermittent and is likely to be referred over a relatively large area of a related dermatomal segment. Erythema, edema, and increased skin temperature may be present depending on the tissues involved.[13]

As the repair process progresses to the chronic stage of inflammation, the pain or discomfort will occur after end feel is felt by the therapist performing passive motion testing. A patient in the chronic stage of inflammation will typically report that an injury occurred more than 72 hours ago. There will be little or no erythema, edema, or skin temperature elevation. Patients will typically describe the pain or discomfort as being over a relatively localized area close to the site of the lesion and as being relieved by rest and changes in position. There is usually no history of insomnia, unless the affected joint is the hip or shoulder, making it difficult for the patient to sleep on the involved side.

The distinction between acute and chronic inflammation has been used by clinicians in the decision process of choosing a therapeutic physical agent.[15] This distinction can also be used in the decision process for determining the most appropriate type of exercise for the patient who is in various stages of the healing process.

When the involved tissues are in the acute phase of inflammation (cellular reaction phase), the following general guidelines are suggested when an exercise program is designed. Avoid activities of daily living (ADL) that cause symptomatic discomfort during or immediately after an activity. Exercise or ADL should be encouraged if the amount is below the level that will produce symptomatic discomfort. Exercise or ADL of adjacent uninvolved tissues should be encouraged. If the inflamed tissue is contractile, passive exercise within a pain-free range is appropriate. If the inflamed tissue is noncontractile, isometric exercise is indicated.

When the involved tissues are in the chronic phase of inflammation (fibro-plasia and maturation), the following guidelines are suggested when the type of exercise is chosen: The patient should begin to participate in activity and exercise that causes a tolerable level of symptomatic discomfort or pain in an attempt to provide controlled progressive stress to the injured tissue so that an organized realignment and hypertrophy of the involved tissue can occur.[16,17] Curwin suggests that symptomatic discomfort is of benefit during the rehabilita-tive process of inflamed tendons because it assures the therapist and the patient that the involved tissue is being stressed.[11] Exercise should be relatively more aggressive and should aim to achieve an optimal load. The therapist and the patient should carefully monitor the program for adverse responses to the applied exercise load such as an exacerbation of symptoms or the development of new symptoms.

STRETCH

If an assessment of the specific limitations reveals that the patient has decreased joint motion, stretching and mobilization techniques are indicated.

Prior to the initiation of a stretching exercise, a careful evaluation and assessment should determine which specific tissues are short as well as if they are acutely or chronically inflamed. Typically, the limitation to joint motion is a result of the influence of both contractile and noncontractile tissues. When a pathology exists, however, one tissue type may have relatively more influence than another on limiting joint motion.

Identifying that a tissue is short requires that the tissue be selectively lengthened and compared against some norm. Table 10-1 lists the reversal of the shortening functions of the muscles (contractile tissue) around the foot/ankle so that positions of maximal length of the muscles can be identified. Little if any normative data specify what normal amounts of motion(s) or length are.[18,19] Fortunately, the patient often has only one involved side, which allows the clinician to compare the amount of motion available on the involved side to the uninvolved side. This should provide a basis from which to assess whether a muscle or other soft tissue is relatively short, long, or normal.

Placing the foot/ankle carefully in a position of maximal muscle length (Table 10-1) and closely assessing the end feel may allow the clinician to inter-pret whether a possible restriction is a result of a shortening of contractile tissue, noncontractile tissue, or both. A bone-to-bone or capsular end feel at the position of maximal stretch implicates a noncontractile tissue as limiting the motion. A markedly restricted passive accessory motion which is assessed in the loose pack joint position implicates that a restriction is secondary to short-ening of noncontractile tissue. A muscle spasm end feel implicates muscle as

Table 10-1. Joint Position for Maximal Stretch of Muscle

Muscle	Talocrural	Subtalar	Midtarsal	MTP	IP
			Joint and Position		
Gastrocnemius	Dorsiflex evert	Dorsiflex evert			
Soleus	Dorsiflex evert	Dorsiflex evert			
Posterior tibialis	Dorsiflex evert	Dorsiflex evert	Dorsiflex evert		
Flexor digitorum longus	Dorsiflex pronate	Dorsiflex pronate	Dorsiflex pronate	Dorsiflex two through five	Dorsiflex two through five
Flexor hallucis longus	Dorsiflex pronate	Dorsiflex pronate	Dorsiflex pronate	Dorsiflex, first	Dorsiflex, first
Tibialis anterior	Plantarflex pronate	Plantarflex pronate	Plantarflex pronate		
Extensor digitorum longus	Plantarflex supinate	Plantarflex supinate	Plantarflex supinate	Plantarflex two through four	Plantarflex two through four
Extensor hallucis longus	Plantar supinate	Plantar supinate	Plantar supinate	Plantar, first	Plantarflex, first
Peroneus brevis	Dorsiflex supinate	Dorsiflex supinate	Dorsiflex supinate		
Peroneus longus	Dorsiflex supinate	Dorsiflex supinate	Dorsiflex supinate	Dorsiflex, first	Plantarflex
Interossei				Dorsiflex	

MTP, metatarsal phalangeal; IP, interphalangeal.

the structure limiting motion. The patient's perception of the sensations of where the limitation of motion is will often assist in determining which tissue(s) may be causing a limitation of motion. A stretching sensation perceived in the area of the muscle belly implicates muscle, whereas a stretching sensation in the area of the joint implicates either tendon or noncontractile tissue (capsule, bone). A passive dorsiflexion of the ankle that results in a sensation that the restriction of the motion is in the area of the Achilles tendon implicates contractile tissue, whereas a sensation of the limitation in the area of the dorsal aspect of the talocrural joint implicates noncontractile tissue.

After careful evaluation, a stretching exercise program can be designed to meet the individual needs of the patient. It is important to stretch only the tissue(s) that is short and not that which is long. If the involved tissue is identified as being in the acute phase of the inflammatory process, stretching exercises should be avoided until end feel occurs simultaneously with symptoms. The stretching technique, however, may dictate the optimal anatomical position for treatment (e.g., tight gastrocsoleus muscle group). To avoid stretching the talocalcaneonavicular ligament, the subtalar joint should be held in slight supination during the weightbearing stretching technique. In the nonweightbearing technique using manual force, a strap, or a cord, however, the gastrocsoleus could be stretched as suggested in Table 10-1.

MacConiall suggests that each joint has a closed pack position, which is defined as the position where the joint surfaces are maximally congruent and the ligaments are maximally taut.[20] According to MacConiall, if one wants to lengthen a short ligament/capsule the joint should be placed in its maximally taut position (closed pack position) while being stretched. When the aim is to lengthen a joint capsule, the pulling sensation should be in the area of the joint. Conversely, if one does not want to lengthen a ligament/capsule, it should be placed on slack (maximum loose pack position) during the stretching exercise and the pulling sensation should be in the area of the muscle belly.

If a muscle is shorter than normal, the joint that the muscle crosses probably cannot be positioned in the maximum closed pack position. Therefore, the muscle can be lengthened without lengthening the ligaments/capsule by avoiding the closed pack position. When the aim is to lengthen a muscle, the pulling sensation should be perceived in the muscle belly of the specific muscle to be stretched and not in the area of the tendon or joint capsule. Stretch what is short, and do not stretch what is of normal length or long.

It has been suggested that stretching exercises should be preceded by general relaxation techniques.[21] Mennell believes that if the underlying bony structure is not aligned properly and the joints are not free to move, exercise therapy will be of little help.[22] Therefore, if limitation to motion is a result of contractile and noncontractile tissue, accessory motion mobilization should precede stretching exercises designed to increase physiologic motion. As much edema as possible should be removed or decreased from the part to be lengthened prior to performing stretching exercises.[23] Edema reduction can be aided with many of the physical agents that are available.[24] Physical agents have additional benefits that make stretching exercise and mobilization techniques more effective. Sapage has proposed that the optimal method to lengthen collagen tissue is to stretch the tissue while it is being heated and then to cool the tissue while the stretch is maintained.[25] There are many ways to heat the tissue, such as hot packs, ultrasound, and/or active contraction of the involved muscle with exercise. Other researchers have advocated proprioceptive neuromuscular techniques as being useful in achieving relaxation, which can aid in the lengthening of short tissues.[26,27]

Most experts agree that slow static stretching with a relatively low force for a long duration is the preferred method.[28,29] Interestingly, some studies have demonstrated that greater increases in ROM occur with ballistic stretching as opposed to static stretching.[30] Data comparing the effectiveness of static vs ballistic type stretching exercises is limited and not conclusive; however, I believe that the preferable method is slow static stretching.

Designing the stretching exercise so that the patients can perform it on their own has some distinct advantages.[31-33] It is conducive for stretching for a relatively long duration as patients can stretch more frequently at their convenience. Self-stretching exercise requires that patients be willing and capable of independently participating in their treatment. It is important that the patients be carefully instructed as to the specific method of stretching, so that they do not lengthen tissue that is already long.

PROGRESSION/OVERLOAD

Many experts suggest that an overload is a necessary ingredient for any exercise program.[34,35] Use of the term overload can be confusing, however. A strict definition of overload is to load to excess.[36,37] Some clinicians may interpret excess to mean a level of exercise that the patient is unable to tolerate. Other clinicians, however, may interpret overload to mean a level of exercise that is greater than the level of activity that is normally encountered. The latter definition is the correct one.

The aim in designing an exercise program is to determine the optimal amount of exercise—that which will stimulate the greatest improvement in a physiologic parameter. The optimal amount of exercise is on a continuum between not enough and too much exercise. The amount of exercise can be more than previously encountered (overload), but it may not be the optimal amount. The challenge is to make the progressive increase in the amount of exercise closer on the continuum of the amount of exercise to the optimal amount. Finding the optimal amount of exercise for a given individual is an ongoing process and requires continual reassessment and modification of the amount of exercise.

SPECIFIC PROBLEMS

Examples of how the concepts of closed kinetic chain exercise, eccentric exercise, the relating of exercise to inflammation, self-stretching, and progression can be applied to some of the more typical patient diagnosis and/or syndromes is presented. The example exercise programs should not be considered the only exercise therapy that is appropriate for that particular pathology. It is hoped that the exercise programs will be used only as an aid to understand the general concepts previously presented in this chapter. Readers are encouraged to use the general concepts and their own creativity to design individualized exercise programs based on the functional demands and limitations of patients. The example exercise programs presented are not supported with data as to their effectiveness with the particular diagnosis; however, they are based on logical rationale. Perhaps, proposing potential exercise programs will stimulate others to develop clinical research to disprove or support their effectiveness for particular syndromes.

HAMMER TOES

Hammer toe deformity results in shortening of the dorsal capsule of the metatarsalphalangeal (MTP) joint, plantar capsule of the interphalangeal (IP) joint, flexor digitorum longus (FDL), lumbercales, and lateral bands of the

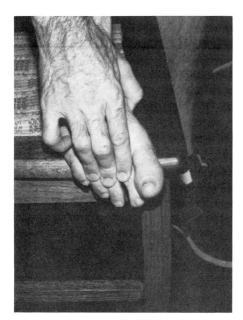

Fig. 10-2. Stretch position for a short dorsal capsule of the metatarsalphalangeal joint without stretching the dorsal capsule of the IP joint.

extensor hood.[33] The dorsal capsule of the IP joint and plantar capsule of the MTP joint become long.[38] Therefore, the exercise program should stretch the dorsal capsule of the MTP without stretching the dorsal capsule of the IP joint (Fig. 10-2). This is accomplished by plantarflexion of the MTP joint and extension of the IP joint. The plantar aspect of the IP capsule and the FDL should be stretched while the plantar aspect of the MTP capsule is maintained in a position of slack. This is accomplished by dorsiflexing the IP joint with the MTP joint maintained in neutral. The lumbercales and lateral bands should be stretched by placing the MTP joint in neutral or slight dorsiflexion and both IP joints in plantarflexion.

Consideration should be given to applying plantar glide mobilization of the MTP to gain motion in the direction of plantarflexion. Careful evaluation is necessary to make sure that the MTP volar plate and capsule has not already been lengthened by the deformity. Despite the fact that the IP joint is restricted in dorsiflexion, dorsal glide mobilization of the IP joint should be avoided as the dorsal capsule is frequently lax in patients with hammer toes.

The muscles that extend the IP joint (lumbercales, interrossi, extensor digitorum longus) should be hypertrophied with exercise. In an open kinetic chain, the intrinsic muscles are believed to function as extensors of the IP joints.[39] In a closed kinetic chain, however, the intrinsics are primarily stabilizers of the intermetatarsal joints.[5] During normal stance and gait, very little muscle activity exists to extend the IP joints.[5] This makes it very difficult to design an exercise to activate the intrinsics of the foot in a closed-chain model that would encourage the muscles to function as IP extensors. The following method is suggested as a possibility. Place the foot on a block on the floor with the metatarsal heads (MTH) on the edge of the block so that toes can flex at the

MTP. Maintain the rearfoot in a neutral position so that the muscles that cross the affected joints are maintained in a more optimal length. Request that the patient actively flex at the MTP while trying to extend at the IP joints.

This type of exercise program is likely to be more successful if it is instituted early in any disease process that may predispose a patient to the development of hammer toes (rheumatoid arthritis). An exercise program can be a valuable adjunct to orthotic and splinting therapy for hammer toes.

PLANTAR FASCIITIS/FLEXOR HALLUCIS BREVIS/ABDUCTOR HALLUCIS TENDINITIS

Plantar anteromedial heel and arch pain is frequently associated with a diagnosis of plantar fasciitis. It is difficult, however, to diagnose differentially whether pain in this area is flexor digitorum brevis (FDB) tendinitis, abductor hallicus brevis (AHB) tendinitis, or plantar fasciitis. The following discussion is based on the assumption that the mechanism causing the inflammation is similar among the three diagnoses. Therefore, the exercise program will be similar for all three diagnoses. Jahass believes that patients with plantar fasciitis could benefit from an exercise program but provides no data supporting the effectiveness of the use of exercises in this patient population.[40] The following information is presented as a possible program of exercise for patients with plantar fasciitis.

The windlass phenomenon as originally proposed by Manter states that when the toes are dorsiflexed the plantar fascia becomes taut and causes the arch to raise.[41] Manter attributed this phenomenon to the anatomic attachment of the fascia to the proximal end of the first phalanx. The AHB and FDB muscles have a similar anatomic attachment. Therefore, the windlass phenomenon can not be attributed solely to plantar fascia.

Jahass suggests that plantar fasciitis should respond positively to stretching.[40] I believe, however, that not all patients with a diagnosis of plantar fasciitis have a short plantar fascia. Indeed, in some patients with plantar fasciitis, the fascia is assessed as being too long. Careful clinical examination of the amount of first ray dorsiflexion that occurs with and without restricting the plantarflexion motion of the MTH may aid the clinician in determining whether the plantar fascia and associated muscles are short or long. I have seen some patients with excessive dorsiflexion of the first MTP (greater than 65° without MTH stabilized and greater than 35° with the MTH stabilized), and some patients with restricted dorsiflexion (less than 60° without the MTH stabilized and less than 35° with the MTH stabilized). It is not yet clear why some patients with plantar fasciitis have excessive first MTP dorsiflexion and some have limited first MTP dorsiflexion. The relative amount of motion of the first MTP dorsiflexion may be a function of the stage of inflammation, of the bony deformity (forefoot equinus), or of the relative use of the fascia.

A short plantar fascia, FHB, or AHB can be stretched by having the patient place the foot flat on the floor and by passively pulling the relaxed toes into dorsiflexion (Fig. 10-3).

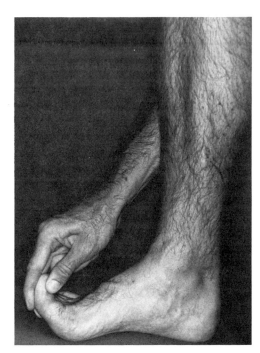

Fig. 10-3. Stretch position for a short plantar fascia, flexor hallucis brevis, and/or abductor hallucis brevis.

If the plantar fascia is long, the intrinsic and/or long toe flexors may also be long and therefore weaker in their normal functional ROM. In this example, the toe dorsiflexors are likely to be short. Stretching of the toe dorsiflexors and strengthening of the toe flexors are indicated in this case. The tension-generating capability of the toe flexors can be improved by performing an exercise of curling or bunching up a towel that is placed under the foot while it is on a supporting surface.

Patients with a diagnosis of plantar fasciitis often exhibit an asymmetrical biomechanical relationship at joints proximal to the ankle. Kapandji states that the biceps femoris and iliotibial (IT) band act to rotate the tibia externally.[39] In a closed kinetic chain, this action is reversed and the biceps and IT band decelerate internal rotation of the tibia.[5] If there is an adaptive shortening or lengthening of these tibial rotators, particularly the short head of the biceps femoris (monoarticular tibial rotator), the amount of pronation during gait will probably be affected.

Inman has documented a mechanical relationship between subtalar motion and tibial rotation. This relationship is based on the orientation of the axis of the subtalar joint and the intimate fit of the talocrural joint.[42] The action of the muscles that cause pronation/supination and tibial internal/external rotation should influence this relationship.

Excessive length or weakness in the external tibial rotators (muscles that eccentrically contract to limit internal rotation) could predispose the person to a relative inability to decelerate pronation. Excessive pronation has a high correlation with the incidence of plantar fasciitis.[43] Conversely, short tibial external rotators (muscles that contract eccentrically to limit internal tibial rotation) could predispose the person to a relative inability of the tibia/fibula to rotate internally and of the subtalar joint to pronate. If, there is less than the normal amount of pronation at the subtalar joint, the body may compensate by pronating excessively at the midtarsal joint. Excessive motion at the midtarsal joint may place abnormal stress on the plantar fascia and associated muscles.

It is important to distinguish whether the influence of the tibial external rotators are causative or compensatory in a patient with plantar fasciitis. If the biceps is short and is believed to be causing excessive midtarsal pronation, the biceps femoris should be stretched. If a short biceps femoris is believed to be compensatory (i.e., it is attempting to control excessive pronation), it should be stretched only after the primary cause for the excessive pronation has been identified and treated.

If the biceps femoris muscle (which is an external tibial rotator, hip extensor, and adductor) is short, an antagonist hip flexor internal rotator such as the tensor fascia is probably longer than normal and weak in a functional range. In this case, a strengthening program for the hip abductor internal rotator (tensor fascia latea) is indicated. Both the tensor and the biceps femoris are tibial external rotators but have antagonist functions at the hip. Therefore, care must be taken to stretch the tibial external rotator that is short but not to stretch the tibial external rotator that is long.

If the symptoms associated with plantar fascia can be attributed to a tendinitis of the flexor or abductor hallucis brevis, a stretching and strengthening exercise program is indicated. Tendinitis should respond well to an eccentric exercise program.[11] Ideally, the exercise should be in a closed kinetic chain if possible. I have not yet been able, however, to design a closed kinetic chain eccentric strengthening exercise program for the intrinsic foot muscles other than progressive walking and running.

ANKLE SPRAINS

A limited number of controlled studies document the effectiveness of exercise programs for the management of sprained ankle.[44] The common mechanism of injury in most ankle sprains is an excessive force in the direction of plantar flexion and inversion.[45] This results in trauma to the soft tissue structures around the lateral ankle, usually involving the anterior talofibular ligament.[46]

If it is determined that the anterior talofibular ligament is partially torn the following guidelines should be considered. During the acute stage of the inflammatory process, ADL that cause symptomatic discomfort during or immediately after the activity should be avoided. Exercises or ADL should be encouraged if the amount of activity is below the level that will produce symptomatic discomfort. Exercise or ADL that stress adjacent uninvolved tissues should be encouraged. Isometric exercises should be encouraged because the involved tissue is noncontractile.

Rest from function can be accomplished with strapping or bracing of the joint with the anterior talofibular ligament in a shortened position (dorsiflexion and eversion). Proper positioning can retard accumulation of excessive edema, especially when combined with external compression, appropriate modalities, and elevation.[47] Isometric resistive exercises can be performed using the uninvolved foot or the patient's own hands to provide the resistance.

The patient should be encouraged to use the ankle for normal functions as long as it does not cause symptomatic discomfort that can be correlated with excessive strain of the involved ligament. Time should be taken to assure that the patient understands which specific activities will cause the symptomatic discomfort that is correlated with strain of the involved ligament. Passive plantarflexion with inversion of the foot or palpation of the anterior talofibular ligament will typically reproduce a particular type of discomfort that is described as a sharp, intense, and well-localized pain. When the patient is asked to perform functional activities in a progressive sequence, the activities that elicit the particular type of discomfort associated with strain of the involved ligament can be identified. The functional activities that are correlated with pain of the involved ligaments should be avoided until the injury has progressed into the chronic stage of inflammation.

The patient may also experience symptomatic discomfort that is distinctly different from the type of discomfort correlated with strain of the involved ligament. Pain that is not sharp, intense, or well localized to the involved tissue may be correlated with the excessive edema that results from macrotrauma of the ankle. Discomfort that is described as an ache or stretching sensation and that is localized to areas distant from the involved ligament are probably correlated with excessive edema formation. When the patient is asked to perform functional activities in a progressive sequence, the activities that elicit the type of discomfort correlated with excessive edema can be identified. The patient is instructed to avoid any activities that cause symptomatic discomfort correlated with strain of involved ligaments and is allowed to participate in activities that cause discomfort correlated with excessive edema formation.

Full weightbearing ambulation with a forceful toe-off during the acute stage of a sprained anterior talofibular ligament will probably cause a symptomatic discomfort that should be avoided, whereas full weightbearing ambulation with a normal heel strike and foot flat but a less forceful toe-off should allow the patient to avoid strain and associated pain of the involved ligament. Ambulation with full weightbearing may cause discomfort that is correlated with excessive edema formation; the patient should be instructed to tolerate this discomfort, as it may facilitate action of the muscle pump and encourage venous and lymphatic return.

The traditional treatment goals for rehabilitation of a partially torn anterior talofibular ligament is to restore ROM and strength.[48] Perhaps therapists should expand their goals to include one that is directed toward the ligamentous tissue repair process. As the repair process progresses to the fibroplasia stage of

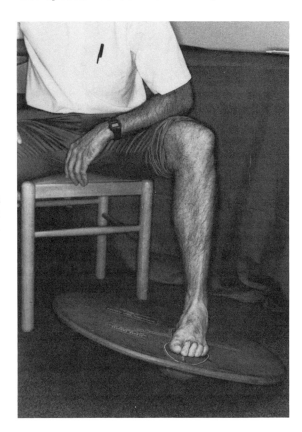

Fig. 10-4. Exercising with a Biomechanical Ankle Platform System Board in a sitting position.

wound repair, the early application of appropriate stresses to the involved ligament may facilitate proper reorientation of collagen structures in the ligament. Often the mutability of the collagen tissue is greatest in the early stages of the repair process prior to the formation of the collagen crossbridges and potential scar tissue.[16] If the patient complains of discomfort prior to end feel during passive ROM, it is too early to initiate passive exercise. When the patient complains of discomfort in the area of the involved ligament at the same time end feel is reached during passive ROM, however, it is probably appropriate to begin passive stretch of the ligament. Theoretically, tensile forces applied to healing collagen tissue should stimulate the proper alignment of the collagen fibers and retard the formation of disorganized scar tissue.[15] This can be accomplished by having the therapist or patient perform passive plantarflexion with inversion within a ROM that is short of producing symptomatic discomfort. A similar effect can be accomplished by exercising with a Biomechanical Ankle Platform System (Camp International Inc., P.O. Box 89, Jackson, MI 49204) (BAPS) in a sitting position (Fig. 10-4). A BAPS board aids the subject in moving the ankle/foot through the normal proportionate ROM.

As the sprained ankle progresses to the chronic stage of inflammation, more emphasis should be placed on maintaining and restoring joint function.

This is best accomplished by using closed kinetic chain exercises and functional activities progressing from easy to more difficult tasks (e.g., starting with normal gait without crutches without a limp, to toe raises on both feet, to toe raises on the affected foot, to jogging, to running a straight line, to running circles with the affected leg on the inside of the circle, to running circles with the affected foot on the outside of the circle, to large figure-eights, to small figure-eights, to running and cutting, etc.).[3] During the progressive functional activities, the presence of symptoms should be carefully monitored so that the stresses do not become excessive. Activities that cause symptoms which would be subjectively rated by the patient as moderate or severe in intensity should be avoided. The patient should not be progressed to the next step of the functional weightbearing activities if mild or moderate intensity of symptoms develop, but should be encouraged to participate in activities that are symptom-free or cause only a mild intensity of the symptom.

The BAPS board or similar device can also be used during the chronic stage of inflammation to progress the amount of exercise. The ground-reactive forces that occur when the patient uses the BAPS board can be increased by adding weight to the body with a back pack or by pulling down on the parallel bars. The ROM that the joint is moved through while the BAPS board is used can also be progressed by increasing the size of the ball used.

MOBILIZATION

Mobilization is passive movement performed by someone on a joint needing treatment.[49] Mobilization can be a passive physiologic motion or a passive accessory motion. A physiologic movement is one that a patient can voluntarily perform. An accessory motion is a normally occurring joint movement that cannot be reproduced by the patient and must be performed by the therapist.[50] Accessory motions are described as slide, spin, and roll.[20] For the purposes of this chapter, mobilization refers to passive accessory motion.

Many excellent texts and articles describe how to perform accessory motions on patients.[50-54] Rather than repeating what these noted experts have already adequately described, this section concentrates on self-mobilization. Self-mobilization is an extension of the traditional mobilization techniques that have been described. It is an attempt to have patients with their own hands glide, spin, or roll the various joints of the foot/ankle. It is still classified as an accessory motion; because patients could not volitionally perform these motions without the use of their hands or assistive devices. The concept of self-mobilization has been proposed by several European therapists.[31,33,34] The published material is not extensive, however, and does not adequately cover the joints of the foot and ankle.

The advantages of self-mobilization are that it can reinforce the mobilization techniques that the therapist performs. If the hypomobility is caused by shortened ligaments and capsule, mobilization therapy may be more effective if treatment can be continued by patients on their own.

Like most therapies, the actual effectiveness of self-mobilization therapy

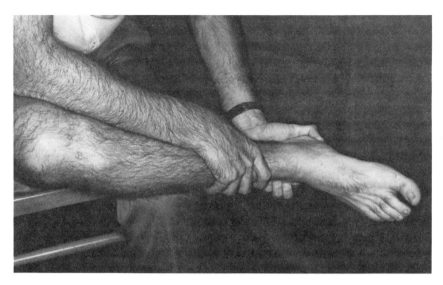

Fig. 10-5. Self-mobilization of posterior glide of the distal fibula on the tibia.

has not been scientifically examined. Its use in the treatment of patients appears to have merit, however, and should be subjected to clinical trials.

POSTERIOR GLIDE OF THE DISTAL FIBULA ON TIBIA

Position

The patient should be sitting in a chair with the affected foot crossed over and stabilized on the unaffected knee. The foot/ankle should be in a loose pack position of 10° plantarflexion (Fig. 10-5).

Fixation

The arm on the same side as the affected foot/ankle may be used to assist in stabilization. The forearm is placed along the shaft of the affected tibia. The elbow presses down on the knee so that the hip assumes a position of flexion, external rotation, and abduction. The hand grasps the tibia to provide a counter or stabilizing force to the mobilization force.

Mobilization Force

The fingers on the side opposite to the affected foot/ankle should grasp the anterior border of the fibula at the distal tibial fibula joint. This is best accomplished by supinating the forearm and approaching from the underneath side of the affected foot/ankle. This necessitates that the anterior border of the fibula be found solely by palpation and not visualization. The thumb is placed on the posterior aspect of the heel parallel to the long axis of the heel and can be used to provide additional counter or stabilizing force. The fingers pull the distal end of the fibula toward the posterior aspect of the ankle.

Indications

Restricted dorsiflexion is indication for this exercise.

ANTERIOR GLIDE OF THE DISTAL FIBULA ON TIBIA

Position

The patient should be sitting in a chair with the affected foot on the floor. The foot/ankle should be in slight plantarflexion either by extension of the knee or by use of a small heel lift (Fig. 10-6).

Fixation

The patient should bend over and place the thumb and thenar eminence of the same side as the affected ankle along the long axis of the anterior crest of the tibia at the level of the joint. The thumb should provide a counter force.

Mobilization Force

With the fingers of the same side as the affected ankle, the posterior aspect of the distal fibula should be grasped and pulled anterior.

Indications

Restricted plantarflexion and/or associated proximal tibial fibula joint problems are indications for this exercise.

LONG AXIS DISTRACTION OF THE TALOCRURAL/SUBTALAR JOINT

Position

The patient should sit on a bed with a sturdy foot board or on the floor with the foot adjacent to a immovable fixture to which a strap can be attached (leg of a couch, radiator, or leg of a utility sink).

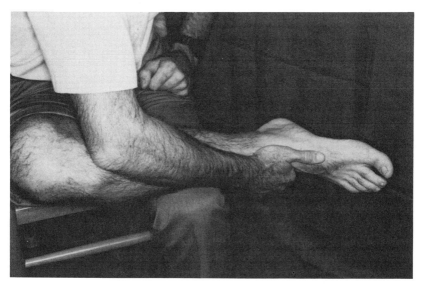

Fig. 10-6. Self-mobilization of anterior glide of the distal fibula on the tibia.

Fixation

A relatively wide belt is carefully wrapped in a figure-eight around the talus and calcaneus. The figure-eight should cross on the dorsum of the foot/ankle, and there should be a loop or a stirrup to allow a second belt to be looped through the first. The second belt is looped through the first and buckled securely around a stable fixture. The dorsiflexors of the affected foot should stay as relaxed as possible, and the foot should be in a loose pack position (10° plantarflexion) (Fig. 10-7).

Mobilization Force

The patient attempts to scoot or slide away from the foot board or stable fixture by pushing with the unaffected leg. The calcaneus and talus are prevented from moving by the belt arrangement.

Indications

A long axis distraction motion is helpful in stretching the joint capsule and preparing a hypomobile joint for other mobilizations.

Comments

It is relatively easy for the patient to control the amount and duration of force applied during this mobilization, but it is difficult to isolate the movement to a specific joint. The subtalar joint, talocrural, knee, and hip joint are affected

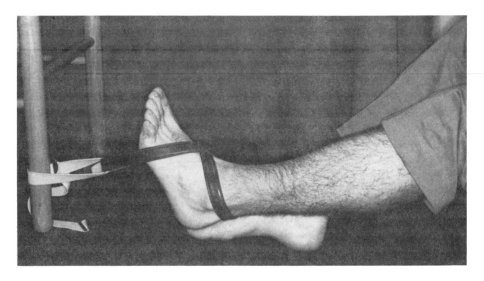

Fig. 10-7.   Self-mobilization of long axis distraction of the talocrural/subtalar joint.

with the method of distraction; therefore, care must be taken to assure that the adjacent joints are not adversely affected by this mobilization.

POSTERIOR GLIDE OF THE TIBIA ON THE TALUS

Position

While in a sitting position, the patient puts the affected heel up on a stool or table with the knee out straight. The foot/ankle should be in 10° of plantarflexion (Fig. 10-8).

Fixation

The calcaneus and talus are fixed against the supporting surface.

Mobilization Force

The unaffected leg is placed across and on top of the affected tibia. This position allows gravity to cause a posterior glide of the tibia on the talus. The amount of the force applied during this technique can be increased by having the patient actively push down on the tibia with the unaffected leg.

Indications

Restricted plantarflexion is indication for this exercise.

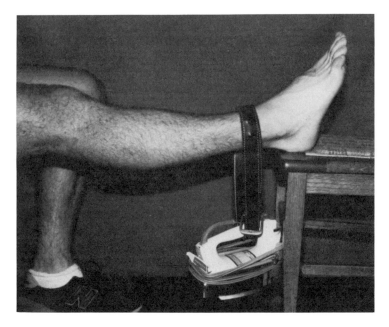

Fig. 10-8. Self-mobilization of posterior glide of the tibia on the talus. An ordinary iron is used to provide a weight to assist with mobilization force.

MEDIAL/LATERAL TILT OR GLIDE OF THE SUBTALAR JOINT

Position

The patient should be sitting in a chair with the affected foot crossed over and stabilized on the opposite knee.

Fixation

The arm on the same side as the affected midtarsal joint may be used to assist in stabilization. The forearm is placed along the shaft of the affected tibia. The elbow presses down on the knee so that the hip assumes a position of flexion, external rotation, and abduction. The hand grasps the tibia at the ankle.

Mobilization Force

The hand on the opposite side of the affected foot/ankle pushes or pulls the calcaneus into inversion or eversion (down or up) (Fig. 10-9). This force can be directed to cause a tilt or a glide. The force can be modified to emphasize the anterior or posterior aspect of the joint.

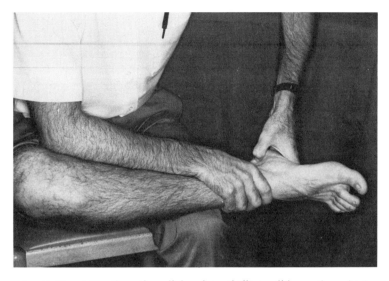

Fig. 10-9.   Self-mobilization of medial or lateral tilt or glide on the subtalar joint.

Indications

Restricted calcaneal inversion or eversion of the subtalar joint is indication for this type of exercise.

DORSAL/PLANTAR GLIDE OF THE INTERMETATARSAL JOINTS

Position

The patient stands with the affected foot flat on an uncushioned stool or chair. The metatarsal that is to be stabilized is placed on the chair edge so that the adjacent metatarsal to be mobilized is off the edge of the chair (Fig. 10-10).

Fixation

Partial body weight should be borne on the affected foot as it placed on the chair.

Mobilization Force

The metatarsal to be mobilized is moved into a dorsal or plantar direction.

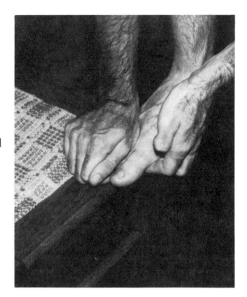

Fig 10-10. Self-mobilization of dorsal glide of the intermetatarsal joints.

Indication

Restricted intertarsal gliding is indication for this exercise.

LONG AXIS DISTRACTION OF THE MTP JOINT

Position

The patient should be sitting in a chair with the affected foot crossed over and stabilized on the opposite knee. The joint should be in a slight amount of plantarflexion.

Fixation

The arm on the same side as the affected MTP joint may be used to assist in the stabilization. The forearm is placed along the shaft of the affected tibia. The elbow presses down on the proximal tibia so that the hip assumes a position of flexion, external rotation, and abduction. The hand grasps the affected metatarsal just proximal to the joint line.

Mobilization Force

The thumb and index finger from the side opposite the affected MTP joint grasps the proximal phalanx close to the affected joint line and pulls in a direction of the long axis of the joint.

Indications

Restricted motion at the MTP joints is indication for this exercise.

Comments

The above description can be used for any of the five MTP joints or the IP joints. An alternative method is to use adhesive tape and make a stirrup and loop similar to the method described for long axis distraction of the talocrural joint (Fig. 10-11).

DORSAL/PLANTAR GLIDE OF THE MTP JOINT

Position

The patient should be sitting in a chair with the affected foot crossed over and stabilized on the opposite knee. The joint should be in a slight amount of plantarflexion.

Fixation

The hand on the same side as the affected joint grasps the metatarsal distally at the joint line. The hand provides a slight counterforce to the mobilization force.

Mobilization Force

The thumb and index finger grasps the proximal phalanx close to the MTP joint line and glides the joint in either dorsal or plantar direction depending on the restriction.

Indications

Dorsal glide is indicated for a limitation of dorsiflexion, and plantar glide is indicated for a limitation of plantarflexion.

Comments

The above description can be used for the IP joints as well. An alternative method is to use the stabilization and fixation as described in dorsal plantar

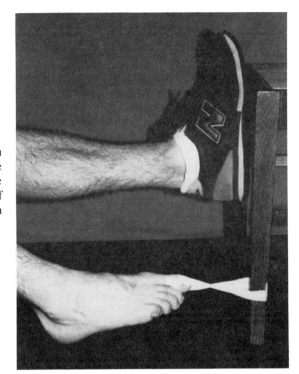

Fig. 10-11. Self-mobilization of long axis distraction of the metatarsalphalangeal joint. The subject is using two loops of tape to assist with mobilization force.

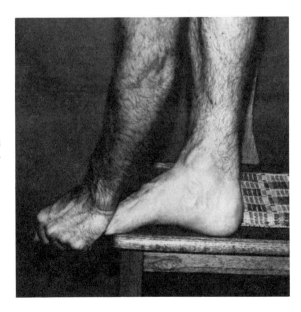

Fig. 10-12. Self-mobilization of plantar glide of the metatarsalphalangeal joint.

glide of the intermetatarsal joint. Care should be taken to assure that the MTP joint is neither abducted nor adducted (Fig. 10-12).

SUMMARY

The use of therapeutic exercise and mobilization for problems about the foot/ankle have been discussed. Few if any controlled clinical trials have documented the effectiveness of exercise in the management of pathologies about the foot/ankle. Therefore, an attempt was made to provide a rationale for using closed kinetic chain exercises, eccentric exercises, stretching exercises, and mobilization techniques in managing foot/ankle problems in hopes that the reader will use the concepts to create exercise programs that are individualized for their patients.

REFERENCES

1. Kisner C, Colby LA: Therapeutic Exercise Foundations and Techniques. FA Davis, Philadelphia, 1985
2. Jesse J: Hidden Causes of Injury Prevention and Correction for Running Athletes and Joggers. Athletic Press, Pasadena, CA, 1977
3. Kegerreis S: The construction and implementation of functional progressions as a component of athletic rehabilitation. J Orthop Sports Phys Ther 5:14, 1983
4. McArdle WD, Datch FI, Datch V: Exercise Physiology Energy Nutrition and Human Performance. Lea & Febiger, Philadelphia, 1981
5. Root MR, Obrein WP, Weed JH: Normal and Abnormal Function of the Foot. Vol. 2. Clinical Biomechanics, Los Angeles, 1977
6. Green DR, Whitney AK, Walter P: Subtalar joint motion—a simplified view. J Am Podiatry Assoc 69:83, 1979
7. Gray G: When the Foot Hits the Ground Everything Changes. Program Outline and Prepared Notes. A Basic Manual. USA Physical Rehabilitation Network, Toledo, Ohio, 1984
8. Ing B: Biomechanics of Running Shoes. Human Kinetics, Champaign, IL, 1986
9. Mann R: Biomechanic. In Jahass M (ed): Disorders of the Foot. WB Saunders, Philadelphia, 1986
10. Wilkie DR: The relation between force and velocity in human muscle. J Physiol 110:249, 1950
11. Curwin S, Stanish W: Tendonitis, Its Etiology and Treatment. Collamore Press, Lexington, MA, 1984
12. Cyriax J: Textbook of Orthopaedic Medicine 8th Ed. Vol. 1. Balliere Tindall, London, 1982
13. Thomas C: Taber's Cyclopedic Medical Dictionary. 5th Ed. FA Davis, Philadelphia, 1985
14. Bryant MW: Clinical Symposia Wound Healing. Ciba, Summit, NJ, 1977
15. Knight K: Cryotherapy Theory Technique and Physiology. 1st Ed. Chattanooga Corp, Chattanooga, TN, 1985

16. Arem AJ, Madden JW: Effects of stress on healing wounds—intermittent noncyclical tension. J Surg Res 20:93, 1976
17. Tipton CM, Mattes RD, Maynard JA, Carey R: The influence of physical activity on ligaments and tendons. Med Sci Sports 7:(3)165, 1975
18. Kendall FP, McCreay EK: Muscle Testing and Function. 3rd Ed. Williams & Wilkins, Baltimore, 1983
19. Janda V: Muscle Function Testing. Butterworth, Boston, 1983
20. MacConiall MA, Basmajian JW: Muscles and Movements. A Basis for Human Kinesiology. Williams & Wilkins, Baltimore, 1969
21. Evjenth O, Hamber J: Muscle Stretching in Manual Therapy. A Clinical Manual. Vol. I. The Extremities. Alfta Rehab Forlag, Alfta, Sweden, 1984
22. Mennell J: Foot Pain. Little, Brown, Boston, 1965
23. Kolb P, Denegan C: Traumatic edema and the lymphatic system. Athletic Training 18:(4) 339, 1983
24. Bardwick PA, Swezey RL: Physical modalities for treating the foot affected by connective tissue diseases. Foot Ankle 3:41, 1982
25. Sapega A, Quedenfeld TC, Moyer RA, Butler RA: Biophysical factors in range of motion exercise. Phys Sports Med 9:(12)57, 1981
26. Kabat H: Studies of neuromuscular dysfunction—the role of central facilitation in restoration of motor function in paralysis. Arch Phys Med 33:523, 1952
27. Holt LE: Scientific stretching for sport. Sport Research, 1973
28. Holt LE, Kaplin HM, Okita T, Hoshiko M: The influence of antagonistic contraction in hip position of the responses of agonistic muscles. Arch Phys Med Rehabil 50:279, 1969
29. Lehaman JF: Therapeutic Heat and Cold. Williams & Wilkins, Baltimore, 1979
30. Light KE, Nazik S, Personius W, Barstrom A: Physical Therapy. 64:(3)330, 1984
31. Holland GJ: The physiology of flexibility—a review of the literature. Kinesiol Rev 49, 1968
32. Rohde VJ: Dei automobilisation der extremitatengelenke teil II—hand und fubgelenke. Z Physiother Jg 28:51, 1976
33. Gustavsen R: Training Therapy Prophylaxis and Rehabilitation. George Thieme Verlag, New York, 1985
34. Lewit K: Manipulative Therapy in Rehabilitation of Motor System, Butterworth, Boston, 1985
35. Fox EL, Mattews DK: Physiological Basis of P.E. and Athletics. WB Saunders, Philadelphia, 1976
36. Anonymous: Websters 7th New Collegiate Dictionary: G and C Merrian, Springfield, IL 1963
37. Hellebrandt FA, Houtz SJ: Mechanism of muscle training in man—experimental demonstration of the overload principle. Phys Ther Rev 36:(6)371, 1956
38. Caillet R: Foot and Ankle Pain. FA Davis, Philadelphia, 1981
39. Kapandji IA: The Physiology of the Joints. Churchill Livingstone, London, 1982
40. Jahass M: Disorders of the Foot, WB Saunders, Philadelphia, 1982
41. Manter JT: Movements of the subtalar and transverse tarsal joints. Anat Rec 80:(4)397, 1941
42. Inman VT: The Joints of the Ankle. Williams & Wilkins, Baltimore, 1976
43. Roy S, Irwin R: Sports Medicine Prevention Evaluation Management and Rehabilitation. Prentice-Hall, Englewood Cliffs, NJ, 1983
44. Tropp H, Askling C, Gillquist J: Prevention of Ankle Sprains. Am J Sports Med 13:(4)259, 1985

45. Anderson KJ, Lecocq JF, Lecocq EA: Recurrent anterior subluxation of the ankle joint. J Bone Joint Surgery [Am] 34:853, 1952
46. Balduini FC, Ktetzlaff J: Historical perspectives on injuries of the ligaments of the ankle. Clin Sports Med 1:(1)3, 1982
47. Wilkerson GB: Treatment of ankle sprains with external compression and early mobilization. Phys Sports Med 13:(6)83, 1985
48. Kay DB: The sprained ankle: current therapy. Foot & Ankle 6:(5)22, 1985
49. Cookson JC, Kent BE: Orthopedic manual therapy—an overview. Phys Ther 59:(2)136, 1979
50. Maitland GD: Peripheral Manipulation. 2nd Ed. Butterworth, London, 1979
51. Cyriax JC: Textbook of Orthopaedic Medicine. 8th Ed. Vol. 2 Balliere Tindall, London
52. Kaltenborn F: Mobilization of the Extremities—Examination and Basic Treatment Techniques. Olaf Norlis Bokhandel, Oslo, Norway, 1980
53. Stoddard A: Manual of Osteopathic Technique. 3rd Ed. Hutchinson, London, 1983

11 | Orthotic Devices, Shoes and Modifications

Joseph K. Reed
Stacy Theriot

HISTORY

History reveals that foot covering was one of the first things made by our ancestors. The wearing of shoes has a tremendous impact on our health and well-being. We wear shoes not only for appearance, but also for comfort and protection. Because they are the only item of our wearing apparel that has contact with the earth on which we live, work, and play, they are present during nearly all our activities of daily living (ADL).

Until about a century ago, all footwear was made by hand. Only a few hand tools (e.g., the knife, the awl, and the hammer) were used until the latter half of the nineteenth century. The shoemaker did well to make one pair of shoes a day. This limited production made shoes scarce and expensive. Only the fortunate few had more than one pair.

Since the invention of the sewing machine in the mid-nineteenth century, the shoe industry has become highly mechanized. Increasing advancements in the industry have made it possible to utilize new materials and to increase production markedly. These new techniques have reduced the price of footwear to a level at which more than three pairs of shoes are purchased each year per person in the United States.[1]

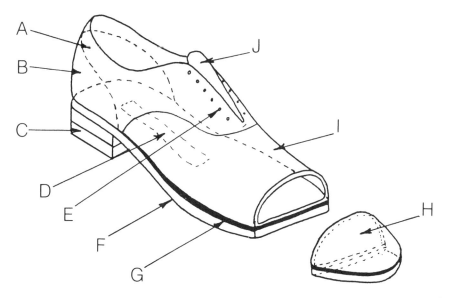

Fig. 11-1.   Major parts of shoe-*A*, quarter; *B*, counter; *C*, heel; *D*, steel shank; *E*, eyelet row; *F*, outsole; *G*, welt; *H*, toe box. (Adapted from Cracchiolo A: The use of shoes to treat foot disorders. Orthop Rev 8:73, 1979.)

PARTS OF THE SHOE

The major parts of a shoe are the upper, the sole, and the heel. Another sole called the insole is also situated next to the foot in most shoes. Most shoe manufacturers consider this insole the backbone or foundation of the shoe. Various areas of the shoe have individual names, some of which are obvious, such as toe, heel, ball, and backseam. The "area" that lies between the heel and the ball of the shoe is known as the "shank." The shank of the shoe is a separate item carefully shaped of spring steel, steel and leatherboard, or wood strips positioned in the shank area between the insole and the outsole. The purpose of the shank is to strengthen the shoe between the heel and ball, thereby preventing it from collapsing, and to provide additional support for the foot (Fig. 11-1).

The upper is divided into four parts: the vamp, tongue, and two rear quarters. The vamp extends from the instep anteriorly. The tongue is an extension of the vamp in a blucher-style oxford, but in a bal-type oxford, the tongue is separate. The toe of the vamp is often covered with a separate piece of leather called the "tip." The rearward line of the tip may be "straight" or "winged." The vamp is joined to the "quarters" which make up the sides and back of the upper. The two quarters are joined at the backseam. Inside and outside quarters differ in shape and size. For the oxford shoe, the outside quarter is cut lower than the inside to avoid contact with the lateral malleolus. In the bal oxford, the back edges of the vamp cover the forward edges of the

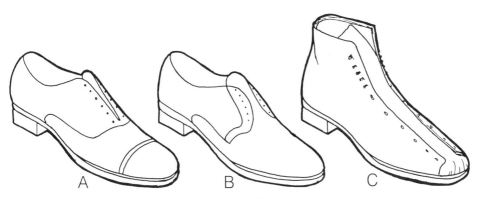

Fig. 11-2. Shoe styles: (**A**) bal, (**B**) blucher, (**C**) lace to toe. (Adapted from Zamosky I: Shoe modifications in lower-extremity orthotics. Bull Prosthet Res 10(2):54, 1964.)

quarters; however, the forward edges or ears of the quarters are on top of the vamp in the blucher style[2,3] (Fig. 11-2).

Three basic types of reinforcements can be made to the upper: the medial counter, the heel counter, and the toe cap. The medial counter helps support the medial arch of the shoe, and the heel counters aid in controlling the rearfoot. The toe cap prevents the anterior portion of the vamp from losing its shape.

Other terms that make up the nomenclature of the shoe with which one should become familiar are: breast or leading edge of the heel, foxing, lining, top line, eyelet row, and welt.[2]

SHOE CONSTRUCTION

Shoes are fabricated over a model, called a "last," which can be made of either wood, plastic, or plaster. Shoe construction can be divided into several basic groups, based on the method used in attaching the outsole to the upper. These basic groups are nailed, sewn, cemented, and direct molded shoes. Sometimes a combination of construction is used depending on the type of shoe or materials used (Fig. 11-3).

Originally, the upper was attached by tacks or staples which penetrated into the substance of the insole. Thus, the insole was covered with some type of lining to avoid injury to the foot. This type of construction was at one time used to a large extent in fabricating men's work shoes, but the sewn construction technique has become increasingly popular. Several techniques are used in sewn construction; however, the Goodyear Welt construction is recognized as the standard for quality. The distinguishing feature of this technique is that the welt, upper, lining, and insole are sewn together using a strong, flexible chainstitch. The outsole is then attached by means of a lockstitch, which passes through the welt and the edge of the outsole. This seam is outside the area of greatest pressure in wear, since it lies in a small extension that juts out from the

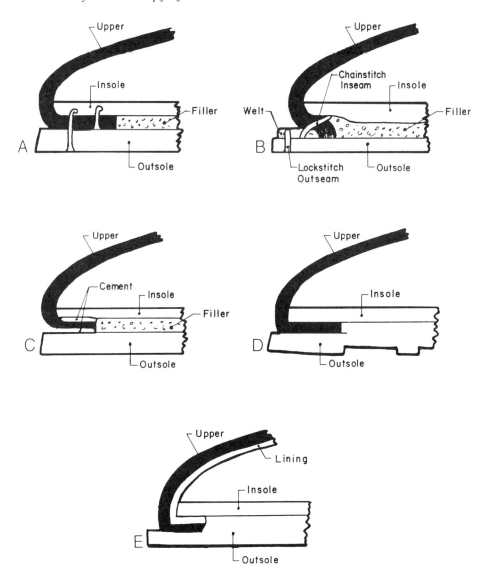

Fig. 11-3. Types of Construction: (**A**) nailed, (**B**) sewn, (**C**) cemented, (**D**) vulcanized, (**E**) injection molded. (Adapted from Rossi W, Tennant R: Professional Shoe Fitting. National Shoe Retailers Association, New York, 1986.)

sides of the main structure of the shoe. The cemented shoe construction is characterized by an absence of stitching, tacking or other visible attachments in the bottom assembly. The upper, insole, and outsole are all connected using contact cement. The newest construction technique is a process of simultaneously molding and attaching sole and heel units to a preassembled upper. This method of construction is frequently used in the fabrication of casual footwear.

The molding process can be subdivided into vulcanizing or injection molding techniques. Machine design and rubber technology have made it practical to mold in place or vulcanize a complete rubber outsole and heel unit on an assembled leather upper in one operation. The sole is bonded to the upper with cement which cures during the vulcanizing process. This method is frequently used in the fabrication of men's leather boots and work shoes with heavy soles. The injected molding process uses a machine equipped with precision molds made for each size of last. A preassembled upper is placed in position in the machine and the mold closed. A molten charge of long-wearing soling compound in a plastic state is forced into the cavity formed between the bottom of the mold and the shoe bottom. As in the vulcanized shoe, the cement that sets during the curing cycle forms the bond between upper and sole.[1,2]

Because of the advancements in synthetic materials, this versatile process is presently playing a major role in modern footwear manufacturing. We suggest that in view of the difficulty with adhesive bonding to synthetic materials, such as PVC soling, and the stretching of uppers made of synthetic material, that this type of footwear be avoided if modification of the upper or outsole is believed necessary in solving a foot problem.

Each construction method fills specific footwear needs: cements appear chiefly in women's shoes, Goodyear Welts chiefly in men's and boy's shoes, nails in workshoes, and injection molding in casual inexpensive footwear. Divisions are not rigid, however, because many women's shoes are fabricated by sewn construction such as Goodyear Welts. Likewise, many men's shoes are fabricated with cements or a combination of sewn and cement construction, and many work shoes are Goodyear Welts.

SIZING

The American shoe industry supplies more than 300 shoe sizes and widths to fit the many different foot sizes and shapes. They range in half sizes by groups from infants' size 0 to a man's size 16. Twelve widths range from AAAAA to EEEE, although not all sizes are made in all widths.[4]

The history of shoemaking reveals that full sizes have been around for centuries. In the late nineteenth century, the Retail Boot and Shoe Dealers National Association set up schedules giving length, ball width girth, waist, and instep girth measurements for each last group. This became known as "The Standard Measurement of Lasts" and provides for $\frac{1}{3}$ inch in length between whole sizes and an increase of $\frac{1}{4}$ inch in girth for each whole size.[5]

About this same time, the American shoe industry introduced a half-size program. There is $\frac{1}{6}$ inch difference in length between half sizes, with adjustments also made in girth measurements. The shoe manufacturers' standard classifications of groups of lasts and shoe sizes are: Boys', sizes $2\frac{1}{2}$ to 6; Growing Girls', sizes $2\frac{1}{2}$ to 9; Women's, sizes 3 to 10; Men's, sizes 6 to 12. Some overlap exists in general size, however, and some groups have been extended to fit extremes.

Table 11-1. Available Shoe Widths

Widths		
AAAAA	A	E
AAAA	B	EE
AAA	C	EEE
AA	D	EEEE

Retail shoe stores that cater to individuals who have foot problems or present a fitting problem stock shoes in widths A through D, with A being the narrow width. A reliable retail shoe store can order from the manufacturer shoe widths to fit the extremes. Table 11-1 illustrates the variations of widths the industry has provided.

In working with the problem foot, it soon becomes evident that the general department store or discount shoe store does not carry appropriate styles or sufficient sizes to obtain proper shoe fit. We suggest that the individual working with the problem foot establish an association with a member of the "Prescription Footwear Association." These members generally deal with orthopedic footwear and have access to a number of shoe styles in a wide variety of sizes. Clinicians can write the association for a list of their members in their area. (Prescription Footwear Association, 1414 Avenue of the Americas, 7th floor, New York, NY 10019).

The following are some standards in shoe sizing worth noting:

1. $\frac{1}{3}$ inch difference in length between full sizes, $\frac{5}{16}$ inch between 9 and 10
2. $\frac{1}{6}$ inch difference in length between half sizes 6 to $6\frac{1}{2}$
3. $\frac{1}{16}$ inch difference in width across ball between widths B to C
4. $\frac{1}{12}$ inch difference in width across ball between whole sizes 9B to 10B
5. $\frac{1}{4}$ inch difference in girth between width same size B to C
6. Three half sizes between women and men; women's size 8 equals men's size $6\frac{1}{2}$

When buying shoes, it is important to remember to try them on in the middle of the day. Feet swell slightly as the day progresses. If you purchase shoes in the morning or evening, you may find that they are not an ideal fit. When purchasing running shoes make sure that the heel counter is balanced. Often when the heel is being glued to the sole, it is inadvertently placed in a varus or valgus attitude.

Fitting

Many of the shoe styles that are now in vogue do not fit the shape of the foot. As a result, comfort and protection of the foot from deformity is compromised by many in lieu of style. Hallux valgus is one such deformity caused by wearing shoes that are not the proper width. Therefore, a wider shoe may have to be purchased to compensate for the differences in space between specific

Table 11-2. Characteristics of Commonly Used Orthotic Materials

Trade Name	Characteristics	Uses
PPT	Polyurethane open-cell foam, non-thermoplastic, very durable, soft durometer. Available in nylon covered, felt covered, uncovered, perforated, smooth skin covered. Thickness $\frac{1}{16}$ to $\frac{1}{2}$ inch.	Nonmolded insoles, line-molded insoles
Spenco	Closed cell neoprene nonthermoplastic, soft durometer, nylon covered. Thickness $\frac{1}{8}$ inch.	Nonmolded insoles, line-molded insoles
Aliplast	Polyethylene closed-cell foam thermoplastic, autoadhesive, high specific heat, memory. Durometers 4E, 6A, 10, XPE. Thickness $\frac{3}{16}$ to $\frac{1}{2}$ inch.	Soft densities (4E, 6A) line. Splints and braces. 10 insoles. XPE—semirigid orthoses
Plastazote	Polyethylene closed cell foam thermoplastic, moderately autoadhesive (P4073, P7093), memory, low specific heat, fine cell structure, not durable. Durometers P4073 (soft), P7093 (medium), H9062 (firm). Thickness $\frac{1}{16}$ to 1 inch.	(P4073, P7093) temporary orthotics, used as tissue interface in combination with firmer materials. H9062—binding for rigid sandal.
Pelite	Polyethylene closed-cell foam thermoplastic, nonautoadhesive, memory, high specific heat. Available in regular perforated and ventilated. Durometers soft, medium, firm, extra-firm. Thickness 3 or 5 mm.	Prosthetic liners, line braces and splints. Base of multilayer orthosis.

toebox styles. Shoes should be wide enough to allow the material of the upper to be rolled between the index finger and thumb. Likewise, there should be at least a half an inch of space between the tip of the longest toe and the front of the toebox. Loafers present a special problem in fitting. For the loafer to stay on the foot, it must be too short. After the upper of the loafer has stretched to the contour of the foot, the heel pistons at the toe-off phase of gait. We suggest that these ideas regarding correct fitting of shoes be implemented when buying conventional or extra-depth shoes.

ORTHOTIC DEVICES

Materials

A wide spectrum of materials is available for use in fabricating insole devices. Each material possesses unique characteristics and properties that make it suitable for specific orthotic applications. As a result of this myriad of new materials, elaborate orthotics can now be made in a relatively short amount of time. Polyethylene foams have simplified orthotic fabrication because of their thermoplastic property. Several polyethylenes are ideal for making molded insoles because they can be molded directly to the patient's foot. Polyurethane foams and microcellular rubber wear well and have low durometer values (measurements of firmness); therefore, they are ideal for simple nonmolded inserts (Table 11-2).

Terminology

Thermoplastic materials are moldable when heated. A material with memory returns to its original state after being molded by reheating. This allows reuse of poorly formed material that would otherwise be wasted. The durometer value describes the measurement of firmness of a material. The larger the durometer value, the harder the material. Compression set is the percentage by which a material will compress after being under a set load for a given period of time. The durability of a material is dependent on its compression set. These are some of the characteristics of a material that should be considered when choosing the best materials for a particular foot problem.

Orthotic devices are used in three ways: (1) to help absorb some of the shock produced by walking or running, (2) to distribute pressure evenly over the entire plantar surface of the foot, and (3) to correct or accommodate biomechanical imbalances of the foot.

INSOLES

Simple nonmolded insoles help dissipate the forces applied to the foot during walking.[6,7] A foot that is biomechanically imbalanced is subjected to the same amount of pressure as a properly aligned foot, but the forces are concentrated on particular areas of the foot. Molded insoles or balanced orthotics effectively distribute the pressures evenly on the plantar surface of the foot.

Nonmolded Insoles

Extra-depth shoes usually have a removable spacer that can be used as a pattern for a nonmolded insert. If a spacer is not supplied, a pattern can be made by tracing the outline of the shoe onto a sheet of paper. Trim approximately $\frac{1}{4}$ inch from around the tracing. Place the pattern into the shoe and trace along the interior border of the shoe with a pencil. Next, remove the pattern and trim accordingly. The arch area is formed by drawing a reflection of the medial arch of the pattern (Fig. 11-4). A medial arch support can be incorporated into this insole by gluing a schaphoid pad to this area of the finished insole. The pattern or template is then traced onto one of the polyurethane foams or microcellular rubber insole materials commonly used for non-molded

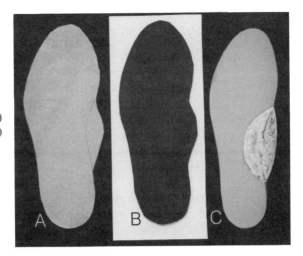

Fig. 11-4. Simple insole: (**A**) template, (**B**) reflected arc, (**C**) scaphoid pad.

insoles (see Table 11-2). The edges of the cutout insole are ground smooth and the area under the toes is buffed to provide sufficient room in the toe box.

This nonmolded insole can be modified to help correct biomechanically imbalanced feet. One such variation is the "cobra pad," which can be used to manage patients with a mild forefoot varus deformity. This orthosis consist of a nonmolded insole with a cobra-shaped felt pad glued to its underside along the medial border. The felt pad pattern is made by drawing a parabola on the insole template that connects the points that correspond to the five metatarsal heads (MTHs). This line is extended back toward the medial arch and around the entire heel $\frac{1}{2}$ inch from the edge of the template (Fig. 11-5). The pad is glued in

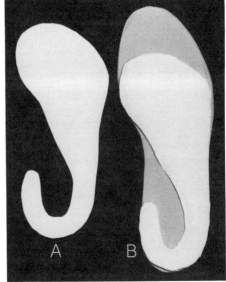

Fig. 11-5. Cobra pad: (**A**) template, (**B**) finished insole.

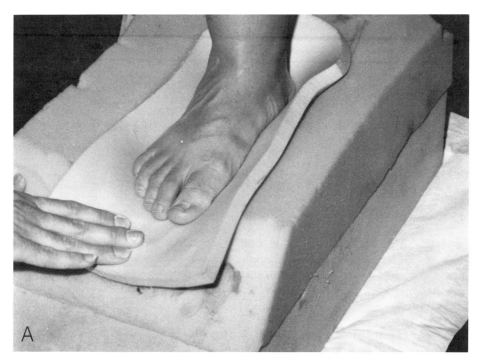

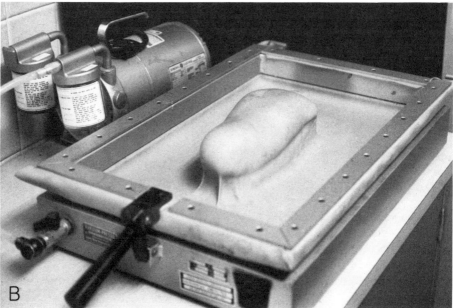

Fig. 11-6. Molding techniques: (**A**) foam block, (**B**) vacuum press.

place just behind the metatarsal heads. The inner edges of the pad are skived (cut so that the edge is tapered) to eliminate edge pressures. The felt is sloped from full thickness behind the medial MTHs to zero thickness under the most lateral MTH. Pads of varying thickness can be used depending on the number of degrees the insole is being posted. The cobra pad can also be modified for a valgus deformity.[8]

Molded Insoles

If a patient has a particular area of high plantar pressure, a molded insole is needed to help maximize the amount of surface area receiving the pressure.[9–11] There are several methods of molding. The simplest entails molding a low temperature thermoplastic material, such as Plastazote (Cascade Orthopedic Service, 46 Galli Drive, Novato, CA 94947), directly to a person's foot using a 6-inch-thick foam rubber block approximately 2 feet long, with one end angled at 60°. This angle allows the material to be molded to the foot but prevents the material from curling up in front of the toes. The person is seated with the knee and ankle bent to 90°. The warmed material is placed on the foam, and the patient's foot is positioned on the block so that the toe cleft is aligned with the point where the foam begins to slope downward. The foot is pushed down into the material with moderate force and held there until the orthotic material has cooled (Fig. 11-6A). Only low-temperature thermoplastics can be molded directly to the patient's foot using the aforementioned procedure. A high-temperature thermoplastic like Pelite (Durr-Fillauer Medical, Inc., 2710 Amnicola Highway, Chattanooga, TN 37406) can be molded using a positive cast model and the foam block technique; however, a more effective choice for molding these materials around a positive model is the vacuum press method (Fig. 11-6B). The positive model of the foot is made from a neutral position cast.

The neutral position cast is taken with the patient in the prone position. The subtalar joint is palpated using the third finger and thumb. Subtalar neutral position can be determined by palpating for congruity of the calcaneus with the head of the talus just anterior to the malleoli. The medial side of the head of the talus can be palpated just anterior and distal to the medial malleoli; the lateral side is found on the anterior surface of the ankle joint beneath the extensor tendons.[11] While the foot is maintained in this position, five layers of 6-inch-wide plaster are draped over the foot from the top of the malleoli over the ends of the toes (Fig. 11-7A). A tuck is made on each side of the ankle, and the plaster is molded well to the plantar surface of the foot. The foot can be held in the proper position by finding the neutral position of the subtalar joint and applying a dorsiflexion and abductory force on the fourth and fifth metatarsal heads. After the cast has dried sufficiently, the edges of the skin are pulled away from the cast. The cast is loosened from the heel and then slipped down off the toes. While the cast is still moist, the impression at the fourth and fifth MTHs is smoothed.

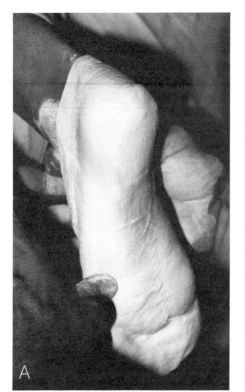
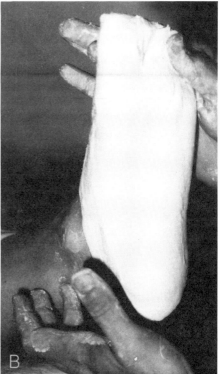
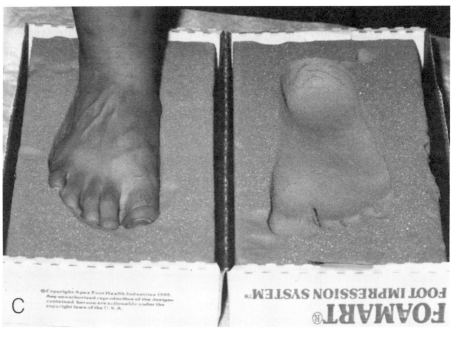

Fig. 11-7. Neutral position casting techniques: (**A**) prone, (**B**) suspension, (**C**) foam impression tray. (Foamart Foot Impression System, © Apex Foot Health Industries, 1985).

Suspension casting is another technique commonly used in making neutral position casts. The patient is positioned in the supine or sitting position. The fourth and fifth toes are grasped between the thumb, third, and fourth fingers. Traction is applied to the fourth and fifth toes to hold them in a neutral position. The foot is placed in the subtalar neutral position, and a mild dorsiflexory and abductory force is applied to the forefoot, which locks the midtarsal joint.

Two 5 × 30 inch plaster splints are folded in half. The resulting four-ply bandage is draped over the medial side of the foot, and a similar piece of plaster is placed over the lateral side of the foot. The plaster is smoothed well to decrease the amount of wrinkles and prevent bowstringing. If these two pieces do not overlap on the plantar surface, an additional piece of plaster can be added. The foot and leg are raised off the supporting surface by an upwardly directed force through the fourth and fifth toes, thus theoretically allowing elongation of the soft tissues. (Fig. 11-7B).[12,13] The foot is held in the position outlined above until the plaster is dry. The edges of the plaster are loosened from the skin, and the cast is slipped off the foot.

Two layers of plaster are placed along the superior edge of the neutral position cast to raise the sides of the cast to the same height as the heel of the cast. Next, a parting agent such as sodium silicate, talcum powder, or liquid soap is applied to the entire inner surface of the cast. The negative cast is allowed to dry and is then filled with molding plaster.

Another option used to obtain a plaster last of the foot is the foam impression tray technique. The tray can be found in the catalogues of most orthopedic suppliers. The foot is pressed into a tray filled with an open cell foam, and the impression that results is filled with plaster (Fig. 11-7C). This technique has some negative aspects. The foot cannot be held in subtalar neutral position when this system is used; therefore, a balanced orthosis cannot be constructed from the plaster model. Furthermore, there is no way of referencing the position of the foot to the remainder of the leg.

After the model has dried, the plaster bandages or surrounding foam are removed from the positive model. The plantar surface is smoothed using Carborundum Sand Screen abrasive (Apex Foot Products, 330 Phillips Ave., South Hackensack, NJ 07606) or a piece of metal screening and a file. A mark can be drawn using a felt-tip pen, which bisects the calcaneus of the positive model. This line is used as a reference in determining the number of degrees posting needed to compensate for a biomechanical malalignment of the forefoot.

When the model has been modified and dried completely, it is ready to be used. The model is placed in a vacuum press. The insole material is heated and then placed over the model, and an airtight rubber bladder is pulled down over the cast while suction is applied. Care must be taken to cut materials so that a large amount of excess material does not prevent intimate molding of the material to the sides of the cast. The foam block technique is simple and inexpensive when time, equipment, and materials are taken into consideration. The vacuum press achieves a better molding of the materials, however, and is more practical high-temperature thermoplastics are used.

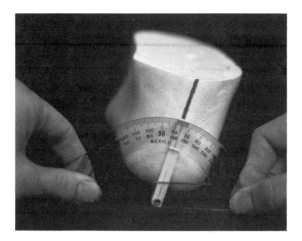

Fig. 11-8. Measuring the degree of forefoot deformity from the bisected heel of a neutral position cast.

Balanced Orthosis

The cobra pad, which has been previously discussed, is an example of the simplest form of a balanced insole. Unlike the cobra pad, most balanced orthotic devices are molded insoles. A balanced orthosis is a device that realigns the foot so that it is in proper biomechanical alignment. The amount of correction and the number of degrees posted depend on how large the deformity is and whether the patient has wore some type of correction before. If the deformity is large, a full correction may not be tolerated by the patient. It is recommended that the orthosis not be posted any more than 8 to 10 degrees.[15] The heel of the positive mold, which is made from the neutral position cast, is bisected using a felt-tip pen. This bisection is used to measure in degrees the extent of the deformity (Fig. 11-8).

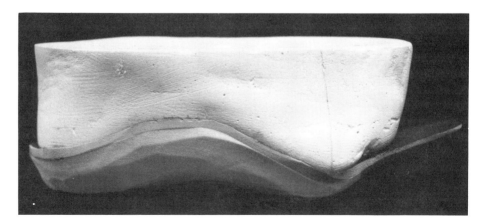

Fig. 11-9. Trim lines for a nonrigid insole: low at the ball of the foot and raised around the heel area.

After the materials have been molded to the model, the material is ground so that the calcaneal bisect forms a perpendicular when resting on a level surface. The sides of the insole should be reduced to a thickness of about $\frac{1}{16}$ inch. The medial arch area is ground to fit the curve of the shoe. There should be no abrupt changes in the thickness of the material, a smooth transition from the post to the remainder of the insole is desired. Trim lines should be low at the anterior part of the insole to prevent the shoe from being too tight at the ball of the foot. Posterior trim lines can be brought up higher to form an arch support and help control the heel (Fig. 11-9).

A semirigid insole is ideally composed of a matrix of materials. A soft frictionless interface such as nylon covered PPT (Professional Protective Technology, 21 East Industry Court, Deer Park, NY 11729) or Spenco (Spenco Medical Corporation, P.O. Box 8113, Waco, TX 76710) is often desirable next to the skin. The middle layer is usually one of the medium durometer polyethylenes which is backed with a firm durometer material such as Aliplast XPE (Ali Med, 68 Harrison Ave., Boston, MA 02111). This type of semirigid insole tends to be durable; thus, it is good for heavy patients or very active patients who tend to "bottom-out" their insoles quickly.

EXTRA-DEPTH FOOTWEAR

If a foot disorder must be managed using an accomodative or balanced insole, it may be necessary to use extra-depth shoes. Extra-depth footwear are manufactured with a $\frac{3}{16}$- to $\frac{5}{8}$-inch-thick removable insole. When the insole is removed, an additional vertical height inside the shoe is available. Newly fabricated insoles can replace the original insole. The extra-depth shoe is of great benefit in accommodating hammer or clawed toes.

A large selection of extra-depth shoes for both men and women are sold commercially under the trade name Treadeasy shoes. (P.W. Minor Sons, 3 Treadeasy Ave., Batavia, NY 14020). The Treadeasy shoe has a stiff counter and a $\frac{3}{16}$-inch-thick removable inlay of sponge rubber and fiber board backing that is covered with a thin, loose vinyl sock lining. The Treadeasy shoe line is now offering an extra-depth shoe for both men and women that affords more than 25 percent additional depth and 13 percent additional ball room than does the ordinary extra-depth shoe. It is fully leather lined with a $\frac{3}{4}$-inch crepe wedge sole. It is marketed as the Madam X for women and the Super X for men (Fig. 11-10A). It comes in a variety of widths up to 5E in both styles. The Treadeasy shoe offers a variety of styles and materials in upper design, including a lace-to-toe style that permits easy access of the foot into the shoe as well as adjustability of the shoe over the toes. This shoe is also available with velcro closures for individuals who have hand disabilities.

The Drew Shoe Company (Irving Drew Corporation, Lancaster, Ohio 43130) also offer extra-depth shoes for women. The newer Drew shoes have a long medial counter and long vamp, whereas the older Drew shoes are similiar in design and style to the Treadeasy shoe. Shoes with deerskin uppers are

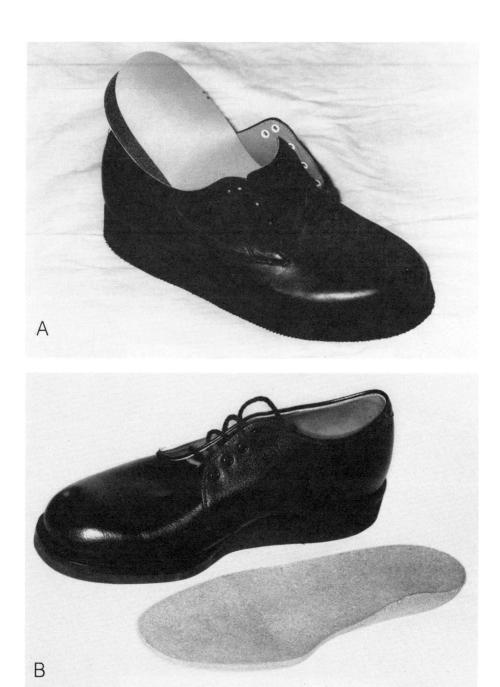

Fig. 11-10. Types of extra-depth shoes. (**A**) Super X. (**B**) Contour Depth Inlay. (*Figure continues.*)

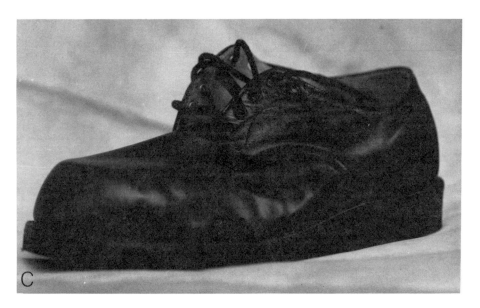

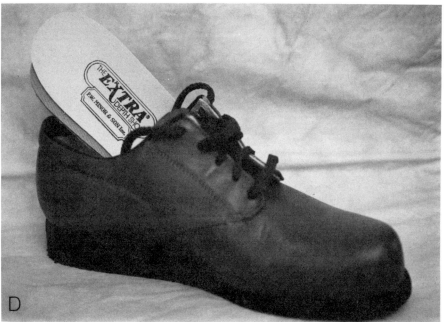

Fig. 11-10 (*Continued*). (**C**) Super D. (**D**) Miss Contour Pillowtop.

available from Treadeasy for both men and women and from Drew for women only. We believe that one must be extremely selective when choosing this type of upper. Deerskin is a very soft leather that tends to stretch easily with wear, and the shoe quickly loses its shape and support. Frequently, with use of a soft semirigid balanced insert, the shoe shape is modified and control of the foot by the insert is lost.

The Alden Shoe Company (Alden Shoe, Taunton Street, Middleborough, MA 02346) manufactures two typs of extra-depth shoes for men. The Contour Depth Inlay (CDI) (Fig. 11-10B) shoe has a stiff counter and an inlay of graded depth with the greatest depth under the tarsal bones, which affords support to the vulnerable MTHs. It is not necessary to purchase the nonallergenic cork inlay. The contour depth concept affords greater depth under problem areas such as MTHs and less depth under the toe tips, which usually present less of a problem.

The SUPER D is the other depth inlay shoe available from the Alden Shoe Company (Fig. 11-10C). This shoe is constructed over a last that allows up to $\frac{5}{8}$-inch insert depth clearance. The pattern is a four-eyelet, plain toe blucher of soft nappa tanned leather uppers and linings. Because the shoe is fully leather lined, with a specially designed toe box, it is easily reshaped to accommodate the deformed foot or the foot with hammer or clawed toes. The outsole is a wedge of lightweight microcell soling. It is estimated that the shoe is 47 percent lighter than other shoes. The SUPER D and CDI shoes are similar in appearance.

A complaint frequently expressed by wearers of extra-depth shoes is that the heel is constantly lifting out of the shoe. Several manufactures of extra-depth shoes have added a cushion around the top of the heel of the shoe. This is called a "pillow top." The pillow top aids in heel control and minimizes the heel-pump, often experienced when the ball of the foot is properly fitted and the heel remains slightly loose (Fig. 11-10D).

A good modern jogging shoe can also serve as an extra-depth shoe. Many of the better quality jogging shoes come with insoles that can be removed and replaced with a corrective or accommodative insert. These shoes have soft cloth or mesh uppers that minimize pressure over the dorsum of the foot and toes. The jogging shoe is a flexible shoe; however, one can modify the sole to make it rigid so that the rocker or roll-over sole concept can be used. In selecting a jogging shoe, one should choose a shoe with a stiff heel counter. Recently, several manufactures have incorporated rigid heel counters in their shoe design in an attempt to improve heel control. Several manufactures are also offering jogging shoes in a selection of widths, thereby affording beter fit and improved foot control. The Prescription Footwear Association (see p. 290) can provide information on the different types of footwear available.

CUSTOM-MADE FOOTWEAR

A foot that cannot be fitted with conventional or extra-depth shoes presents a special problem. Several companies manufacture custom footwear, however.

A wide variety of styles, from jogging shoes to hiking boots, is available. Most custom shoes are made of leather or suede because these materials have the ability to stretch and mold to the individual's foot. The conventional blucher or bal patterns can be ordered, as can unilateral or bilateral side openings with tie, buckle, or velcro closures. Slip-on loafers and clogs are also available. A choice of materials, such as leather, fur, cotton fabric, or plastazote is available for the shoe lining. Leather is the most popular lining, but a patient's unique needs should be studied to determine the best suited material (e.g., a patient with hyperhydrosis would benefit from a cloth-lined shoe that would absorb some of the excess moisture).

For individuals who are allergic to the cements, dyes, or chemicals used in the tanning of some leathers, the dermapedic shoe is specially manufactured. The shoe is fabricated using hypoallergenic cement and leather tanned by a method that eliminates irritating chemicals. For women, these shoes are retailed under the trade name Foot-So-Port Shoes. (Available through Musebeck Shoe Co., 803 Westover Street, PO 247, Oconomowoc, WI 53066). The Alden Shoe Company retails a dermapedic shoe for men.

Custom shoes are made using casts of an individual's feet, thus accommodating any deformity the person may have. Manufacturers specify how they want the casts made and shipped. A list of special instructions and modifications along with any pertinent patient information should accompany the casts.

Casting for Shoe

To cast the foot for a shoe one must have the person sit with the knee and ankle bent to 90°. A foam rubber pad approximately 2 × 6 × 14 inches, which is covered with a plastic bag, is placed under the foot. Elevate the person until the foot is resting lightly on the foam rubber.[16] Petroleum jelly is applied to all surfaces of the foot and leg that the cast will cover. For persons with no hair on their legs, this step can be omitted. Next, 8-inch fast-setting plaster is folded into a five-ply splint that extends from just above the malleoli to 2 inches past the toes. Another piece of plaster is precut in this same fashion, large enough to cover the entire top of the foot. Wet the first piece of plaster, wring out excess water, and lay it on the foam pad. Smooth out any wrinkles, and place the foot on the plaster splint in the position described above, with the toes approximately 2 inches from the end of the bandage. Mold plaster around the foot and ankle. Roll the edges of the plaster back to form a ledge. After this piece has dried, apply petroleum jelly along the entire ledge. This will allow the cast to be separated once completed. Apply the top piece of plaster in the same fashion as the bottom, making sure that the two pieces are in contact. If 6-inch plaster is used, the posterior piece of plaster is measured in the same fashion. The anterior part of the cast, however, will have to be made of two pieces of plaster, one that extends between the malleoli and another that fits over the forefoot (Fig. 11-11). Allow the cast to dry thoroughly. Pull the skin away from the top of the cast, loosen the plaster along the edges of the cast, and remove the top portion. Have the person wiggle the toes; gently lift the foot off the foam rubber.

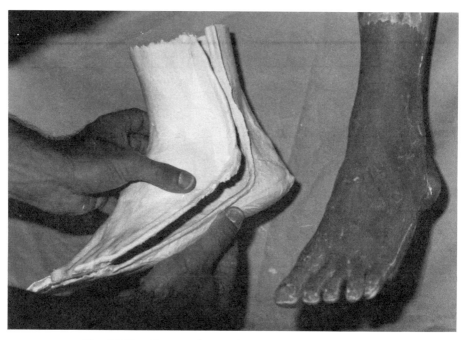

Fig. 11-11. Cast used to construct a custom-made shoe.

Remove the bottom of cast by grasping the heel of the cast and pulling down and forward. A positive model(last) of the foot is made from the above cast, and the custom footwear is fabricated over this model.[17-19]

INTERNAL AND EXTERNAL SHOE MODIFICATIONS

Internal Modifications

Besides putting an orthotic device into a shoe to help relieve pressure on a specific area, the clinician can remove part of the innersole of the shoe to help decrease localized pressure. This technique is known as "welling" and is used

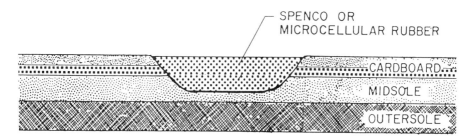

Fig. 11-12. Cross-sectional view of welling.

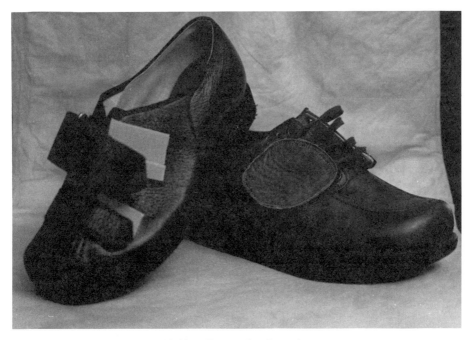

Fig. 11-13. Types of velcro closures.

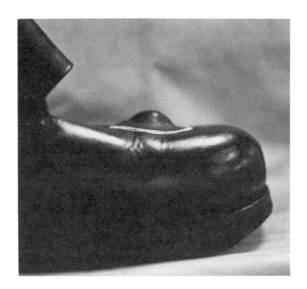

Fig. 11-14. Gusset.

typically to help manage a prominent MTH.[20,21] The procedure entails digging out a piece of the innersole of the shoe that is slightly larger than the area of pressure. The sides of the hole should be sloped inward, and a soft material such as PPT or microcellular rubber should be used to fill the indentation (Fig. 11-12). This soft material helps decrease pressure by spreading the forces over time and space.

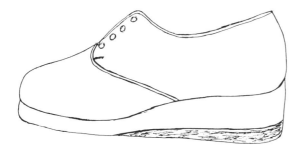

Fig. 11-15.   Heel wedge.

EXTERNAL MODIFICATIONS

Types of Shoe Closures

For the person who has trouble lacing and tying shoe strings, several optional types of shoe closures are available, usually some type of velcro closure system. Ortho-lace closures (available through most health-care catalogues) are a combination of shoe laces that are secured to a flap that fastens with velcro (Fig. 11-13).

Gusset

Occasionally an extra-depth shoe does not provide sufficient space to accommodate a claw or hammer toe deformity. If pressure on the toe is not relieved by spot stretching, the area of the upper that covers the toe can be

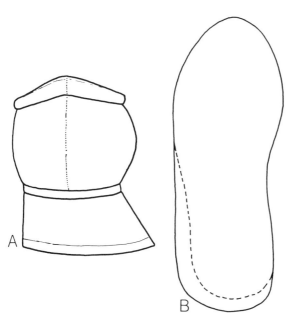

Fig. 11-16. Heel Flare. (**A**) Posterior view of shoe. (**B**) Sole of shoe with heel flare marked by dotted line.

removed and replaced with a soft leather gusset (Fig. 11-14).[20,21] The gusset should be cut slightly larger than the hole in the toebox. The edges of the patch are skived, and the perimeter of the opening in the shoe is roughened with sand paper to facilitate bonding of the contact cement used to secure the gusset in place. In addition to modifications to the shoe upper, many changes can be made to the outer sole of the shoe to help relieve plantar pressures and accommodate biomechanically malaligned feet.

Heel Wedge

A heel wedge is often used to help relieve the forefoot of increased pressures caused by a fixed equinus deformity.[22,23] This practice does not correct the deformity but merely accommodates the plantarflexed position of the foot. The height of the wedge is dependent on the degree of deformity. The wedge is usually made of neoprene crepe and is extended posteriorly from the midpoint of the medial arch (Fig. 11-15).

Lateral Heel Flare

Another biomechanical deformity that can be treated by making modifications to the heel of the shoe is rearfoot varus. The lateral heel is flared helping to decrease the incidence of inversion injuries.[3,20] The flare is formed by attaching a piece of ½-inch crepe along the lateral side of the heel from just anterior to the lateral arch extending approximately one inch past the center of the heel (Fig. 11-16). Both ends and the superior edge of the crepe are skived so that the addition will blend into the sole smoothly.

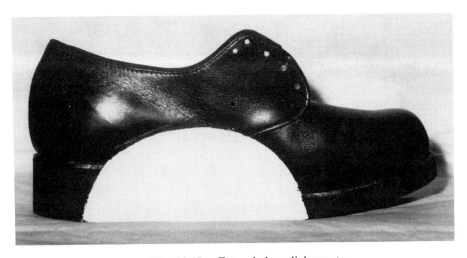

Fig. 11-17. Extended medial counter.

Extended Medial Counter

A patient whose gait exhibits excessive pronation gait often has a shoe that shows signs of wear on the medial counter. The medial sole of the shoe can be extended upward to aid in preventing the shoe counter from collapsing, thus helping to realign the foot. The shoe should be worn for several weeks so that the medial counter is broken-in before the medial extension is applied. Excessive pressure to the medial arch from a medial counter that is too rigid is thus eliminated. The material should be extended three-fourths of the way up the medial counter from the first metatarsal head to the breast of the heel. A piece of $\frac{1}{2}$-inch crepe is cut in a semicircular pattern. The edge along the arch is skived so that the material will conform to the indention in the medial counter of the shoe. This also allows the extension to be flush with the upper (Fig. 11-17). The reinforcement is glued into place using contact cement.

Metatarsal Bar

Several modifications can be made to the sole of the shoe to help redistribute pressures on the plantar surface of the foot during walking. A metatarsal bar is used to relieve pressure from the MTHs. It is analogous to the metatarsal pad used in making orthotic devices. The shoe being modified in this way should have at least a 1-inch heel and a flexible sole.[5,23] The thickness of the material used to make the bar is dependent on the heel height. On the average, a $\frac{1}{4}$-inch-thick piece of neoprene crepe is suitable. The bar is placed just behind the MTHs and extended back $2\frac{1}{2}$ to 3 inches. The bar corresponds to the width of the shoe. The anterior edge can be skived or left full thickness, while the bar is rounded posteriorly (Fig. 11-18).

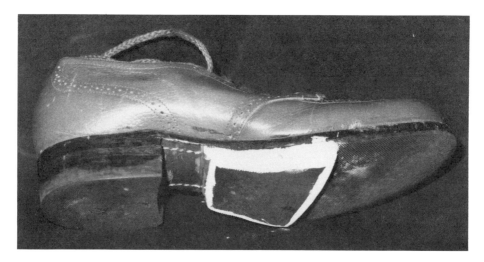

Fig. 11-18.   Metatarsal bar.

Rigid Sole

Rigid sole shoes are commonly used to manage hallux rigidus deformities. As a result of the limited range of motion (ROM) at the first metatarsalphalangeal (MTP) joint, the great toe receives a large amount of pressure in a flexible sole shoe during the push-off phase of gait. Pressure reduction is achieved by making the sole rigid, thus eliminating the bending of the shoe at the toebreak.[11] A metal corset stave, bent to match the contour of the sole, is glued to the sole of the shoe (Fig. 11-19). If a shoe with a crepe wedge sole is used, a space for the stave can be welded out of the sole. It is impossible to have a heel-toe gait with a flat rigid sole shoe; therefore, the sole is fashioned into a "roller" sole. This enables the person to have a more normal gait, as opposed to walking flat-footed. To form a roller sole, the crepe under the toebox is beveled off to the midsole. After the metal stave is glued in place, a $\frac{1}{2}$-inch piece of crepe is used to cover the stave and finish forming the roller.

If a shoe with a conventional heel is made rigid, the heel must be removed. A crepe wedge can then be added to the sole before the corset stave is secured, or the corset stave can be glued to the original sole and then covered with a crepe wedge. A $\frac{1}{4}$-inch piece of crepe is then added to the shoe and ground to form a roller sole (Fig. 11-20A).

Rocker Sole

The rocker-bottom shoe is another type of rigid sole shoe used specifically to help alleviate pressure under the MTHs.[5,9,18] The toe of the shoe is bent upward, approximately 15°, until a slight crease is formed in the toebox. One factor that must be taken into account, when deciding the angle at which to bend shoe, is the amount of available toe extension. The crepe under the toebox is ground down to the midsole following the angle of the toebox. When the toebox is not bent and beveled initially, more soling material is needed to form the rocker. A higher sole height results, which will increase instability and the weight of the shoe. Next, the sole is made rigid as outlined previously. Instead of rolling the sole, a sharp-angled sole is constructed (rocker sole). The apex of the rocker is placed just posterior to the MTHs (Fig. 11-20B).

Fixed Ankle Boot

Severely shortened feet as well as feet with a history of neuropathic fractures of the tarsal bones require custom boots to prevent further deformity and eliminate motion in the affected joints.[11,24] The fixed ankle boot (FAB) was developed to manage feet that need maximum protection. A FAB may be constructed using an over-the-counter workboot or a custom-made boot. The counter of the boot is extended to just below the knee by sewing a piece of leather of sufficient length to the brim of the boot. The outer sole of the boot is

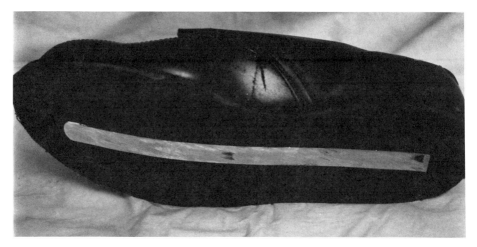

Fig. 11-19. Corset staves glued to shoe sole to provide rigidity.

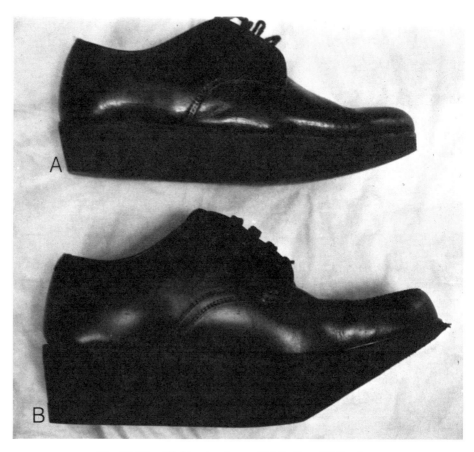

Fig. 11-20. Rigid sole shoes. (**A**) Roller. (**B**) Rocker.

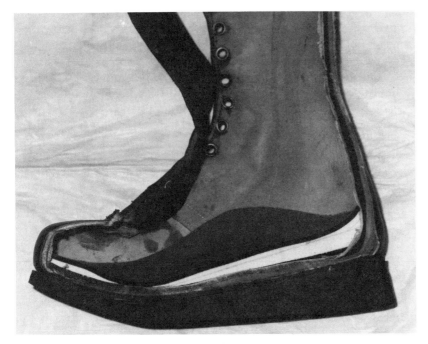

Fig. 11-21.   Cross section of fixed ankle boot.

removed down to the welt. A piece of polypropylene is vacuum-formed over the boot and positive model, then trimmed in the pattern of an ankle foot orthosis (AFO). The polypropylene is then glued to the sole and upper of the boot (Fig. 11-21). A patch of leather is sewn over the AFO to finish the upper of the boot. The final step in constructing the boot is forming a rigid (rocker or roller) sole.

FITTING THE SHORTENED FOOT

A foot that is shortened due to bony reabsorption or surgery is certainly a challenge to manage successfully. Because the weightbearing surface is reduced, the pressures of walking are concentrated, thereby increasing the likelihood of tissue breakdown.

The type of protective footwear used for a shortened foot depends on the amount of deformity and reduction in size of the foot. A mild deformity can usually be managed in an over-the-counter extra-depth shoe. If both feet are relatively equal in size, the feet are fit in a normal fashion. Men with shortened feet often cannot find extra-depth shoes in their size. Several shoe styles, however, are available in both men's and women's sizes. There is a difference of three half-sizes between women's and men's shoes. Therefore, men can usually be fit with a women's size if the shoe is not marketed in a men's size small enough to fit.

When the feet are of unequal size, it is more difficult to fit the feet without buying two pairs of shoes or having custom footwear made. If the difference between the feet is no more than one size in length, the larger size can be used. Many times, the shorter foot is also the wider foot. Because the shoe is measured to fit the longer foot, some of the difference in width is compensated for by the additional length of the shoe. An all leather shoe is preferable because it can be stretched if additional room is needed. A difference in width greater than two sizes can not be accomodated by stretching, however.

If the feet cannot be fitted with conventional extra-depth shoes, custom footwear must be fabricated. For example, severely shortened feet require custom-made low-quarter boots or FAB. Many times, a shortened foot is fitted with a larger shoe for cosmetic reasons. A toefiller, which is usually made of some type of foam material, is used to prevent the foot from slipping back and forth in the shoe. Toefillers are potentially dangerous. Care must be taken to assure that no pressure is being imposed on the foot by the toefiller. Of greater importance is the fact that the first metatarsophalangeal (MTP) joint and the toe break of the shoe should match. If the foot falls posterior to the toe break, stress is concentrated at the distal end of the foot, thus increasing the chance of further complication.

SUMMARY

Shoes are an important part of our daily wardrobe. A multitude of styles is available, but some styles are not suitable even for the "normal" foot. Thus, one must be judicious in selecting footwear. Shoes should afford both protection and comfort, which becomes of paramount concern when a person has "problem feet."

Patients with diabetes, arthritis, and injuries caused from biomechanically malaligned feet are a sample of the wide variety of patients who can benefit from protective footwear. In an effort to familiarize health care professionals with the importance of shoe selection and modification, the numerous types of orthopedic and custom-made footwear available have been discussed. Basic shoe terminology and construction has been reviewed. Types of orthotic insoles along with characteristics of materials commonly used for insole fabrication were outlined, and instructions on fabricating orthotic devices, casting the foot for a shoe or balanced insole, and making shoe modifications have been given.

REFERENCES

1. Anonymous: How American Shoes are Made, United Shoe Machinery Corporation, Boston, 1966
2. Rossi WA, Tennant R: Professional Shoe Fitting. National Shoe Retailer Association, New York, 1984

3. Zamosky I: Shoe modifications in lower-extremity orthotics. Bull Prosthet Res 10-2:54, 1964

4. Anonymous: The True Story of Shoe Sizes, Sterling Last Corporation, New York Island

5. Jahss MH: Shoes and shoe modifications. p. 267. In American Academy of Orthopedic Surgeons (eds): Atlas of Orthotics. CV Mosby, St. Louis, 1975

6. Smiler I: Foot problems of elderly diabetics. Geriatr Nurs 3:177, 1982

7. Seymour RJ, Clark S, Ruhl M, Leichter SB: Management of the diabetic foot. Physiother Can 32:25, 1980

8. McPoil TG: The cobra pad—an orthotic alternative for the PT. J Orthop Sports Phys Ther 5:30, 1983

9. Hampton GH: Therapeutic footwear for the insensitive foot. Phys Ther 59:21, 1979

10. Doxey GE: The semi-flexible foot orthotic: fabrication guidelines for use. J Orthop Sports Phys Ther 5:26, 1983

11. Enna CD, Brand PW, Reed JK, Welch D: The orthotic care of the denervated foot in Hansen's disease. Orthot Prosthet 30:33, 1976

12. Burns MJ: Non-weightbearing cast impressions for the construction of orthotic devices. J Am Podiatry Assoc 67:790, 1977

13. Valmassy RL: Advantage and disadvantages of various casting techniques. J Am Podiatry Assoc 69:707, 1979

14. Sgarlato TE: A compendium of podiatric biomechanics. California College of Podiatric Medicine, San Francisco, 1971

15. Langer S: Posting—theory and practice. Langer Lab Biomech Newlett 1:3, 1973

16. Anonymous: ACOR Casting Instructions, Acor Molded Shoes, South Euclid, OH

17. Reed JK: Footwear for the diabetic. p. 360 In Levin ME, O'Neal LW (eds): The Diabetic Foot. CV Mosby, St. Louis, 1983

18. Barrett JP: Plantar pressure measurements—rational shoe-wear in patients with rheumatoid arthritis. J Am Podiatry Assoc 235:1138, 1976

19. Jacobson MA: Simple footgear corrections useful in office emergencies. Orthop Rev 8:63, 1979

20. Cracchiolo A: The use of shoes to treat foot disorders. Orthop Rev 8:73, 1979

21. New York University Prosthetics and Orthotics: Lower-Limb Orthotics. New York University Post-Graduate Medical School, New York, 1981

22. Edwards CA: Orthopedic shoe technology for the orthopedic shoe technician. Precision Printing, 1981

23. Milgram JE, Jackson MA: Footgear—therapeutic modifications of sole and heel. 3:57, 1978

24. Girling J: Footwear for anesthetic feet. p. 313. In McDowell F, Enna C (eds): Surgical Rehabilitation in Leprosy. Williams & Wilkins, Baltimore, 1974

12 | Surgical Overview

Shepard Hurwitz

Pain, instability, and deformity are the major reasons for considering surgical treatment of the ankle. Nonoperative means of management should be the first approach for all nonacute and nontumor conditions. If a generous trial with conservative treatment does not bring the desired relief or improvement, and if the patient is willing to accept the risks, surgery may be an acceptable choice.

The goals of surgery are (1) to preserve or improve function, (2) to relieve or reduce pain, and (3) to remove a disease process. Ideally, all these goals can be met with a single well-planned and well-executed surgical procedure. At times, the surgical goals are mutually exclusive, (e.g., a malignant process that requires a below-knee amputation). These special cases require case-by-case analysis. Often a successful result depends on the original decision to preserve life instead of function, and rehabilitation services play a major role in functional substitution and return.

The decision-making process in surgery is crucial—and is becoming even more so. Patients are now consumers and want to make their choices with a great deal of information about the particulars of various possible procedures.

PREDICTING POSTOPERATIVE RESULTS

From the physician's viewpoint, the patient first must be able to withstand the surgery before any thoughts of elective reconstruction are entertained. The patient must be healthy enough to survive the physiological stress of surgery in general. In ankle surgery in particular, there must not be any local factors to contraindicate a procedure. There should be adequate blood flow and existing protective sensation, but no active infection or destructive bony lesion.

Assessment of the patient's potential for rehabilitation also is of great pedictive value and is a decision often best made by those who know the patient

315

well. A carefully selected and competently performed operation is of little value to a patient who loses ankle motion or whose ankle swells because he or she cannot comply with postoperative routines and instructions. Corrective bone or joint surgery may not help the patient with neuromuscular disease whose control, strength, and endurance fade irreversibly in the postoperative healing period.

Postoperative pain is difficult to predict and even more difficult to explain in meaningful terms to a patient preoperatively. Preparing the patient who experiences more intense pain than was expected for a difficult rehabilitative process may represent preoperative failure.

Widespread pathology may complicate the surgeon's preoperative ability to predict postoperative problems. For example, the rheumatoid patient with multiple joint difficulties may not tolerate the traditional rest and elevation after an ankle fusion because of either lower or upper extremity symptom exacerbation. Generally, in the patient with several major joint problems, one should attack the most symptomatic joint first and then reevaluate the entire patient after the full benefit of the surgical procedure is reached.

PLANNING THE OPERATIVE PROCEDURE

Surgery is a means of helping people reach their potential. It is not, for the most part, a substitute for careful evaluation and medical treatment. Once surgery is chosen to treat an ankle problem, planning the operative procedure is the next step.

Elements of planning include the physical examination, radiographs and special studies such as computed tomography (CT) scans. The surgical exposure selected should minimize soft tissue trauma which may cause postoperative swelling and/or skin necrosis. All attempts must be made to preserve nerves and blood vessels during surgery; incisions should be planned to minimize the chance of damaging nerves or arteries in gaining exposure to the bones or ankle joint.

The ankle can be approached from four basic directions: anterior, medial, posterior, and lateral. Combinations of these four are possible but should not compromise the intervening structures. Simultaneous approaches such as anteromedial should be avoided; this jeopardizes the bridge of skin between the two areas and unnecessarily threatens the deep peroneal and saphenous nerves. The mediolateral or anteroposterior combinations are safer.

The following list matches frequently seen ankle conditions with the preferred approach:

Anterior (Figs. 12-1 and 12-2)
    Lateral osteochondritis of talus
    Removal of anterior osteophyte
    Removal of loose body

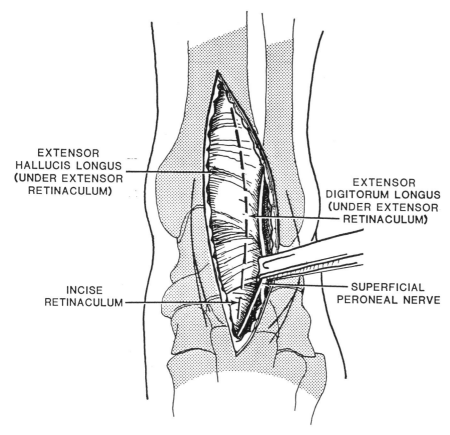

Fig. 12-1. Anterior surgical approach to the ankle joint. This is the most common way to perform reconstructive ankle surgery. Anterior scarring may limit postoperative plantar flexion.

    Fusion
    Replacement
  Medial (Figs. 12-3 through 12-5A and B)
    Ligament repair/reconstruction
    Tendon release
    Arthrotomy to repair osteochondritis
    Fracture repair
  Posterior (Figs. 12-6 and 12-7)
    Release
    Removal of os trigonum fragment
  Lateral (Figs. 12-8 and 12-9)
    Ligament repair/reconstruction
    Removal of osteophyte
    Tendon release or stabilization
    Fusion
    Fracture repair

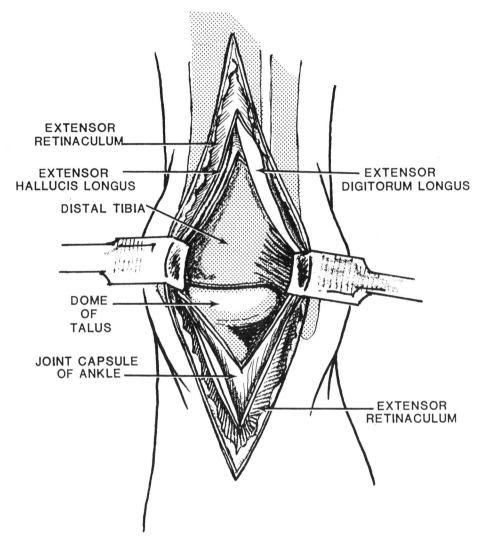

Fig. 12-2. Exposure of the anterior ankle joint. Care is taken to protect the superficial peroneal nerve and the anterior tibial artery with the deep peroneal nerve.

PHASES OF HEALING

Ankle surgery has in common with all trauma the wounding process, which in turn triggers the body's healing response. Wounding produces pain, swelling, and motor inhibition ("splinting"). The wound evokes an inflammatory response in the tissues. This response heightens the pain produced by nerve trauma but is the necessary first step to increase local blood flow and infest the wound with scavenger and immune cells that remove debris and inhibit infection.

The inflammatory phase gradually gives way to a reparative phase marked

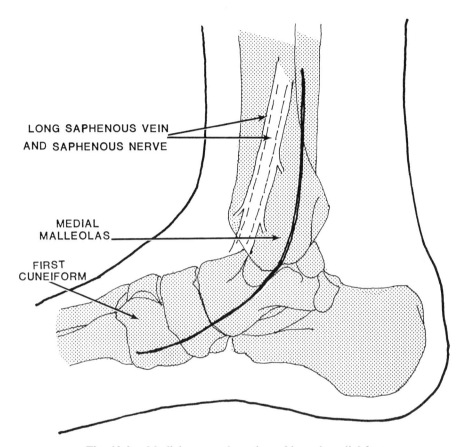

LONG SAPHENOUS VEIN
AND SAPHENOUS NERVE

MEDIAL
MALLEOLAS

FIRST
CUNEIFORM

Fig. 12-3. Medial approach to the ankle and medial foot.

by ingrowth of new blood vessels and the appearance of cells trying to rebuild
the damaged structures. These cells begin to specialize in producing the materials needed: bone, cartilage, dense connective tissue (ligament), loose connective tissue, and skin. Much of this new tissue is collagen heaped together and
called callus (from the Latin: ''hard'').

The repair phase ends with remodeling of the various callus tissues into
more perfect tissue types and regaining of the mechanical properties of
strength, lubrication, and elasticity. One way in which the healing process fails
is through creation of dense adhesions between all moving parts and surfaces.
This is a biological attempt to fuse the region and prevent motion. Another
problem is failure of the structures to reunite (called non-union for bone),
causing mechanical failure of the system.

The remodeling phase is very long and may even be a constant process
going on at a very low level of cell activity, as witnessed by the opening up of
old wounds in malnourished patients or scurvy victims. Conceptually, we add
another phase—maintenance of function. This underlines the importance of
neuromuscular and cardiovascular elements, which not only contribute to func-

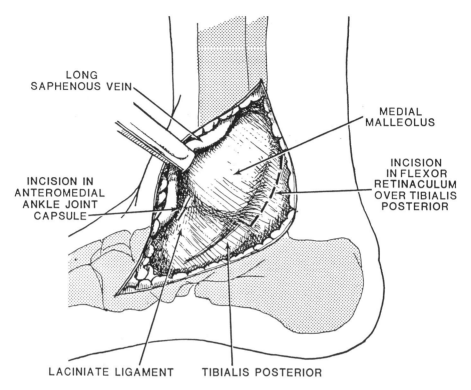

LONG
SAPHENOUS VEIN

MEDIAL
MALLEOLUS

INCISION
IN FLEXOR
RETINACULUM
OVER TIBIALIS
POSTERIOR

INCISION IN
ANTEROMEDIAL
ANKLE JOINT
CAPSULE

LACINIATE LIGAMENT   TIBIALIS POSTERIOR

Fig. 12-4. Medial ankle approach illustrating surgical access to the joint, the flexor tendons, and the tarsal tunnel. Distal extension gives access to the navicula and medial cuneiform.

tion but have been shown to affect repair and remodeling favorably. The maintenance phase also helps preserve the outcome of remodeling and should delay the combined destructive effects of age and trauma on joints and tendons.

POSTOPERATIVE CARE AND MANAGEMENT

The postoperative position of the ankle is neutral. Equinus contractures begin with postoperative immobilization in the plantarflexed position. A compressive dressing—either a cast or a bulky dressing with splints—is used along with physiologic elevation for 48 hours. Early motion is possible at 48 to 72 hours if pain allows. The ankle still is splinted at neutral except during exercise periods.

We now recommend early active exercise. There is a growing body of experience with continuous passive motion (CPM) in the immediate and early postoperative periods, but results are not yet conclusive.

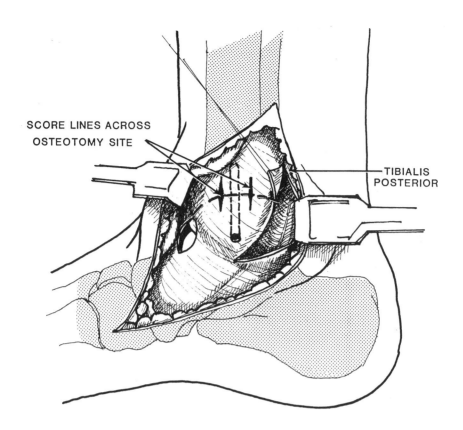

SCORE LINES ACROSS
OSTEOTOMY SITE

TIBIALIS
POSTERIOR

Fig. 12-5. (**A**) Osteotomy of the medial malleolus to enter the tibiotalar joint. (**B**) Frontal view of medial osteotomy; a screw will be placed in the bone hole to reattach the medial malleolus.

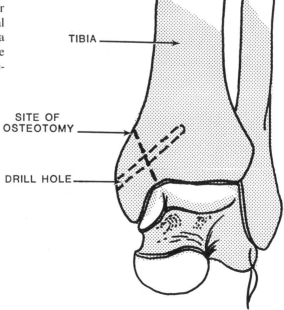

TIBIA

SITE OF
OSTEOTOMY

DRILL HOLE

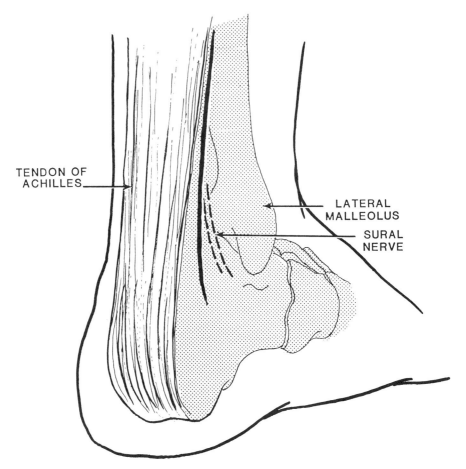

Fig. 12-6.   Posterolateral approach to the ankle. This is a useful approach for surgery of the Achilles tendon and posterior calcaneus.

Sutures are removed at 10 days to 3 weeks postoperatively. This is a decision point: whether to immobilize or not. An ankle fusion will be rigidly immobilized for 12 weeks, perhaps longer. If a bone graft is used for an ankle reconstruction, nonweightbearing is enforced for 12 weeks although active range of motion (ROM) can start at 2 to 3 weeks. Fractures usually are protected from weightbearing for 6 weeks, but early motion may begin during this phase. Ankle replacements are splinted, weightbearing is allowed but protected for 4 to 6 weeks, and early motion is begun during the hospital stay.

ROM is the first priority of joint function. In the absence of proper ROM, the patient may suffer pain, weakness, and failure of other related joints. The notable exception is ankle fusion, in which we attempt to preserve hip, knee, and toe function. Once the fusion is solid, subtalar motion is enhanced, and the patient is evaluated for optimum heel height and/or compression modification.

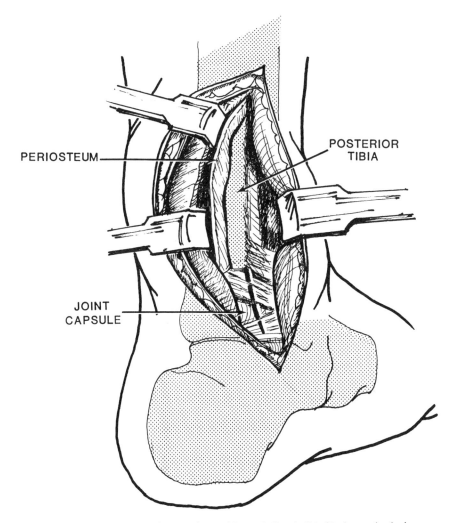

Fig. 12-7. Exposure of posterior ankle and distal tibiofibular articulations.

Early motion is a determinant of the intensity and duration of ROM exercises. The importance of the type of exercise used to regain motion is being reconsidered, in part due to new emphasis on passive motion machines. Joint motion then enables the muscles to retrain, however, using isotonic or isokinetic machines.

With strength comes endurance and, it is hoped, the ability to walk unaided for an unlimited distance. Sports retraining requires a more goal-oriented strengthening program combined with a controlled reentry into sports activity. Exercises to retrain complex neural processes such as balance or reaction time may be indicated on an individual basis.

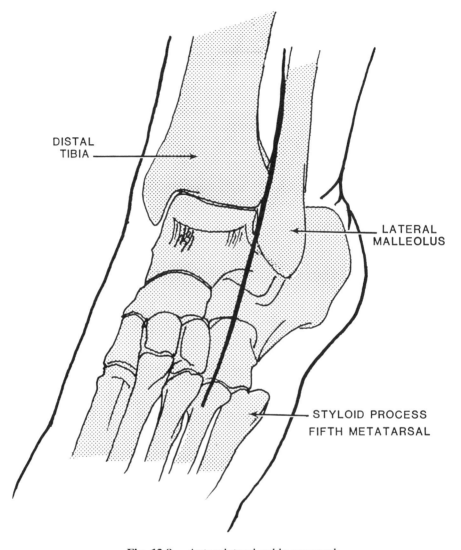

Fig. 12-8.   Anterolateral ankle approach.

Maintenance exercise or maintenance therapy may combine various modalities depending on the problems anticipated. Stiffness requires diligent stretching, heat, and perhaps forced manipulation under anesthesia. Swelling requires compressive hose with judicious use of ice, elevation, and diuretic medication. Laxity or latent instability may require bracing. Antiinflammatory medication may be helpful to reduce pain and unwanted synovitis in the various recovery phases and may be needed periodically to treat "flares" of an ankle that has previously undergone operation.

Finally, surgery often begets surgery, as in the case of a failed ankle replacement salvaged by an extensive procedure to graft and fuse the joint. The

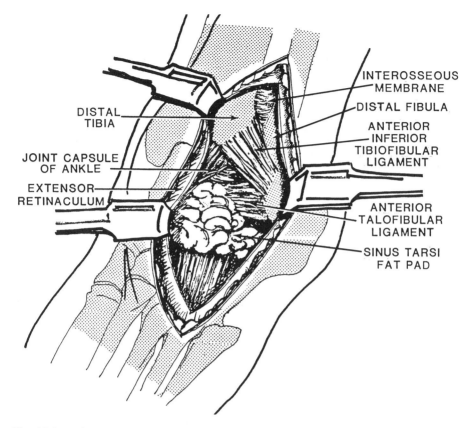

DISTAL TIBIA

JOINT CAPSULE OF ANKLE

EXTENSOR RETINACULUM

INTEROSSEOUS MEMBRANE

DISTAL FIBULA

ANTERIOR INFERIOR TIBIOFIBULAR LIGAMENT

ANTERIOR TALOFIBULAR LIGAMENT

SINUS TARSI FAT PAD

Fig. 12-9. Dissection anterolateral approach; useful for entry into the lateral tibiotalar joint, anterior ligament repair, and exposure of the sinus tarsi.

multiply operated ankle is rehabilitated in a similar manner, but the time frame is determined by the extensiveness of the procedure. Early motion is critical because scarring will proceed much more aggressively after multiple surgeries. Often, however, the multiply operated patient has a tenuous wound, and mobilization must be delayed to ensure healing.

HINDFOOT SURGERY

Stabilization of the calcaneus was once a very common procedure because of poliomyelitis. Today, most hindfoot stabilizations are performed because of trauma-induced subtalar arthritis. Rheumatoid arthritis is a very common disorder of the hindfoot that requires stabilization. Neurologic disorders such as meningomyelocele, Charcot-Marie-Tooth disease, and permanent peroneal palsy often necessitate hindfoot stabilization as well as motor transfers.

The triple arthrodesis is the basic procedure: the talocalcaneal joints, talonavicular joint, and calcaneocuboid joint are the requisite three joints that

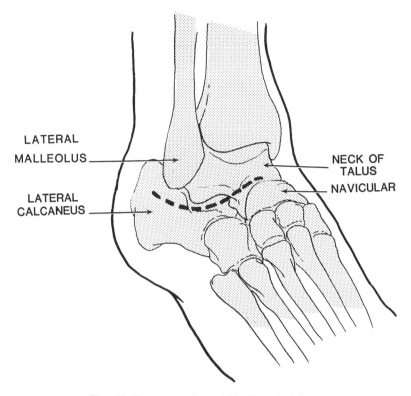

Fig. 12-10.   Anterolateral hindfoot incision.

must be fused. Limited fusion of the talus to the calcaneus or to the navicular have been reported to be successful in certain medical centers but do not enjoy universal acceptance as durable hindfoot procedures. The triple arthrodesis has the reputation for durability and allows the surgeon greater latitude in planning correction of deformity in the frontal and sagittal planes. The triple arthrodesis can eliminate painful joint motion and change the characteristics of heel strike and ankle load-bearing (see Figs. 12-10 and 12-11).

Correction of calcaneal valgus is the easiest realignment of the valgus heel through a triple arthrodesis. Varus deformity, as well as cavus and equinus, likewise can be treated by corrective osteotomy as part of the arthrodesis. Calcaneal osteotomy to correct medial or lateral heel strike has limited indications in hindfoot surgery.

A controversial hindfoot procedure is partial fasciotomy or exostectomy for heel pain believed to be associated with plantar fasciitis/heel spur syndromes. The orthopedic literature does not support this type of surgery because of a 50 percent failure rate. Podiatrists perform more heel surgery for plantar pain than do orthopedists.

Rehabilitation following hindfoot surgery involves preserving knee and toe ROM early in the postoperative period. Cast immobilization lasts 6 to 8 weeks, and I believe this should be followed by bracing in an ankle-foot orthosis for

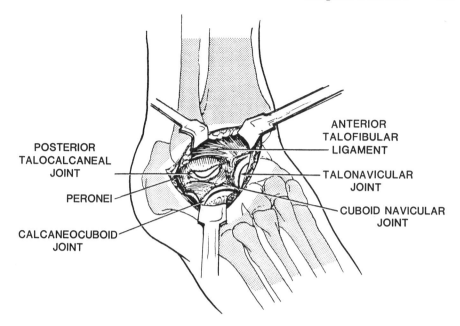

Fig. 12-11. Dissection of hindfoot. Exposure of the joints fused in a triple arthrodesis: talocalcaneal, calcaneocuboid, and talonavicular. Care is taken to avoid injury to the anterior ankle joint.

another 6 weeks. During the period of bracing, active ankle ROM should be started and knee strengthening should be continued. Ankle strengthening cannot begin until the surgeon determines that a solid bony fusion exists in the hindfoot. Swelling is often a problem involving both foot and ankle. Compressive stockings, frequent elevation, and ice may be needed to control swelling. Accommodative changes in shoewear usually are needed.

MIDFOOT SURGERY

Surgery to correct malalignment or to remove painful dorsal exostoses or ganglia are the most common operations. Pes cavus can be reduced by a closing wedge osteotomy of the midfoot (Fig. 12-12). Bony prominences on the dorsum of the foot can cause pain from contact with shoes.

Rehabilitation following midfoot surgery depends on whether bone healing is needed and whether cast immobilization is used. Once the protected healing phase is over, ROM is restored to the ankle and subtalar complex. Strengthening is started when pain has subsided and ankle range has been obtained.

FOREFOOT SURGERY

Corrective forefoot surgery concerns three areas: the great toe, the lesser toes, and the metatarsals. Great toe surgery is most commonly performed for painful bunion/hallux valgus, hallux rigidus, and osteoarthritis of the metatar-

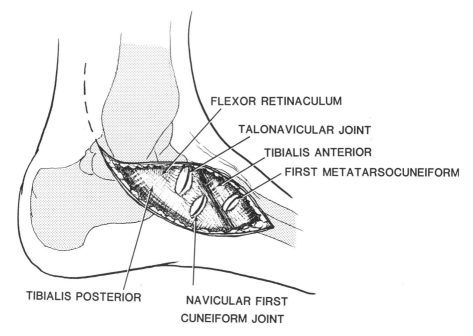

FLEXOR RETINACULUM

TALONAVICULAR JOINT

TIBIALIS ANTERIOR

FIRST METATARSOCUNEIFORM

TIBIALIS POSTERIOR

NAVICULAR FIRST
CUNEIFORM JOINT

Fig. 12-12.   Joints of the medial foot.

sophalangeal (MTP) joint (Figure 12-13). Lesser toe surgery is done to correct hammertoe (cock toe), deformity, or painful corns (Figure 12-14). Metatarsal surgery includes resection of digital (Morton's) neuromas and realignment of metatarsals to reduce plantar pain. Much of forefoot surgery today is toe or metatarsal amputation in diabetic patients. Rheumatoid patients frequently have reconstruction of the forefoot involving resection of the metatarsal heads (MTHs).

The greatest problem following surgery of the great toe is medial forefoot swelling and MTP joint stiffness. Bunionectomy often involves metatarsal osteotomy to realign the metatarsal with a soft tissue realignment of the MTP joint. If osteotomy is included, a period of 4 to 6 weeks must elapse before assisted ROM can be started; clinical healing of the bone should precede vigorous attempts to regain MTP joint extension. Persistent swelling is difficult to eliminate, but ice and elevation are recommended as is a limited level of activity.

Longitudinal toe stretching and heelcord stretching should be part of the rehabilitation of the great and lesser toes. Functionally, MTP joints should extend to accommodate heel rise: flexion serves little purpose. Ankle dorsiflexion should be adequate to allow for gentle heel rise and thereby lessen the floor reaction forces under the MTHs during late stance.

Metatarsal surgery usually produces swollen feet and stiff toes. If osteotomies are done, they must be allowed to heal before maximal force can be used to regain toe MTP joint range.

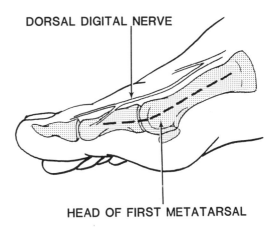

DORSAL DIGITAL NERVE

HEAD OF FIRST METATARSAL

Fig. 12-13. Medial approach to the metatarsophalangeal joint of the great toe. This is a common incision for bunion surgery but may be used to correct metatarsal and phalangeal deformity as well as route for joint surgery (e.g., joint replacement or fusion).

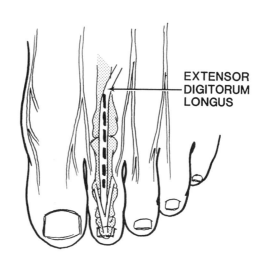

EXTENSOR DIGITORUM LONGUS

Fig. 12-14. Dorsal midline incision for lesser toe procedures. This approach gives access to the extensor tendons and all the joints of the toe.

Tendon transfers in the foot are done rarely. Once healing has occurred, active use and assisted ROM are started. Foot tendons belong to muscles that are pattern-governed, and the muscles cannot be individually retrained during gait. Transferred tendons often act through a tenodesis effect because of adhesions and poor tension characteristics after the transfer (e.g., posterior tibial transfer for peroneal palsy dropfoot.

After *all* foot surgery, there is a need to reevaluate shoewear and gait characteristics. The goal of therapeutic footwear is to achieve balance of the foot with regard to varus, valgus, heel strike, and toe-off characteristics. Foot surgery usually will not restore balance, and the postsurgical foot may require shoe modification, orthotic supplements, or ongoing gait retraining in addition to restoration of motor strength and joint motion.

CONCLUSION

Foot and ankle surgery is restorative in its ability to provide stability, eliminate pain, and aid shoewear. Postoperative healing and rehabilitation should complement one another to restore function of the lower extremity in a timely manner. The remodeling and rehabilitation phases of healing take the longest and often require the greatest skill on the part of the health team.

Index

Page numbers followed by f indicate figures; page numbers followed by t indicate tables.